## Texts in Statistical Science

# Introduction to Randomized Controlled Clinical Trials

## Second Edition

# CHAPMAN & HALL/CRC
## Texts in Statistical Science Series

Series Editors
Bradley P. Carlin, *University of Minnesota, USA*
Chris Chatfield, *University of Bath, UK*
Martin Tanner, *Northwestern University, USA*
Jim Zidek, *University of British Columbia, Canada*

# Texts in Statistical Science

# Introduction to Randomized Controlled Clinical Trials

## Second Edition

John N.S. Matthews

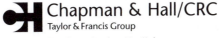

## Chapman & Hall/CRC

Taylor & Francis Group

Boca Raton   London   New York

Chapman & Hall/CRC is an imprint of the
Taylor & Francis Group, an informa business

Chapman & Hall/CRC
Taylor & Francis Group
6000 Broken Sound Parkway NW, Suite 300
Boca Raton, FL 33487-2742

© 2006 by Taylor and Francis Group, LLC
Chapman & Hall/CRC is an imprint of Taylor & Francis Group, an Informa business

International Standard Book Number-10: 1-58488-624-2 (Softcover)
International Standard Book Number-13: 978-1-58488-624-2 (Softcover)

**Visit the Taylor & Francis Web site at**
**http://www.taylorandfrancis.com**

**and the CRC Press Web site at**
**http://www.crcpress.com**

# Dedication

*To the memory of my father*

# Preface to the First Edition

Clinical trials are experiments performed on human subjects, usually patients, in order to assess the efficacy of a treatment that is under investigation. Over the last two to three decades randomized concurrently controlled clinical trials have become established as the method which investigators must use to assess new treatments if their claims are to find widespread acceptance. The methodology underpinning these trials is firmly based in statistical theory, and the success of randomized trials perhaps constitutes the greatest achievement of statistics in the second half of the twentieth century. As such it is important that students of statistics should be able to study this area of their subject as soon as possible in their courses.

Whereas there are many excellent books on clinical trial methodology, almost all are written for the practitioner, whether statistician or doctor, who is about to participate in the running of a trial. There is a natural tendency in such books both to cover administrative issues and to keep to a minimum any mathematical passages. However, while trial administration is of undoubted importance, too much emphasis on it is unnecessary and an unwelcome distraction for students making their first acquaintance with the underlying principles. Moreover, for a readership whose knowledge of mathematics is likely to be substantially greater than their knowledge of medicine, many of the principles involved can be introduced more precisely and succinctly by the appropriate use of mathematics. This book is intended as an introduction to the statistical methodology that underpins randomized controlled trials, and is aimed primarily at the student of statistics. Administrative aspects receive little emphasis and, if it is believed that it would help the primary readership, a mathematical approach is adopted.

Although it is hoped that many will find the book useful as an introduction to the subject, the needs of final-year undergraduate or postgraduate students at British universities have been my main concern. However, there is considerable variation within this group in the statistical techniques they already know, and I have attempted to rely only on a few basic prerequisites. This has led to a slight distortion of the subject matter. For example, so that a knowledge of logistic regression is not needed for this book, trials with binary outcomes are given less prominence than might be expected from their prevalence in practice. The complete avoidance of survival analysis perhaps leads to an even greater distortion. However, I believe these distortions are justified by the wider accessibility that results.

The view of clinical trials embodied in this book is, of course, my own. This has been formed over many years through collaboration and contact with many colleagues, both doctors and statisticians and so many people have been involved that it would be impossible to list them all. However, I must acknowledge, in particular, the tremendous debt I owe to Peter Armitage, Michael Healy, and David Appleton. I am also most grateful to Peter Farr for permission to use his data in the exercises in Chapter 8.

**JNSM**
*Newcastle upon Tyne*
*Autumn 1999*

# Preface to the Second Edition

The change of publisher between editions, from Edward Arnold to Chapman & Hall/CRC, has given me the opportunity to make corrections and add some new material. The aim, to write a book for students of statistics focusing on statistical rather than administrative aspects of clinical trials, remains the same. Some extra material on more sophisticated methods for balancing treatment allocations has been added to Chapter 4. The main change is the addition of Chapter 7, which is largely concerned with the analyses of clinical trials with binary or survival time outcomes. Many trials have outcomes of this kind, and in the preface to the first edition I acknowledged that the exclusion of outcomes of these forms was a distortion of the subject. This was done to ensure that the book did not require the reader to be familiar with more sophisticated methods of analysis, such as logistic regression and proportional hazards models. On reflection, this was an unnecessary restriction. None of the chapters in the book depend on Chapter 7, so those wishing to avoid this material can still avoid it. The chapter is quite long because an attempt has been made to provide brief introductions to the required techniques.

I am grateful to all those who have commented on the previous edition, whether informally or in book reviews. The errata supplied by Craig Borkowf and Miland Joshi were especially useful. I am also very grateful to Professor Peter Farr for his permission to use the data from the PUVA vs. TL-01 trial to illustrate much of Chapter 7.

**JNSM**
*Newcastle upon Tyne*
*Winter 2005*

# Contents

# 1

## What Is a Randomized Controlled Trial?

### 1.1 Definition and Key Features

A randomized concurrently controlled clinical trial is simply an experiment performed on human subjects to assess the efficacy of a new treatment for some condition. It has two key features, which in the simplest case are as follows:

1. The new treatment is given to a group of patients (called the *treated group*) and another treatment, often the one most widely used, is given to another group of patients at the same time — this is usually called the *control group*. This is what makes the trial concurrently controlled.

2. Patients are allocated to one group or another by randomization. This can be thought of as deciding on the treatment to be given by the toss of a coin, although more sophisticated methods are usually employed, as we shall see.

It is often understood that the controls are concurrent and these trials are referred to simply as *randomized controlled trials* or, in this book, RCTs. The following should be noted:

1. It is possible, and often desirable, to compare more than two treatments in a single trial. However, much of the exposition herein is restricted to this simple case because most of the essential ideas behind RCTs are then most transparent.

2. Trials are applied to many different modes of treatment. Most of this book will use examples of drug trials, in which the patients are given tablets. However, RCTs are used to compare all manner of interventions, for example, new surgical procedures, screening programs, diagnostic procedures, etc. Some examples are given in the next section.

1

3. It may seem unnerving that a visit to the doctor could result in your being given a treatment, not on the basis of the doctor's knowledge or expertise, but on the toss of a coin. Not only is it unnerving, but you may well be given what turns out to be the inferior treatment. For these, and other reasons, there is an important ethical aspect to the conduct of RCTs, which sets them apart from experiments in areas such as agriculture or industry.

## 1.2    Historical Context and the Nature of RCTs

### 1.2.1    Historical Background

Throughout history, mankind has been afflicted by disease and has attempted to devise treatments to cure or ameliorate the suffering of the afflicted. It is assumed that this is a desirable aim, and it is also desirable to know which treatments work, which do not, and whether one treatment is better than another. As will be seen later in the book, some of these questions are rather simplistic, but they are, in essence, what RCTs are about.

In the past, the effectiveness of treatments has often been decided by reference to *ad hoc* usage in the hands of some eminent authority. Indeed, this approach was widespread until quite recently: RCTs — as we know them today — made their entrance only in the period since the Second World War. However, since medieval times, there have been isolated attempts to obtain empirical evidence on the effectiveness of treatments.

## Example 1.1: Some Early Trials

| Condition Being Treated | Treatments Compared and Results | Investigator, Date, and Reference |
|---|---|---|
| Wounds sustained in battle to capture the castle of Villaine | Boiling oil vs. a digestive of egg yolks, oil of roses, and turpentine. The latter, a new treatment, was found to be superior | Ambroïse Paré, 1537. Quoted in FR Packard, *The Life and Times of Ambroïse Paré*, Hoeber, New York, 1921, pp. 27,163. |
| Treatment of scurvy on board HMS Salisbury | Two patients allocated to each of cider, elixir vitriol, vinegar, nutmeg, sea water, and oranges and lemons. Those given oranges and lemons showed "… the most sudden and visible good effects" | James Lind, 1747. Lind, J., *A Treatise of the Scurvy*, Sand Murray Cochran, Edinburgh, 1753, pp. 191–193. |

## 1.2.2 Impact of RCTs and Importance of Statistics

The RCT is the introduction of the scientific method into the process of comparing treatments. As with the cases in Example 1.1, empirical evidence is sought to settle the question of whether one treatment works better than another, that is, we observe the effects of the treatments on the groups and compare them. The following should be noted:

1. Our test of whether one treatment is better than another is based on observing the treatments when they are applied to patients.
2. It is not based on any theory of how the treatments might work (although that presumably played a role in bringing the treatments to trial in the first place).
3. It is not based on anecdotal evidence, perhaps gained from a doctor "trying out" the treatment in an uncontrolled manner.
4. It is not based on any appeal to authority or on the basis of anyone's opinion.

Over the last 50 years, RCTs have become established as the primary and, in many instances, the only acceptable source of evidence for the efficacy of new treatments. So much so that claims for the efficacy of a treatment on the basis of points 3 or 4 in the preceding list, which used to be commonplace, now are seldom heard, are treated with scorn, and, in the case of point 3, may even be illegal or unprofessional. An excellent source for information on the evolution of trials (and much other material on trials) is the James Lind Library, found at http://www.jameslindlibrary.org.

The use of empirical evidence to settle the matter is what makes statistics important in RCTs. Not all patients will react to treatment in the same way, and whether the difference between the two treatment groups is important, given the variation in the response observed within each group, is clearly a statistical question. Indeed, the RCT is of little value unless the results obtained can be generalized to as yet untreated patients; this inference from the sample to the population is a statistical exercise. As with any inferential process, the quality of the inference will be higher if the data used are collected appropriately. Again, statistical ideas are of the utmost importance in the design of RCTs, although the use of classical designs, such as randomized blocks and split-plots are not often used in RCTs.

RCTs are used to gather empirical evidence about differences between treatments. However, in this area there is a delicate balance between evidence and belief. It is unlikely that a treatment will ever be subjected to the rigors of an RCT if no one believes it represents an improvement on the *status quo*. You therefore will find people involved in the conduct of RCTs who believe that one treatment (usually the new one) may be superior. However these people will also acknowledge that their beliefs are essentially unsupported and might be even be mistaken. Simply believing that one treatment is superior to another is not a justification for acting on that belief: such justi-fication requires you to collect evidence to prove or refute your beliefs and the RCT is the currently accepted tool for doing this.

RCTs are therefore of the utmost importance to modern medicine and statistics, and statisticians are of the utmost importance to RCTs. However, none of the preceding discussion explains what it is about RCTs that have given them this position of importance. This omission will be rectified if answers can be given to the following, and this will be attempted in the course of Section 1.3 of this chapter.

1. Why do you need to compare groups anyway?
2. What is so important about randomization?
3. How do you compare groups?

### 1.2.3   Ethical Issues

RCTs are essentially experiments and, though these may not have been commonplace in medicine until recently, scientists have been performing experiments for centuries; so is there anything new about RCTs? In the sense of the scientific logic that underlies the use of RCTs, the answer is probably no. Nevertheless, even if the logical basis of the experimental method is common to most scientific disciplines, many methods and matters of detail are often peculiar to a new field of enquiry, and much of this book will be concerned with techniques largely encountered only in RCTs.

However, there is one fundamental feature of RCTs that sets them apart from virtually all other experiments: the experimental units are people. This places various ethical responsibilities on the investigator. We will not con-sider the ethical implications of RCTs in detail, but will note three issues that are of utmost importance.

1. A patient must never be given a treatment that is known to be inferior.
2. Patients must be fully informed about all the circumstances sur-rounding the treatments in the trial, including possible adverse reac-tions and side-effects they may experience. Once informed, patients must only be entered into the trial if they give their consent, prefer-ably in writing. Withholding consent must not compromise their further treatment in any way. Only in very exceptional circumstances does the investigator not need to obtain informed consent and, in some countries, even these cases are proscribed.
3. Patients who have entered a trial may withdraw at any time and they must then receive the most appropriate treatment available outside the trial.

Other ethical issues that have implications for points of methodology are mentioned when the relevant methodology is discussed.

The interests of patients are safeguarded by the Declaration of Helsinki, which outlines the ethical constraints that surround experimentation on human subjects. This is an international statement of principle and different countries implement it differently. In the U.K., each health authority has an ethics committee that must approve all proposals for experiments involving human subjects. No reputable medical journals will publish the description of research that has not obtained such approval. The Declaration of Helsinki is a statement of the policy of the World Medical Association with regard to medical research involving human subjects. It was first adopted in 1964 and has been revised and amended from time to time since then: the latest version can be found at the organization's website, http://www.wma.net.

## 1.3   Structure and Justification of RCTs

Figure 1.1 is a schematic diagram of an RCT. It possesses five key items:

1. A population of eligible patients.
2. A group of patients recruited from this population.
3. Existence of (at least) two treatment groups.
4. Allocation to treatment is by randomization.
5. Outcome measures in the treatment groups are compared at the end of the trial.

The reason for each of these components is considered in the following text: 1 and 2 in Subsection 1.3.1, 3 in Subsection 1.3.2, and 4 and 5 in Subsection 1.3.3 of this chapter.

### 1.3.1   Eligible Patients

In order to conduct an RCT you need a supply of patients who may benefit from the treatment under investigation. These will usually be recruited from a hospital clinic, ward, or a general practice as they present with, or attend for treatment of, their condition. It may be thought that any such patient might profitably be recruited into the trial. However, such a casual approach has a number of disadvantages.

1. The type of patients recruited in this way will be difficult to describe. Many early trials in the treatment of cancer created confusion because different trials admitted patients with widely differing characteristics. Some recruited patients with advanced disease and reported disappointing rates, whereas other trials considered such

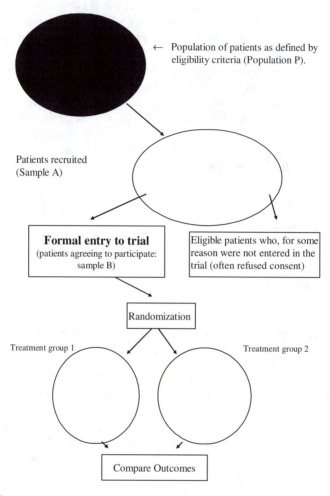

**FIGURE 1.1**
Recruitment to a randomized controlled clinical trial.

patients to be beyond treatment with the agent concerned and recruited only patients with less advanced disease. This resulted in widely varying estimates of the cure rate. The problem was made worse because the trial reports were often not explicit about the types of patients who were treated. It is therefore important that the report of any trial should describe precisely which patients it was intended to treat.

2. Most trials need to enroll so many patients that the trial has to run for many months, possibly even years. Patients are usually recruited to a trial as they present. With such sequential recruitment, it is possible that without clear criteria for recruitment, the type of patient recruited changes over the duration of the trial. Some trials, known

as *multicenter trials*, recruit from several centers, which may be in different parts of a city, different parts of a country, or even from several countries, and achieving consistency between centers without a set of clear criteria would be especially difficult.

3. The aim of the trial is to generalize its results to all patients who are similar to those treated in the trial. Without a strict set of eligibility criteria it is more or less impossible to describe to which types of patients the results of the study can be applied. Even with a clear set of eligibility criteria this is not a simple matter.

## Example 1.2: Example of Eligibility Criteria (Brandjes et al., 1997, *Lancet*, 349, 759–762)

Following a deep vein thrombosis (DVT), a blood clot in the veins of the leg, complications and recurrence known as *postthrombotic syndrome* can arise. A randomized trial was performed to determine if wearing sized-to-fit graded elastic compression stockings reduced the incidence of post-thrombotic syndrome. The eligibility criteria for the trial were as follows.

Patients were included if they were attending the center running the trial with venogram-proven DVT.

Patients were excluded if they also had the following:

A life expectancy of less than 6 months
Paralysis of the leg
Bilateral DVT (i.e., thrombosis occurred in both legs)
Leg ulcers or extensive varicosis (e.g., varicose veins)
Already using compression stockings

Patients were entered into the trial if they satisfied the inclusion criterion, satisfied none of the exclusion criteria, and gave informed consent. The investigators considered 315 consecutive cases that satisfied the inclusion criterion and excluded 20 patients with life expectancy less than 6 months, 11 with leg paralysis, 10 already wearing stockings, and 3 with leg ulcers. A further 77 refused to give consent so the trial proceeded with the remaining 194 patients.

The purpose of eligibility criteria is thus to define clearly the patients who might enter the trial and so allows consistent recruitment and clear description of the scope of the trial.

Broadly speaking, the eligible population is the group of patients to whom we would like to generalize our results. However, it should be noted that no formal attempt is made to ensure that the patients actually recruited are representative of the population of eligible patients. This is, at least in part, because there will seldom be an adequate sampling frame for this population: put simply, we are generally unaware of the eligible patients until they appear at the clinic. Moreover, as Example 1.2 shows, not all potentially eligible patients who arrive at the clinic enter the study, as many may refuse to give their consent.

It follows that, even with carefully defined eligibility criteria, the group of patients to whom we may generalize our results is not easily delineated. However, judgments on this issue would be much more difficult in the absence of eligibility criteria.

### 1.3.2    The Need for Concurrent Controls

If you want to see if a new treatment works, why not give it to a patient and see if he or she gets better? If the outcome of the disease is invariable, then this approach might be tenable. Hill (1962, Chapter 1), writing of the pre-streptomycin era, pointed out that tuberculous meningitis was always fatal, so the recovery of any patient treated with streptomycin provided evidence of the value of the drug. However, instances in which the outcome of a disease is invariable are, these days, extremely rare and can, for practical purposes, be ignored. Instead, patients, their disease, and their reaction to treatment are all variable to some extent. Measuring and accounting for this variability is what gives statistics its central role in RCTs.

If recovery is uncertain, and we give all our patients the new treatment, then we will not know which of the patients who recover do so because of the treatment or because they would have done so anyway. The solution is to include a second group of patients, often called a *concurrent control group* or simply *a control* group, in the trial who do not receive the new treatment. At the end of the trial the aim is to ascribe any differences between the two groups to the new treatment. As in the uncontrolled study, some patients given the new treatment would have recovered anyway, but there will be a similar subgroup in the control group and their effect cancels out in the comparison of the groups. The following points about the use of a concurrent control group should be noted.

1.  The control group may receive any treatment, except the new one. In fact, if there is an effective treatment (on which you hope to improve with the new treatment), then it would be unethical to withhold this from the control group. The trial is then a comparison of the new treatment with the best currently available treatment. If there is no accepted treatment available, then the control group may receive no treatment at all (that is, what they would usually have received), or they may receive a sham treatment known as a *placebo*. The use of placebos raises a number of important issues and will be considered more fully in Chapter 5.

2.  The treatment groups are usually assessed on the basis of suitable summaries, such as their means. That is, we examine the data to see

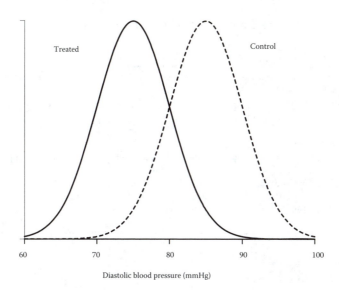

**FIGURE 1.2**
Hypothetical distribution of blood pressure in treated and control groups.

if there is evidence that the mean of the treated population differs from that of the control population. We do not look at the effectiveness on a patient-by-patient basis, so there may well be instances in which some individuals do worse on the "superior" treatment than some others on the "inferior" treatment.

Figure 1.2 shows the distribution of diastolic blood pressure in a group treated with a new drug intended to reduce blood pressure and in a control group. Although the new drug appears to work well insofar as the average blood pressure of the treated group is lower than that of the control group, a reasonable proportion of the control population has lower blood pressure than the treated population. Of course, this may just reflect the distribution of blood pressure in the population as a whole: those with low blood pressure in the control group may well have had even lower blood pressure if they had received the new drug.

3. A treated group and a control group is the simplest possible arrangement for an RCT. Trials with more than two groups are often used. For trials involving conditions for which there is no accepted treatment, you may have two control groups — one receiving a placebo and the other receiving the current treatment, i.e., nothing at all. More elaborate arrangements, such as factorial treatments are possible, as are groups in which different doses of the same treatment are used.

4. It is important that the groups be as alike as possible in all respects other than treatment. This is an issue of the utmost importance and is considered more fully in the next section.

## Example 1.3: Some Examples of Control Groups

| Condition | Treated Group | Control |
|---|---|---|
| Obstructive coronary artery disease (*Lancet*, 1996, 347, 79–84) | Excimer laser coronary angioplasty | Balloon angioplasty |
| Cytomegalovirus (CMV) prophylaxis in liver transplant patients (*Lancet*, 1995, 346, 69–74) | Ganciclovir | High-dose acyclovir |
| Neonatal hypocalcemia (*BMJ*, 1980, 281, 11–14) | Antenatal vitamin D supplements | Placebo supplements |
| Diabetes mellitus in childhood and adolescence (*Arch. Dis. Child.*, 1989, 64, 997–1003) | Special education classes in addition to usual clinic visits | Usual clinic visits only |

### 1.3.3 Allocation at Random

Figure 1.1 shows that having defined a population of eligible patients (population P) and having recruited a group from this population (sample A), the subset of these who formally enter the trial (sample B) are allocated at random to the treatment groups. There are three primary justifications for the use of this method of allocation.

1. In principle at least, it ensures that the groups to be given the different treatments are comparable.
2. The allocation to treatment is unknown at the time of entry to the trial.
3. There is a statistically sound estimate of error available for the comparison of the two treatment groups.

#### 1.3.3.1 Comparable Groups

The aim of an RCT is to assess the relative merits of the treatments being studied. If the treatment groups differ at the end of the trial, it is important that we should be able to assert that this is because of the different treatments. Clearly, if the treatment groups differed systematically before the trial ever started then this would be impossible. Randomization is the means by which the ability to state that the difference in treatment groups is caused by the difference in treatments is achieved.

An important point to bear in mind when considering RCTs is that the aim of randomization is to make the two treatment groups comparable with one another. They are not, individually, necessarily representative of the population of eligible patients. To be more specific, suppose the following:

1. The outcome measured on an individual patient formally entered into the trial is a random variable $X$

2. Neither treatment has any effect
3. We measure the difference in effect of the treatments by comparing means, with the mean in group $i$ ($i = 1, 2$) being $\overline{X}_i$

Now, if $E(X)=\mu$ then, because each of the treatment groups is a random sample from the group entered into the trial, it follows that $E(\overline{X}_1) = \mu = E(\overline{X}_2)$, so the difference in treatments is measured by $\overline{X}_1 - \overline{X}_2$, which has zero expectation, i.e., we have an unbiased estimate of the effect of treatment.

Notice how this formulation depends only on the expectation of $X$ within the group entered into the RCT. No attempt is made to ensure that sample A, those recruited from the population P, is actually a random sample from P. Moreover, sample B is not a random subsample of sample A — those agreeing to take part in a trial will usually be systematically different from those not agreeing. If the mean of the variable $X$ in population P is $\mu'$ it is likely that $\mu' \neq \mu$. However, none of this affects the preceding argument, which simply ensures that the treatment groups are comparable with one another.

Of course, the hope is that, in some sense, $|\mu - \mu'|$ is not too large, otherwise it will be very difficult to generalize the results of the trial. However, it is important to note that no formal attempts are made to ensure that $|\mu - \mu'| = 0$ and that this does not affect the validity of the RCT.

Randomization is intended to ensure that groups are comparable: for example, in two randomized groups the proportion of female patients should be similar, the proportion of patients with blue eyes should be similar, and the distribution of the severity of disease should be similar. The range of prognostic factors, i.e., features of the patient that are related to their outcome (see Chapter 4, Section 4.5) should be similarly represented in the two groups. An important feature of randomization is that it should achieve comparability with respect to all prognostic factors, including those that are unknown to the investigators.

It should be noted that several methods of randomization are possible and that, especially in smaller studies, some of these are more effective than others in achieving comparable groups. This issue will be considered in more detail in Chapter 4.

### 1.3.3.2    *Allocation Unknown at Entry to the RCT*

If the treatment a patient is to receive is known to the doctor before the patient is formally entered into the study, then the decision as to whether or not the patient is actually entered may be affected. This can cause bias and will be considered more fully in Chapter 2, Subsection 2.2.1.

### 1.3.3.3    *Valid Estimate of Error*

Under very general conditions, two groups can be compared using methods that can be justified by the act of randomization. The usual assumptions, such as normality, are not then necessary. This will be mentioned in more detail in the final section of Chapter 7.

---

## Exercises

1.  In a clinical trial, outcomes are measured in 100 patients, 50 having been randomized to treatment 1 and 50 to treatment 2: the outcomes are continuous but not normal. This can be represented in Minitab using column C1 to contain 100 numbers drawn from a nonnormal distribution (e.g., try generating them using Calc -> Random Data -> Lognormal and plotting a histogram or normal probability plot to confirm their nonnormality) and setting fifty 1s and fifty 2s in column C2 (they can be set arbitrarily, but fifty 1s followed by fifty 2s will do). The file RANDCHK.MTB contains the following Minitab code.

```
let k99=k99+1

note apply random permutation to C2 and put results
in C4

random 100 c3;
uniform 0.0 1.0.
sort c2 c4;
by c3.

note copy outcomes for treatment 1 to C11, for 2 to
C12
copy c1 c11;
use c4=1.
copy c1 c12;
use c4=2.

note compute t statistic in k4 [sqrt(1/50+1/50)=0.2]
let k1=mean (c11)
let k2=mean (c12)
let k11=stdev(c11)
let k12=stdev(c12)
```

```
let k3=sqrt((k11**2+k12**2)/2)
let k4=(k1-k2)/(k3*0.2)

note store result in next available row of C5
let c5(k99)=k4
end
```

(a) Explain how the code mimics what happens in a controlled trial in which there is no treatment effect.

(b) If the following were entered in the Session window of Minitab,

```
let k99=0
exec 'randchk' 10000
```

- what would you obtain in c5? What distribution would you expect it to have?

(c) Enter the preceding code into a text file (or use the STOR command in Minitab) and run it. What do you find? Calculate the cumulative distribution function of the $t$-distribution on an appropriate number of degrees of freedom (or of a normal distribution, as it will be very similar), sort these values, and plot them against a column containing 1/10001, 2/10001, ..., 10000/10001. What do you find and what does it mean?

Note that if $X$ is a random variable with cumulative distribution function $F(.)$, then $F(X)$ is uniformly distributed on [0,1].

# 2

## Bias

At the conclusion of an RCT, the investigators are eager to calculate a number that measures the difference between the treatments. The presence of some degree of sampling error in this number is inescapable, but excluding from this number any systematic effect other than the treatment effect is the overriding aim of much of the methodology that surrounds RCTs. Such unwanted systematic effects are called *biases*.

## 2.1   What Is Meant by Bias in RCTs?

Suppose that the outcome variable in treatment group 1 of an RCT is represented by a random variable $X_1$ and that in group 2 by $X_2$. An assumption that is commonly made, and one that will often be made throughout this book, is that the effect of treatment is additive, giving $E(X_1) = \mu + \tau_1$ and $E(X_2) = \mu + \tau_2$, where $\mu$ is the expected value of either $X$ at randomization. In these terms, the main aim of the RCT is to estimate $\tau = \tau_1 - \tau_2$; $\tau$ is often referred to as the *treatment effect*.

Suppose that the mean outcome in group $i$ is $\bar{X}_i$, then if all goes well with a trial, it follows that $\bar{X}_1 - \bar{X}_2$ is an unbiased estimator of $\tau$. However, in practice, many things can happen which ensure that a trial does not go well, leading to the possibility that $\bar{X}_1 - \bar{X}_2$ does not provide an unbiased estimate of $\tau$. Some general remarks are worth making at this point.

1.  The methodology of RCTs is preoccupied with methods for avoiding bias. This is in marked contrast to the aims of classical designed experiments, such as randomized blocks and Latin squares. Here, simple differences between the means of treatment groups are unbiased: the full analysis is needed to ensure that irrelevant sources of variability are excluded from the computations of the standard errors that attend the differences in means. In other words, the emphasis is on increasing precision rather than avoiding bias. In RCTs the design is usually so simple that there is little opportunity

for improving precision (but see Chapter 6 and Chapter 11 for some qualifications of this statement).

2. In saying that problems may lead to $\bar{X}_1 - \bar{X}_2$ being a biased estimator of $\tau$ we are going beyond the usual notion of a biased estimator often encountered in mathematical statistics. If we take a sample of $n$ independent copies of a variable with a normal distribution, mean $\mu$, standard deviation $\sigma$, then we know that $E(s) \neq \sigma$, where $s$ is the sample standard deviation. In other words $s$ is a biased estimator of $\sigma$. However, this is a feature of the estimator we have chosen to use, and an unbiased estimator can be recovered if we use:

$$\frac{\Gamma(\frac{1}{2}(n-1))\sqrt{\frac{1}{2}(n-1)}}{\Gamma(\frac{1}{2}n)} s$$

in place of $s$. In other words, the data are perfectly capable of providing an unbiased estimator of $\sigma$; we just need to use an unbiased estimator. When we speak of a biased estimate of $\tau$ in an RCT, we usually mean that something has gone wrong with the data collection, and the data collected may be incapable of providing an unbiased estimator. In the proofs of $E(\bar{X}_1 - \bar{X}_2) = \tau$ that are widely encountered in textbooks of mathematical statistics, there is usually a preamble that states that the variables forming the means are independent, identically distributed random variables from the respective distributions. In biased trials it is some aspect of this condition that has been violated.

## 2.2   Types of Bias

In the course of conducting an RCT many practical problems that could lead to bias will be encountered. It is useful to describe some of these under the following headings.

1. Selection bias
2. Allocation bias
3. Assessment bias
4. Publication bias
5. Stopping rules

These terms will now be explained in turn. Terms 2, 3, and 5 will be dealt with briefly in this chapter and more fully in subsequent chapters; publication bias will not be considered in detail in this book.

### 2.2.1  Selection Bias

Selection bias can occur when the decision to enter a patient to an RCT is influenced by knowledge of which treatment the patient will receive when entered. In a well-run RCT selection bias should not occur, because the patient will be formally entered into the study before the treatment is chosen. Indeed, it is for this reason that there is a procedure of formal entry to the trial (see Figure 1.1 in Chapter 1); once a patient is formally entered into the trial they are entered in a patient log, and randomized. They cannot then be removed from the trial. Of course, a patient may exercise their right to withdraw from the study at any time but, as far as possible, data from that patient will have to be analyzed at the conclusion of the study (see Chapter 9).

If the doctor admitting patients to the RCT is not happy with a particular eligible patient receiving one or more of the trial treatments, then that patient should not be entered into the trial at all. This causes no problem of bias — selection bias is a problem only if some patients might be entered if they are sure to receive (or not to receive) certain treatments. However, it would be disturbing if many consenting, eligible patients were not entered in this way; in the notation of Subsection 1.3.3 of Chapter 1, it would tend to make $|\mu - \mu'|$ uncomfortably large. It may point to a defect in the specification of the eligibility criteria or the doctor may not be a suitable investigator for this RCT.

It may seem that if a patient is eligible and agrees to enter the trial that is the end of the matter and foreknowledge of the treatment on the part of the admitting doctor cannot affect matters. However, before any patient is entered into any trial, the benefits and adverse effects of all the trial treatments must be fully explained. The doctor may know that if a patient consents to entering the trial they will get a certain treatment. If the doctor has reservations about the suitability of that treatment for that patient, it will be difficult for the doctor, either consciously or more often subconsciously, not to emphasize the negative aspects of the trial. This increases the chance that the patient will not agree to enter the trial. Note that we are not discussing the situation in which the patient is told what treatment they are to receive before obtaining their consent.

Problems of selection bias can occur in nonrandomized studies, for example, in which patients are allocated alternately to one of two study treatments. In general, this cannot happen with randomized studies, unless the person admitting patients to the RCT also prepared the randomization list. Preparing a randomization list in advance can be good practice but should never be done by anyone involved with the recruitment of patients — it is best done by the trial statistician. Some methods of random allocation, if inadequately implemented, can lead to similar problems (see Chapter 4, Section 4.2). Example 2.1 is a hypothetical example which, although rather stylized, illustrates the nature of the problem that can arise.

## Example 2.1: Hypothetical Example of Selection Bias

Consider a trial to compare two treatments for a serious malignant disease. One treatment (N) is nonsurgical and not invasive (it involves a course of tablets with limited side effects), whereas the other treatment (S) involves surgery and most patients take 2 or 3 months to recover from the operation. Eligible patients are to be allocated to N or S alternately by a single doctor.

Patients agreeing to enter the trial have had the severity of their disease graded as 1 or 2 on the basis of a biopsy sample taken earlier: grade 2 indicates more severe disease. The proportion of patients with grade 1 disease is $\lambda$ and that with grade 2 is $1-\lambda$.

The survival time for patients, $X$, has mean $\mu_1$ for patients with type 1 disease: this is expressed as $E(X\mid 1)=\mu_1$ and, similarly, $E(X\mid 2)=\mu_2$. As type 1 patients have less severe disease we suppose $\mu_1 > \mu_2$. Also, $E(X)=\lambda\mu_1 +(1-\lambda)\mu_2$ is the mean survival time for untreated patients. We further suppose that treatment by N changes mean survival by $\tau_N$, with a similar definition for $\tau_S$. It is also supposed that this change affects the mean survival equally for type 1 and type 2 patients. Therefore, in an obvious notation:

$$E(X\mid N,1)=\mu_1 +\tau_N \qquad E(X\mid N,2)=\mu_2 +\tau_N$$

$$E(X\mid S,1)=\mu_1 +\tau_S \qquad E(X\mid S,2)=\mu_2 +\tau_S$$

It follows that if we admitted all patients equally to the trial, the mean survival time in group N would be

$$E(X\mid N,1)\Pr(1\mid N)+E(X\mid N,2)\Pr(2\mid N)=(\mu_1 +\tau_N)\lambda +(\mu_2 +\tau_N)(1-\lambda)=\mu +\tau_N$$

Similarly, that in group S would be $\mu +\tau_S$ so the difference in treatment means would be $E(X\mid N)-E(X\mid S)=\tau_N -\tau_S$, i.e., the estimate would be unbiased.

The nature of the disease is such that all the eligible patients are essentially willing to enter the study. However, the doctor is uneasy about submitting patient with severe disease (type 2) to the risks and pain of a surgical operation. This is reflected in the way the doctor explains some of the risks of the trial to type 2 patients whom he knows will receive S. As a result, there is a probability $p$ that a type 2 patient destined for S will refuse to enter the study. If $A$ denotes the event of being admitted to the trial, this situation can be described by the equations

$$\Pr(A\mid N,1)=1 \qquad \Pr(A\mid N,2)=1 \tag{2.1}$$

$$\Pr(A \mid S, 1) = 1 \qquad \Pr(A \mid S, 2) = 1 - p = q \qquad (2.2)$$

We can only base our calculations on patients admitted to the study, so our estimate of treatment effect is now not $E(X \mid N) - E(X \mid S)$ but $E(X \mid A, N) - E(X \mid A, S)$.

We need to calculate $E(X \mid A, N)$ and $E(X \mid A, S)$. The first step in this is to note that

$$E(X \mid A, N) = E(X \mid A, N, 1) \Pr(1 \mid A, N) + E(X \mid A, N, 2) \Pr(2 \mid A, N)$$

and

$$E(X \mid A, S) = E(X \mid A, S, 1) \Pr(1 \mid A, S) + E(X \mid A, S, 2) \Pr(2 \mid A, S)$$

In order to compute $\Pr(1 \mid A, N)$ we apply Bayes' theorem to Equation 2.1, thus:

$$\Pr(1 \mid A, N) = \Pr(A \mid 1, N) \frac{\Pr(1 \mid N)}{\Pr(A \mid N)} = \frac{\Pr(A \mid 1, N) \Pr(1 \mid N)}{\Pr(A \mid N, 1) \Pr(1 \mid N) + \Pr(A \mid N, 2) \Pr(2 \mid N)}$$

Now $\Pr(1 \mid N) = \Pr(1) = \lambda$ because allocation to N is independent of patient type, as allocation happens before questions of admission to the RCT arise. Substituting from Equation 2.1 gives $\Pr(1 \mid A, N) = \lambda$ and hence $\Pr(2 \mid A, N) = 1 - \lambda$. A similar calculation gives $\Pr(1 \mid A, S) = b = 1 - \Pr(2 \mid A, S)$ where

$$b = \frac{\lambda}{\lambda + q(1 - \lambda)} \, .$$

Also, once the information on the type of patient and the treatment to be allocated is known, the expected value of $X$ is independent of whether or not the patient is admitted to the trial. That is, $E(X \mid N, 1) = E(X \mid A, N, 1)$, etc. This is probably obvious for all types of patients except type 2 patients allocated to S. However, it is assumed that those patients of this type who refuse to enter are selected with probability $p$, independently of the distribution of their survival time. In truth, this is likely to be a little unrealistic, but it will suffice for this example. It follows that

$$E(X \mid A, N) = E(X \mid N, 1) \Pr(1 \mid A, N) + E(X \mid N, 2) \Pr(2 \mid A, N)$$

$$= (\mu_1 + \tau_N) \lambda + (\mu_2 + \tau_N)(1 - \lambda) = \lambda \mu_1 + (1 - \lambda) \mu_2 + \tau_N$$

and

$$E(X \mid A,S) = E(X \mid S,1)\Pr(1 \mid A,S) + E(X \mid S,2)\Pr(2 \mid A,S)$$
$$= (\mu_1 + \tau_S)b + (\mu_2 + \tau_S)(1-b) = b\mu_1 + (1-b)\mu_2 + \tau_S$$

From this, it follows that the estimate of treatment effect that is obtained from the trial is

$$E(X \mid A,N) - E(X \mid A,S) = \tau_N - \tau_S + (\lambda - b)(\mu_1 - \mu_2)$$
$$= \tau_N - \tau_S - \frac{p\lambda(1-\lambda)(\mu_1 - \mu_2)}{\lambda + q(1-\lambda)}$$

Thus, the different way the entry to the trial of patients destined for N and S has been handled has led to a bias in the estimate of treatment effect. Three points should be noted about this result.

1. If all patients of type 2 destined for S are admitted, i.e., $p = 0$, the bias disappears.
2. If patients of type 1 and type 2 have the same mean survival time the bias also disappears.
3. As $\mu_1 - \mu_2 > 0$, $E(X \mid A,N) - E(X \mid A,S) < \tau_N - \tau_S$. If N is the superior treatment, i.e., $\tau_N - \tau_S > 0$ then the bias reduces the apparent size of the benefit N confers relative to S. This has occurred because the manner in which the doctor handled the entry procedure meant that patients who have a poorer mean survival time are relatively under-represented in the S group, which consequently appears to have a superior mean survival time. If S is the superior treatment then for the same reason the trial will exaggerate this superiority.

## 2.2.2   Allocation Bias

Patients have many factors that can affect the outcome of their therapy, regardless of the treatment group they are allocated. These prognostic factors might be, for example: whether the tumor is advanced or not; whether initial disease control was good; higher or lower natural levels of immunity; whether or not a patient can walk (ambulatory status). Randomization will, in principle, lead to groups that are balanced, in the sense that the distribution of these factors will be similar in the different treatment groups. However, simple randomization, in which effectively the allocation to treatment is made by the toss of a coin, is obviously a stochastic phenomenon, and there may be particular trials in which balance on an important prognostic factor may not be achieved. This could lead, for example, to a trial of therapies for multiple sclerosis in which one treatment group has a much higher proportion of nonambulatory patients than the other. The treatment in the group with a higher proportion of nonambulatory patients is very likely to compare poorly with other treatments in the trial, simply because the patients in this group have more severe diseases.

This failure to form comparable treatment groups means that the comparison of treatments is biased and we refer to this form of bias as *allocation bias*. The problem can be addressed, at least for known prognostic factors, by a variety of methods: see Section 4.5 and Section 4.6 in Chapter 4.

### 2.2.3 Assessment Bias

At the end of the trial, and often during its course, observations are made on a variety of outcome variables. Many of these will be entirely objective, such as whether a patient has died or the concentration of hemoglobin in the blood. Other variables are less objective: the proportion of the body covered with plaques of psoriasis is usually assessed by a dermatologist using various rules of thumb; blood pressure (systolic) is usually measured by reducing the pressure in the cuff of a sphygmomanometer until the sound of a pulse can be heard in an artery of the arm. Other variables, such as measures of quality of life, though clinically very important, are necessarily highly subjective.

If the observer knows the treatment being given to the patient and if the measurement of an outcome variable contains an element of subjectivity, then it is possible that the value of an observation might be influenced by the knowledge of the treatment. For example, in a trial of treatments designed to reduce blood pressure, the observer's views on the effectiveness of a treatment may affect his judgment of when the noise of a pulse can be heard. Similar problems can arise when patients know which treatment they are receiving. Even if these problems do not occur, the possibility that they might can affect the credibility of the trial. Measures to deal with such assessment bias are discussed in Chapter 5.

### 2.2.4 Publication Bias

The ultimate aim of an RCT is to influence medical practice. This is generally done by publishing a report of the results of the trial in a medical journal. Reports submitted to a reputable medical journal will be subject to peer review, in which experts in the field are asked to judge the suitability of the paper for publication. On the advice of these experts, and depending on a number of other factors, the decision whether or not to publish a paper rests with the editor of the journal.

In recent years, a view has formed among medical scientists that papers reporting positive findings are more likely to be published than those that do not. More often than not, positive findings means that a statistically significant difference between treatments has been demonstrated. If we take significant to equate to $P < 0.05$, then even if there is no treatment effect, one trial in twenty would be expected to demonstrate a significant effect. If these trials are more likely to be published then the medical literature will clearly be misleading.

This is a genuine problem but not one we will consider further, although some related matters will be mentioned in Chapter 12. Some progress is being made in this area. One example is provided by the leading medical journal, *The Lancet*, which will now review papers reporting RCTs before the study is conducted, and will either reject the submission or give an undertaking to review the report once the trial is complete.

### 2.2.5   Stopping Rules

Once a trial has been started, how will it stop? A crude possibility that is clearly unsatisfactory when assessing the stochastic outcomes of a trial is to keep analyzing the data as the trial continues and stop when a promising result has been obtained. This would obviously induce a bias. Such practices can have ethical advantages but can only be condoned scientifically if they are done as part of a prespecified method for assessing data in this way; some of these methods are discussed in Chapter 8. A simpler way to stop without any suspicion of bias of this form is to run the trial until a specified number of patients have been treated. A method of specifying the number of patients is described in Chapter 5.

---

### Exercises

1. It has recently become apparent that various disorders of the stomach are due to infection with a bacterium *Helicobacter pylori* (*H. pylori*). Thus, for example, stomach ulcers are now treated with a short course of antibiotics that eradicate the *H. pylori*. The presence of *H. pylori* in a person's gut can be detected with reasonable certainty by analyzing a sample of the patient's breath.

   In a general practice, there are many patients suffering from stomach problems for which, despite much investigation, no cause could be found (dyspepsia of unknown origin). These patients are treated by giving tablets *T* to reduce the amount of acid secreted by the stomach: they take these tablets permanently. It was decided to run a trial to see if giving antibiotics to eradicate *H. pylori* was preferable to a maintenance dose of *T*. The outcome would be the amount of indigestion remedy (a simple antacid) used by the patient in the year that the trial would last.

It is proposed to randomize patients to two groups, one receiving $T$ for the whole year and the other receiving antibiotics for the first three weeks of the year. In the group randomized to receive the antibiotics, it was suggested that the breath test should be administered and the antibiotic given only to those who gave a positive test. Those patients given antibiotics could then be compared with those given tablets. Explain why this would give a biased comparison and suggest alternatives that would be unbiased.

# 3

## How Many Patients Do I Need?

### 3.1 Criteria for Sample Size Calculations

An RCT is used to gather evidence about the relative merits of two or more treatments. In order to do this we recruit eligible patients, allocate them randomly to the treatments under investigation, and then assess their outcomes. How do we know when to stop? There are broadly two possibilities.

1. You keep recruiting until the question of which treatment is superior is settled.
2. You decide beforehand how many patients you need to recruit and you only analyze when this number has been recruited.

Superficially, alternative 1 seems much the more attractive and such so-called sequential methods have long been scrutinized by statisticians. However, the implementation of this method is fraught with difficulty, especially from the frequentist (i.e., non-Bayesian) point of view adopted in this book, and further discussion is postponed until Chapter 8.

Alternative 2 is, in fact, the approach most often used in practice. By having a fixed target for recruitment, however that is set, you immediately acquire the advantage that you have a known and objective stopping rule. One way of causing a problem with the interpretation of a trial is not to have an explicit stopping rule. If you do not specify at the outset of the trial how and when you will stop the trial, detractors could raise the objection that you stopped when you did because you thought it might favor your preferred treatment. Although this may not be the case at all, the inability to rebut any such allegation would weaken the trial report.

However, you also need to specify a total number of patients that is, in some sense, adequate for your purposes. In rather nonspecific terms, an RCT is about gathering evidence about the difference between the treatments, and the more patients you recruit, the more evidence you obtain. There are problems with obtaining both too much as well as too little evidence.

1. If you recruit too few patients, then you may be unable to settle questions that are central to the aim of the RCT. This is not only scientifically inadequate, it is ethically unsound. An RCT exposes one group of patients to an inferior treatment, which is partly justified because the evidence thereby obtained will be of benefit to future patients. If your trial produces no such evidence, then you have exposed some patients to an inferior treatment and have gained nothing for future patients.

2. On the other hand, it is also unethical to recruit many more patients than you need to settle the primary question asked in the RCT. If you could have decided that treatment A was better than treatment B on the basis of data from 100 patients, but recruited 200, then the patients allocated to treatment B from the final 100 recruits could have been saved from exposure to an inferior treatment.

This is the background to why we need to set a sample size in an RCT. However, it is very vague: what is the primary question, what do we mean by adequate evidence to settle the question? These notions need to be made more precise.

### 3.1.1   The Primary Question

Most RCTs record many variables on each patient. However, at the outset of the trial, there are advantages to designating one of these variables as the primary outcome variable. One of the advantages is that we can focus on this variable when we try to decide how large the trial ought to be: we aim to gather sufficient evidence to settle questions about this variable.

### Example 3.1: Outcome Variables and Primary Outcome Variables

| Trial | Some Outcome Measures | Primary Outcome |
|---|---|---|
| Zanamivir vs. placebo for treatment of influenza A and B (*Lancet*, 1998, 352, 1877–1881) | 1. Amount of cough mixture used<br>2. Days to alleviation of symptoms<br>3. Amount of paracetamol used | Days to alleviation of symptoms |
| Comparison of "hospital at home" vs. acute hospital care (*BMJ*, 1998, 316, 1796–1801) | 1. Quality of life measures<br>2. Physical functioning at 4 weeks and 3 months<br>3. Time in hospital/"hospital at home"<br>4. Mortality at 3 months | Time in hospital/ "hospital at home" |

*Continued.*

| Trial | Some Outcome Measures | Primary Outcome |
|-------|----------------------|-----------------|
| Scandinavian Simvastatin Survival Study on the lowering of cholesterol on patients with coronary heart disease (*Lancet*, 1994, 344, 1383–1389) | 1. Serum LDL cholesterol<br>2. Serum triglyceride<br>3. Mortality<br>4. Whether patient needed bypass surgery | Mortality |

### 3.1.2   Adequate Evidence

If the primary outcome variable $X$ is distributed with mean $\mu$ in the control group and mean $\mu + \tau$ in the treated group then the aim is to learn about $\tau$, the treatment effect, either by estimating it or testing the null hypothesis that it is zero. One could think of adequate evidence in terms of making the standard error of some estimator of $\tau$ small in some sense. However, the difficulty of defining small, combined with the strong interest that is usually focused on the test of the null hypothesis $H_0$: $\tau = 0$, means that adequate evidence is usually thought of in terms of having adequate power to test $H_0$. Therefore, before proceeding to the details of how we calculate a sample size, it will be useful to review some general features of hypothesis tests.

## 3.2   Hypothesis Tests

### 3.2.1   General Remarks

The result of performing a hypothesis test is a probability, universally known as the $P$-value of the test. It is important to be clear what the $P$-value does mean and, perhaps more importantly, what it does not mean. A definition, appropriate to a test comparing groups, is as follows:

> If the null hypothesis is true, the $P$-value is the probability of obtaining a difference between the groups (as measured by the test statistic $T$) as large as or larger than that observed.

More informally, if we assume there is no treatment effect (i.e., $\tau = 0$), then differences between the treatment groups that are very extreme are unlikely to occur by chance and their improbability is reflected in small $P$-values. If a $P$-value smaller than 0.05 is obtained, then this is generally accepted as providing evidence that the null hypothesis is false. A $P$-value less than about 0.01 would provide stronger evidence against the null hypothesis. A $P$-value of 0.1, and certainly of 0.5, would not provide such evidence, as the observed data would be entirely compatible with data drawn from populations in which the null hypothesis was true.

It is of the utmost importance to understand that a $P$-value compatible with the truth of the null hypothesis does not mean that the null hypothesis is true. It is obvious that any dataset compatible with the truth of $\tau = 0$ is also compatible with the truth of $\tau = \varepsilon$ for any sufficiently small, but nonzero, $\varepsilon$. If we do not have enough evidence to demonstrate that $\tau \neq 0$, then this might be because $\tau = 0$ but, in practice, it is much more likely to be because we have not gathered sufficient evidence.

This is a convenient place to note that $P$-values are sometimes interpreted by noting whether they are above or below one of several conventional thresholds. So, for example, a difference between two treatment groups might be said to be significant at the 5% level if $P < 0.05$, or at the 1% level if $P < 0.01$, etc. This method was almost universal when $P$-values had to be obtained from tables; space constraints meant that it was only practical to tabulate the critical values of test statistics at these conventional levels of significance. This is not wholly satisfactory because there is, in practice, likely to be little difference between studies yielding $P = 0.04$ and $P = 0.06$, and it would not be sensible to deem that one study showed evidence of a treatment effect whereas the other did not. Now that computers are widely available, we are no longer restricted simply to quoting whether $P$-values are above or below given thresholds, and reports of RCTs should quote the $P$-value to two significant figures (unless it is very small, when one significant figure may suffice). However, the practice of deeming that a difference is significant at the $100\alpha\%$ level (with $\alpha$ usually 0.05 or 0.01) is also applied in the calculation of samples sizes, as will be seen in the next section. This is necessary because it is needed to define a fixed rejection region for a test, without which the sample size calculation could not proceed.

### 3.2.2   Implication for RCTs

Suppose we conduct an RCT and perform a hypothesis test on the primary outcome variable. If this leads to a $P$-value that is less than about 0.05, we would conclude there was evidence of a treatment effect (i.e., $\tau \neq 0$) and all would be well. However, what can be concluded from the trial if a nonsignificant $P$-value is obtained, say $P > 0.05$? The preceding discussion shows that we cannot conclude that there is no difference between the treatments. The $P$-value indicates the data are consistent with no treatment effect, but they are also consistent with some effect. Clearly, by itself, this is useless. We need to design the RCT in such a way that we avoid making such an unhelpful statement.

If the data are compatible with $\tau = 0$ then we observed that they would also be compatible with $\tau = \varepsilon$ for sufficiently small $\varepsilon$. So, a nonsignificant result in our trial means we have failed to distinguish between "no effect of treatment" and "a small, but nonzero, effect of treatment." However, failure to distinguish between no effect and a very small effect may be of no interest. For example, if a new drug for lowering blood pressure actually achieved a mean reduction 0.1 mmHg (mm of mercury, the usual unit for blood pressure) greater than that of the standard treatment then this would not represent a therapeutic advance. Failure to detect such a small treatment effect would be unimportant. What we must do is ensure that our trials have a reasonable chance of detecting differences that are clinically important. In fact, the term small is ambiguous and we should talk about differences that are clinically important and clinically unimportant. In order to do this, we must ensure that the size of the trial is sufficiently large to detect clinically important treatment effects, and the means of doing this will be described more precisely in the next few sections.

### 3.2.3   One-Sided vs. Two-Sided Tests

Suppose we have measured blood pressure in patients randomly allocated to one of two drugs designed to reduce blood pressure. At the end of the study, we could test the null hypothesis of no treatment effect by performing an unpaired $t$-test. Suppose the calculated statistic is $t$, the $P$-value is usually computed as

$$P = \Pr(|T| > |t|) = F(-|t|) + \{1 - F(|t|)\}$$

where $T$ is a random variable with a Student's $t$-distribution having the appropriate number of degrees of freedom and $F$ is the cumulative distribution function of this distribution. This is a two-sided $P$-value. Thus values of $t$ that are large in absolute size, whether positive or negative, lead to small $P$-values. In other words, differences between the treatment groups in either direction (treatment A better than treatment B, or treatment B better than treatment A) provide evidence against the null hypothesis. Put more formally, this form of the test corresponds to testing

$$H_0 : \tau = 0 \quad \text{versus } H_{alternative} \, \tau \neq 0 .$$

At the outset of an RCT, there may be a good deal of optimism that the new treatment (A) will be an improvement over the standard treatment (B). If treatment A being better than treatment B corresponds to $\tau > 0$, then there may be a temptation to perform the test of:

$$H_0 : \tau = 0 \quad \text{versus } H_{alternative} \, \tau > 0 .$$

The $P$-value would then be

$$P = \Pr(T > t) = 1 - F(t)$$

with $T$ and $t$ defined as before. This is the one-sided $P$-value and if $t > 0$, it will be a half of the two-sided $P$-value (because $T$ is symmetrically distributed about 0). Superficially, this may be rather attractive — we have halved our $P$-value and so appear to have a greater chance of obtaining a conclusive result in our RCT. We have achieved this by altering the alternative hypothesis and this is not as innocuous as it may seem. Small $P$-values will be obtained from large positive values of $t$. Large negative values of $t$ do not result in small $P$-values and provide no evidence against the null hypothesis. Suppose that in our trial, contrary to prior expectation, the group receiving A fared much worse than the group receiving B. Our specification of $H_{alternative}\, \tau > 0$ effectively means that we must accept this as a chance event which casts no doubt at all on our null hypothesis of no difference between treatments. Prior expectations for new treatments are notoriously overoptimistic and few medical statisticians would be prepared to dismiss such an outcome so lightly. Consequently, one-sided hypothesis tests are seldom used; in this book, unless otherwise stated, hypothesis tests are taken to be two-sided.

## 3.3  Sample Size for a Normally Distributed Variable

Suppose we have randomly allocated $n$ patients to treatment group 1 and $m$ patients to treatment group 2. Suppose also that the primary outcome variable, $X$, has a normal distribution with mean $\mu$ in group 1, mean $\mu + \tau$ in group 2, and common standard deviation $\sigma$. We wish to test the null hypothesis $H_0 : \tau = 0$ vs. $H_0 : \tau \neq 0$, and if $\bar{x}_1, \bar{x}_2$ are the sample means and $s$ is the pooled estimate of standard deviation, we compute:

$$D = \frac{\bar{x}_2 - \bar{x}_1}{s\sqrt{\frac{1}{n} + \frac{1}{m}}}$$

which under $H_0$ has a $t$ distribution with $n + m - 2$ degrees of freedom. The difference between the groups would be said to be significant at the $100\alpha\%$ level if:

$$|D| > t_{\alpha/2}(n + m - 2)$$

where $t_\xi(v)$ is such that $\Pr(T > t_\xi(v)) = \xi$ when $T$ has a Student's $t$ distribution with $v$ degrees of freedom.

As $v$ tends to infinity, the distribution of $T$ tends to that of a standard normal variable $Z$, and $t_\xi(v)$ tends to the corresponding quantile, $z_\xi$, of the standard normal distribution where, to be specific, $\Pr(Z > z_\xi) = \xi$. For all practical purposes this limit is achieved when $v \approx 40$. As it is rare for sample sizes for RCTs to be less than 40, we approximate the limits based on the $t$-distribution by those based on the normal distribution, so a difference is said to be significant at the $100\alpha\%$ level if $|D| > z_{\alpha/2}$.

Thus, given the data, we can compute $D$ and we reject $H_0$ if $D$ lies outside the interval $[-z_{\alpha/2}, z_{\alpha/2}]$ or, equivalently, if $\bar{x}_2 - \bar{x}_1$ falls outside the interval

$$[-z_{\alpha/2}s\lambda(m,n), z_{\alpha/2}s\lambda(m,n)]$$

where $\lambda(m,n) = \sqrt{\dfrac{1}{m} + \dfrac{1}{n}}$ . What is the probability of this event? If $H_0$ is true, then by construction, the answer is $\alpha$; this is sometimes referred to as the type I error rate of the test. However, what if $H_0$ is false and $\tau$ takes some nonzero value? This quantity,

$$\Pr(\text{Reject } H_0 \mid \tau) = \psi(\tau)$$

is the power function of the test. The standard notation for power is $1 - \beta$, as $\beta$ is usually reserved for $\Pr(\text{Accept } H_0 \mid \tau) = 1 - \psi(\tau)$, the type II error rate. We can compute $\Pr(\text{Reject } H_0 \mid \tau)$ if we continue to use a normal approximation for the distribution of $D$, and note that its variance and mean are approximately 1 and $\tau/(\sigma\lambda(m,n))$, respectively. The situation is illustrated in Figure 3.1: we simply need to compute the probability that a normal variable with this mean and variance falling outside the acceptance region $[-z_{\alpha/2}, z_{\alpha/2}]$, shown as the shaded box in Figure 3.1.

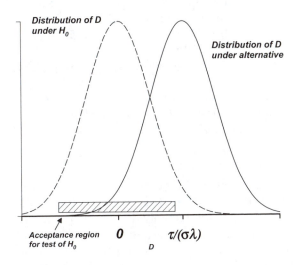

**FIGURE 3.1**
Distribution of test statistic under null and alternative hypotheses.

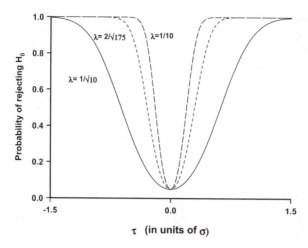

**FIGURE 3.2**
Plot of power function.

If we use $\Phi$ to denote the cumulative distribution function of the standard normal distribution, this is simply:

$$\Phi(-z_{\frac{1}{2}\alpha} - \frac{\tau}{\sigma\lambda}) + \left(1 - \Phi(z_{\frac{1}{2}\alpha} - \frac{\tau}{\sigma\lambda})\right) = 1 - \beta = \psi(\tau) \tag{3.1}$$

The plot of $\psi$ against $\tau$ is known as the *power curve* of the test. This is illustrated in Figure 3.2 at the 5% level of significance for three circumstances: first, a trial with 20 patients in each group, so $\lambda = 1/\sqrt{10} \cong 0.32$; second, a trial with 200 patients in each group, so $\lambda = 1/10 = 0.1$; the third example is another trial with a total of 400 patients but with 50 in one group and 350 in the other, so $\lambda = 2/\sqrt{175} \cong 0.15$.

The graph in Figure 3.2 has the following features:

1. All the curves pass through (0, 0.05), as $\tau = 0$ corresponds to $H_0$ and the probability of rejecting the null hypothesis must then be the significance level of the test.

2. As the value of $\tau$ moves away from 0, the probability of rejecting the null hypothesis increases.

3. For a given nonzero value of $\tau/\sigma$, the probability of rejecting the null hypothesis is smallest for the trial with 40 patients and largest for the trial with 400 patients, equally divided between the groups. The trial with 350 patients in one group and 50 in the other has lower power than that with 400 patients who are equally divided between the groups. In general, the power increases as $\lambda$ decreases, and the power depends on sample size only through the quantity $\lambda$.

4. At any given value of $\tau/\sigma$, we can make the power of the trial any value ($> \alpha$) we choose simply by selecting the appropriate value of $\lambda$, which in turn corresponds to recruiting the appropriate number of patients.

Equation 3.1 allows any one of $\alpha$, $\beta$, $\tau/\sigma$, and $\lambda$ to be found once the other three have been specified. When planning a study, the significance level, $\alpha$, is the easiest to deal with as it is usually set at 0.05 or 0.01. As illustrated in Figure 3.2, for any test, the power will be high for high values of $\tau/\sigma$ and low for low values, so the next step is to decide what is the smallest value of this ratio of interest. In practice, few doctors will be able to specify the ratio directly, and this step actually has two parts: (1) specification of the minimum clinically important difference, $\tau_M$ and (2) obtaining an estimate of $\sigma$. We then decide the power our test ought to have: often values of 90% or 80% are chosen, i.e., $1-\beta = 0.9$ or $1-\beta = 0.8$. We then solve Equation 3.1 for $\lambda$ to obtain the sample size of the study.

Equation 3.1 could be solved numerically, but an approximation is possible that yields a solution in closed form. Without loss of generality we may assume $\tau_M > 0$. In practice, the first term in Equation 3.1 is negligible as it is the probability that the test rejects $H_0$ because $D$ is improbably large, not in the direction of $\tau_M$ but in the opposite direction (indeed, such cases would lead to $H_0$ being rejected but with the wrong inference being drawn about the sign of the treatment difference). Finding $\lambda$ then amounts to solving:

$$\Phi(z_{\frac{1}{2}\alpha} - \frac{\tau_M}{\sigma\lambda}) = \beta = 1 - \psi(\tau) , \qquad (3.2)$$

and as by definition $\Phi(z_\beta) = 1 - \beta$ and by symmetry $\Phi(-z) = 1 - \Phi(z)$, we can use the monotonicity of $\Phi$ to obtain:

$$\frac{\tau_M}{\sigma\lambda} = z_\beta + z_{\frac{1}{2}\alpha} . \qquad (3.3)$$

Of course, we are interested in the sample sizes, and so it is useful to recast Equation 3.3 in terms of $n$ and $m$. If a given value of $\lambda$ yields the desired power, then we would usually (but not invariably; see Chapter 4, Section 4.4) want to ensure that we obtained $\lambda$ subject to using the minimum total number of patients, say $m + n = 2N$. From the definition of $\lambda$ we have

$$\lambda^{-2} = \frac{mn}{2N} = \frac{1}{2}N - \frac{k^2}{2N}$$

where $k = \frac{1}{2}(m - n)$ (such that $m = N + k$, $n = N - k$). Any $N$ which solves this will obey $N \geq 2\lambda^{-2}$, with equality when $k = 0$. Thus, any given value of $\lambda$ is achieved for a minimal total number of patients by using two groups each of size $N$. In this case $\lambda^{-1} = \sqrt{\frac{1}{2}N}$, and substituting in Equation 3.3 gives:

$$N = \frac{2\sigma^2(z_\beta + z_{\frac{1}{2}\alpha})^2}{\tau_M^2} \tag{3.4}$$

This is the formula that is widely used to determine the size for an RCT when the outcome variable is, at least approximately, normal. The "noisier" the measurements, i.e., the larger $\sigma$, the larger the trial needs to be. Also, you need a larger trial to detect a smaller difference in treatment means, $\tau_M$.

## Example 3.2: Determining the Size of a Trial (MIST study group, *Lancet*, 1998, 352, 1877–1881)

A randomized trial to assess the effectiveness of zanamivir, a new treatment for influenza, compared a group randomly allocated to the new treatment with a group randomly allocated to a sham (or placebo) treatment. When planning the trial the investigators decided that the primary variable would be the number of days to the alleviation of symptoms (with alleviation and symptoms defined precisely elsewhere in the plan of the study).

A previous study suggested that a sensible value for $\sigma$ was 2.75 d and the minimal clinically relevant difference that the trial should have good power to detect, $\tau_M$, was taken to be 1 d.

The investigators used a significance level of 5% and specified a power of 90%, so $\alpha = 0.05$ and $\beta = 0.1$. These figures give:

$$z_{\frac{1}{2}\alpha} = 1.96$$

$$z_\beta = 1.28$$

$$\frac{\sigma^2}{\tau_M^2} = 7.56$$

Substituting in Equation 3.4 gives $N = 2 \times 7.56 \times 3.24^2 = 158.8$. Thus the study requires about 160 patients to complete the trial in each group.

## 3.4 Sample Size for a Binary Variable

### 3.4.1 Formulation

In many trials the outcome variable cannot be said to be normally distributed, even approximately. Similar formulae to those in Section 3.3 of this chapter can be derived for many types of outcome. One of the most important is when the outcome variable is binary, i.e., success or failure, yes or no, 0 or 1. Examples include: "The transplanted kidney produced urine within 30 d" or it did not; "The patient was alive 3 years after the procedure" or they died within that period; "The patient was clear of psoriasis within a month" or not. In general discussion, we will often refer to outcomes as positive or negative, success or failure, or 0 or 1 if it is convenient to attach numerical values to these attributes.

In such trials, the groups are compared by considering the proportion of positive outcomes in each group. The number of successes in the group given treatment A, $R_A$, will have a binomial distribution $Bi(n_A, \pi_A)$, where $n_A$ patients are allocated to this treatment group, and similarly for treatment B. The size of the trial will be calculated to give adequate power to test the null hypothesis $H_0 : \pi_A = \pi_B$. The observed proportion of positive outcomes in the group given X is $p_X = R_X / n_X$, where X is A or B.

In this formulation, there is no free parameter corresponding to $\sigma$ as in the case of normal outcomes. This is because $p_A$ has variance $\pi_A (1 - \pi_A) / n_A$, i.e., it is determined by the same parameter that defines its mean. This dependence between mean and variance complicates the calculation of a sample size and it is preferable to transform the data in such a way that there is no longer any such dependence. This requires an approximation technique known as the *delta method* and this will now be explained before we proceed to developing a formula for binary outcomes analogous to Equation 3.4.

### 3.4.2 The Delta Method

Suppose the random variable X has mean $\mu$ and variance $\sigma^2 = \sigma^2(\mu)$, what is the mean and variance of $f(X)$ for a general "well-behaved" (e.g., differentiable as often as we like) function $f$? An exact answer requires evaluation of a sum or integral and often these will not have a closed form. Application of a number of seemingly crude approximations gives a formula that works remarkably well. First, expand $f(X)$ in a first-order Taylor series about $\mu$, giving

$$f(X) \approx f(\mu) + (X - \mu) f'(\mu) \tag{3.5}$$

and hence:

$$\left( f(X) - f(\mu) \right)^2 \approx \left( X - \mu \right)^2 \left[ f'(\mu) \right]^2 \tag{3.6}$$

Taking expectations of Equation 3.5, we get $E(f(X)) \approx f(\mu)$; this can be used in the left-hand side of Equation 3.6, so that when we take expectations of this equation we obtain:

$$\mathrm{var}(f(X)) \approx \sigma^2(\mu)\left[f'(\mu)\right]^2$$

This series of approximations, which works well in practice, is known as the *delta method*.

A common application of the technique is to find a transformation to a scale on which, at least approximately, the variance is unrelated to the mean. This is done by solving the differential equation $\sigma^2(\mu)[f'(\mu)]^2 = \text{constant}$. We illustrate this using the case of interest in the present application, namely in which $R$ has a binomial distribution with parameters $n$ and $\pi$. If we set $X = R/n$ then $X$ has mean $\pi$ and variance $\pi(1-\pi)/n$. If $f(X)$ is to have constant variance we need to solve:

$$\frac{\pi(1-\pi)}{n}\left[f'(\pi)\right]^2 = K = \text{constant},$$

that is, we need to evaluate

$$f(\pi) \propto \int \frac{1}{\sqrt{\pi(1-\pi)}} d\pi$$

Substituting $u^2 = \pi$ in the integral, we obtain the solution $f(\pi) = \arcsin(\sqrt{\pi})$ where of course the arcsin is evaluated in radians. As $[f'(\pi)]^2 = 1/[4\pi(1-\pi)]$ it follows that $\arcsin(\sqrt{X})$ has variance $1/(4n)$, approximately. This transformation is sometimes referred to as the *angular transformation*.

### 3.4.3   Sample Size Formula

If a success is coded as 1 and a failure as 0, then $p$ is the mean of these $n$ variables, so the central limit theorem applies and $p$ has an approximate normal distribution. The approximation is usually tenable provided $n$ exceeds about 30 and $\pi$ is not near its extremes, say between 0.15 and 0.85.

Also, the linear approximation in Equation 3.5 shows that if $X$ is normally distributed then, to the approximation in Equation 3.5, $f(X)$ is also normally distributed. Consequently, we have that $\arcsin(\sqrt{p_A})$ is approximately normally distributed with mean $\arcsin(\sqrt{\pi_A})$ and variance $1/(4n_A)$. We could then test $H_0 : \pi_A = \pi_B$ at the $100\alpha\%$ level by observing if

$$D = \frac{\arcsin(\sqrt{p_A}) - \arcsin(\sqrt{p_B})}{\frac{1}{2}\lambda(n_A, n_B)}$$

falls within $[-z_{\alpha/2}, z_{\alpha/2}]$, with $\lambda$ defined as in Section 3.3. This is analogous to the definition of $D$ in Section 3.3. The analogue of $\sigma$ is $1/2$ and of $\tau$ is $\arcsin(\sqrt{\pi_A}) - \arcsin(\sqrt{\pi_B})$, so the required formulae for sample size are

$$\frac{2\left(\arcsin(\sqrt{\pi_A}) - \arcsin(\sqrt{\pi_B})\right)}{\lambda(n_A, n_B)} = z_\beta + z_{\frac{1}{2}\alpha}$$

and, if we take two groups each with $N$ patients,

$$N = \frac{(z_\beta + z_{\frac{1}{2}\alpha})^2}{2\left(\arcsin\sqrt{\pi_A} - \arcsin\sqrt{\pi_B}\right)^2}$$

Although there is no $\sigma$ to specify, we still need to specify the same number of items when planning a trial as in the normal case. This is because $\arcsin(\sqrt{\pi_A}) - \arcsin(\sqrt{\pi_B})$ is not a function of $\pi_A - \pi_B$, so we cannot just specify the treatment difference, we need to specify the expected success rates on both treatments in order to calculate $\arcsin(\sqrt{\pi_A}) - \arcsin(\sqrt{\pi_B})$. In practice, this is often convenient because you have a good idea of the value of one, as it is likely to correspond to the standard treatment, and the other can be found by specifying a clinically important difference that you wish your trial to be able to detect.

## Example 3.3: Determining the Size of a Trial with a Binary Outcome (*Lancet*, 1994, 344, 1655–1660) (Smith et al., 1994)

Two methods for the management of malignant low bile duct obstruction are surgical biliary bypass and endoscopic insertion of a stent. An RCT was performed to compare these approaches.

The primary outcome of the trial was the binary variable: "Did the patient die within 30 d of the procedure?" The trial was designed to test the null hypothesis at the 5% significance level with 95% power, i.e., $\alpha = 0.05$ and $\beta = 0.05$. The trial wanted to be able to detect a change in mortality rate from 20% to 5%. This gives the figures:

$$z_{\frac{1}{2}\alpha} = 1.96$$

$$z_\beta = 1.65$$

and hence

$$N = \frac{(1.65 + 1.96)^2}{2\left(\arcsin(\sqrt{0.2}) - \arcsin(\sqrt{0.05})\right)^2} = 114.9$$

So we should aim to allocate 115 patients to each treatment.

Note that if we had wanted to detect a change from 0.45 to 0.3, i.e., the same change $\pi_A - \pi_B$, we would have needed 269 patients in each group. This clearly demonstrates that, unlike the normal case, we need to specify not simply the difference in means, but where that difference is located.

This method, using the angular transformation, is entirely respectable and follows easily from the method adopted for normally distributed outcomes. Alternative methods are available and one which is quite widely used is described in Section 4.6 of Armitage et al. (2002).

## 3.5  General Remarks about Sample Size Calculations

Calculating the number of patients needed for an RCT is one of the tasks that the medical statistician is called on to do frequently. Many clinical colleagues believe that this is an entirely objective and routine piece of arithmetic requiring little judgment. Obviously, once $\alpha$, $\beta$, $\sigma$, and $\tau_M$ have been specified in Equation 3.4, then it is just a matter of arithmetic. Also, the values of $\alpha$ and $\beta$ are chosen by the investigator and usually present few difficulties. However, obtaining an estimate of $\sigma$ is often quite difficult: values can sometimes be found from the literature; in other cases it is necessary to execute a small pilot study to obtain an estimate. Of course, if the pilot study is small then the confidence interval for $\sigma$ will be wide. The value of $N$ is quite sensitive to changes in the value used for $\sigma$.

It is often more difficult than might be imagined for the doctor to know what is a clinically important difference and hence specify $\tau_M$. This is likely to be a greater difficulty when the outcome variable is something that has just been identified as being of potential importance, but there is little clinical experience in measuring this quantity. It is sometimes sensible to pick a feasible sample size and then plot the curve similar to that in Figure 3.2 to see how the power of the study changes with $\tau_M$. However, this practice has its dangers, because it gives the investigator the opportunity to decide that a given value should be ascribed to $\tau_M$ simply because a study of convenient size would then have adequate power, and not because there was a good biological or clinical reason to support the choice of $\tau_M$. Even without plotting this graph doctors are often overoptimistic about the value of the new treatment and run trials that are too small because they specify a value of $\tau_M$ that is unrealistically large.

In practice, recruiting an adequate number of patients for a trial is often the most difficult aspect of clinical research. RCTs cannot continue indefinitely: technology and treatments change and your study will become outdated: staff running the trial will leave and motivation may fall: financial resources are limited (staff have often to be recruited to work full-time on the running of the trial). One approach is to determine how many patients are likely to be recruited over the period that it is feasible to run the trial and using this value of $N$, together with values for $\alpha$, $\sigma$, and $\tau_M$ use Equation 3.4 to find the power, $1-\beta$, that can be achieved. If the largest feasible trial has too little power then it may be best to abandon the trial, at least in its current form. Unfortunately, this approach can lead to trials that are too small because, rather than abandon a study altogether, investigators may persuade themselves that an unacceptably low power, say 60% or 65%, may after all be adequate.

When designing a study, it is important for the statistician to perform sensitivity analyses so that they are aware how sensitive their recommendations for $N$ are to uncertainty in the specification of parameters such as $\sigma$. Designing studies with binary outcomes can be a little easier, as there is often a good deal of information about the success rate on one of the treatments, thereby reducing the uncertainty in the formulation.

The preceding methods for determining sample size are probably the ones most widely used in practice. However, for virtually all other aspects of RCTs, statisticians have emphasized the need to focus on estimation of the treatment effect, rather than hypothesis testing. In many respects, it is unfortunate that sample size calculations have become dominated by ones that ensure hypothesis tests have good properties. This is particularly the case for variables whose novelty makes it difficult to specify a clinically important difference — such difficulties often arise because the science is insufficiently mature for hypothesis testing to be an appropriate way to proceed. In these cases, it may be more sensible to determine a sample size that tries to ensure that the width of a confidence interval is below some specified value.

## Exercises

1.

   (a) Celiac disease is a condition that impairs the ability of the gut to absorb nutrients. A useful measure of nutritional status is the biceps skinfold thickness, which has standard deviation 2.3 mm in this population. A new nutritional program is proposed and is to be compared with the present program. If two groups of equal size are compared at the 5% significance level, how large should each group be if there is to be 90% power to detect a change in mean skinfold of 0.5 mm? How many would I need if the power were 80%?

(b) Suppose I can recruit 300 patients, what difference can I detect with 80% power?

(c) Suppose I decide that a change of 1 mm in mean skinfold is of interest after all. How many patients do I need for a power of 80%?

(d) What would be the effect on this value if 2.3 mm underestimates $\sigma$ by 20%? If it overestimates $\sigma$ by 20%?

(e) Assuming that 2.3 mm is a satisfactory estimate of $\sigma$, what sample sizes would we need to achieve 80% power to detect a mean difference of 1 mm, if we opted to allocate patients to the new and control treatments in the ratio 2:1?

2. In a trial of a new treatment for stroke, a thrombolytic (blood-thinning) agent was compared with placebo. The outcome was whether or not there was a favorable outcome (i.e., a binary variable) as assessed with the aid of a scale widely used by physicians in the field. The trial was designed to have 80% power to find an improvement (at the 5% significance level) of 0.1 in the proportion with favorable outcome. How many patients, $n$, would be needed in each group if the proportion responding favorably in the placebo group was 0.3? How would this change if the proportion responding on the placebo group was thought to be 0.2? What would be the number if the proportion responding on placebo were 0.6? Comment on your final answer. (cf. Hacket et al., 1998.)

3. For $x, y \in [0,1]$ define $f(x,y) = \arcsin(\sqrt{x}) - \arcsin(\sqrt{y})$. Prove that $f(x,y) = f(1-y, 1-x)$ and explain the relevance of this result to the determination of sample sizes for RCTs with a binary primary outcome.

4. In an RCT in which the outcome has a normal distribution, a trial was designed to have power 90% to detect a difference in mean treatment effect of $\tau$ with a two-sided test at the 5% level. If the trial results in treatment means such that $\bar{x}_1 - \bar{x}_2 = \tau$, what $P$-value do you obtain? (You may assume that the trial is sufficiently large that the $t$-distribution can be closely approximated by a normal distribution and that the pooled sample standard deviation is essentially equal to the value of $\sigma$ used to plan the study.) What is the $P$-value if $\bar{x}_1 - \bar{x}_2 = \frac{1}{2}\tau$?

5. An RCT is planned to have the size needed to detect a clinically important difference at the 5% significance level. The trial recruits this number and the analysis of the trial gives $P < 0.05$. Does this mean that a clinically important difference has been found?

6. The *t*-statistic for comparing two normal outcomes is $D = (\bar{x}_A - \bar{x}_B)/s\lambda$ where $\lambda = \sqrt{\frac{1}{m} + \frac{1}{n}}$ with $m$ and $n$ are the group sizes, $s$ is the pooled standard deviation, and the numerator is the difference in sample means. If the population standard deviation is $\sigma$ and the true mean treatment difference is $\tau$, the expectation of $D$ is stated to be approximately $\tau/(\sigma\lambda)$. Show this, stating why it is only an approximation.

7. Find the error in the approximation in Question 6 when there are 30 patients; 100 patients in the trial and each group has the same size.

   (You are reminded that the density of a $\chi^2$ variable on $N$ degrees of freedom is $x^{1/2(N-1)}e^{-(1/2)x} / K(N)$, where $K(N) = \Gamma(\frac{1}{2}N)2^{1/2(N)}$, and

   that $\dfrac{\Gamma(\frac{1}{2}N - \frac{1}{2})}{\Gamma(\frac{1}{2}N)} \approx \dfrac{1}{\sqrt{\frac{1}{2}N - 1}}$ .)

8. Use a method analogous to the delta method to derive an approximate formula for $E(\arcsin\sqrt{R/N})$ when $R$ has a binomial distribution with parameters $N$ and $\pi$.

9. Use Minitab to generate 10000 random variables $R$ from a binomial distribution with parameters $N$ and $\pi$. Calculate $\arcsin\sqrt{R/N}$ and find its variance. Compare this with its approximate theoretical value. Do this for all combinations of $N = 10, 30,$ and $100$ and $\pi = 0.05, 0.2,$ and $0.5$. Comment.

# 4

## Methods of Allocation

### 4.1 Simple Randomization

#### 4.1.1 Chance Imbalance of Group Sizes

The archetypal view of a two-group RCT is of the doctor flipping a coin in order to decide how to treat a patient. In principle, this is indeed what random allocation to treatment calls for. There are several practical reasons why this precise method is, perhaps, not ideal. It might be difficult to assure oneself that the coin is unbiased; it may be inappropriate for the doctor to know what treatment is allocated; flipping the coin in front of the patient may overemphasize the aspect of uncertainty in their management. However, all these are practical matters and the essential statistical feature of this view is correct, namely that each patient is allocated to one of the trial treatments with a fixed probability, independently of all the previous allocations. This method is, effectively, the one that is used in many large trials.

However, at least in small trials, there are statistical defects with this method. Suppose there are two treatment groups, A and B, and each of $2n$ patients is allocated to either group, independently with equal probability. The number in group A, $N_A$, then has a binomial distribution, $\text{Bi}(2n, \frac{1}{2})$. The size of the larger group, $N_{\max}$ takes values in the set $\{n, n+1, \ldots, 2n\}$ with probabilities:

$$\Pr(N_{\max} = n) = \binom{2n}{n} \left(\tfrac{1}{2}\right)^{2n}$$

$$\Pr(N_{\max} = r) = 2\binom{2n}{r} \left(\tfrac{1}{2}\right)^{2n} \quad r = n+1, \ldots, 2n$$

These probabilities are plotted in Figure 4.1 for $n=15$. For $n = 15$, $\Pr(N_{\max} \geq 20) = 0.10$, so there is a substantial chance that the two groups will end up with markedly differing sizes. This is disadvantageous from a prac-

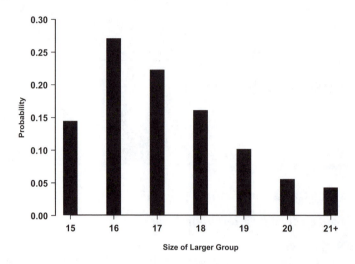

**FIGURE 4.1**
Distribution of larger group size in a trial of 30 patients with two treatment groups formed by simple randomization.

tical point of view, as it may mean that less experience is gained with the new treatment. It also has a statistical disadvantage in that the factor $\lambda$ in Equation 3.3 in Chapter 3 achieves its minimum when the groups have equal size and values of $\lambda$ greater than the minimum reduce the power of the study unnecessarily.

## Example 4.1: The Effect of Unequal Sample Sizes on Power

Suppose we are designing an RCT to detect a clinically important difference equal to a standard deviation, i.e., $\tau_M/\sigma = 1$, at the 5% significance level. If the study recruits 30 patients then the power $1 - \beta$ can be found from Equation 3.3 of Chapter 3 as

$$1 - \beta = \Phi\left( \sqrt{\frac{n_1 n_2}{30}} - 1.96 \right)$$

where $n_1$ patients are allocated to one group and $n_2$ to the other (so $n_1 + n_2 = 30$).

If the group sizes are equal, $n_1 = 15 = n_2$ then we find the power is 78%.
If one group has size 20 and the other 10 then the power is 73%.
If one group has size 6 and the other 24 then the power is 59%.

Thus, an imbalance of 2:1 has not resulted in serious loss of power, whereas more marked imbalance has given rise to a more noticeable loss. However, if it can be avoided, it would be better not to lose any power in this way.

### 4.1.2  Distribution of $\lambda$

The distribution of $\lambda(N_A, N_B)$ is clearly important in determining the effect of unequal allocation on power. In fact the distribution of $\lambda^{-2}$ is easier to handle. Now,

$$\lambda^{-2} = \frac{N_A(2n - N_A)}{2n} = \frac{n^2 - X^2}{2n},$$

where $X$ has been written for $N_A - n$. The normal approximation to the binomial distribution is good, even for quite small values of $2n$ when the probability of success is $1/2$. If we apply this approximation to $N_A$ and then transform to $X$ we find that, approximately, $X$ has a normal distribution with mean 0 and variance $\frac{1}{2}n$. Consequently, we can write $X = Z\sqrt{\frac{1}{2}n}$ where $Z$ has a standard normal distribution (i.e., mean 0, variance 1) and hence:

$$\lambda^{-2} = \frac{n^2 - X^2}{2n} = \frac{1}{2}n - \frac{1}{4}Z^2$$

As $Z^2$ has a $\chi^2$ distribution on one degree of freedom, we can readily describe the approximate distribution of $\lambda^{-2}$. The probability that $\lambda$ exceeds any given $\lambda_0$ can be approximated using this result.

### 4.1.3  Practical Consequences

The loss of power caused by imbalance in the sizes of the treatment groups is not serious unless the imbalance is marked. Indeed, we will take advantage of this observation in Section 4.4 of this chapter. However, the difficulty in recruiting sufficient patients is widely encountered in practice and no loss in power should be tolerated because of an avoidable artifact that brings no benefits.

Simple randomization to treatment groups A and B can be thought of as generating a sequence of As and Bs, each entry in the sequence being equally likely to take either value and is independent of all other elements of the sequence. For example, the following sequence was generated using the random number generator in Minitab:

| 1 | 2 | 3 | 4 | 5 | 6 | 7 | 8 | 9 | 10 |
|---|---|---|---|---|---|---|---|---|----|
| A | A | A | A | A | A | B | B | B | B  |

The first patient entered into the trial receives treatment A, patient 2 gets A, patient 7 gets B, etc. (of course, the practical implementation of this sequence would be such as to conceal the next treatment to be allocated from the admitting doctor). This unrestricted approach, which allows any random sequence to be used for allocation, can lead to groups of markedly different sizes.

---

## 4.2   Random Permuted Blocks

### 4.2.1   Random Permuted Blocks of Fixed Length

The problem of unbalanced group sizes can be solved by a form of restricted randomization known as *random permuted blocks,* or RPBs. The following are all the sequences of length 4 that comprise two As and two Bs:

| | | | | | | | | | | | | | | |
|---|---|---|---|---|---|---|---|---|---|---|---|---|---|---|
| 1. | **A** | **A** | **B** | **B** | 2. | **A** | **B** | **B** | **A** | 3. | **A** | **B** | **A** | **B** |
| 4. | **B** | **B** | **A** | **A** | 5. | **B** | **A** | **A** | **B** | 6. | **B** | **A** | **B** | **A** |

These short sequences are referred to as *blocks.* A list of independent identically distributed random numbers is then generated, each element being chosen from {1, 2, 3, 4, 5, 6} with equal probability. Each number in this list is then replaced by the block of two As and two Bs that corresponds to that number in the preceding key. See Example 4.2 for how this is done.

This results in a sequence in which each patient is equally likely to receive A or B but the randomization has been restricted to allow only sequences of As and Bs such that at no stage along that sequence does the foregoing number of As and Bs differ by more than 2. Indeed after every fourth patient the two treatment groups must have the same size.

The use of blocks of length four is arbitrary but constitutes a sensible compromise between blocks of length two and longer blocks. Blocks of length two impose too great a restriction on the randomization, for reasons which will be mentioned in section 7.6. Blocks longer than eight have two disadvantages: (1) they can allow the difference between group sizes to become too large and (2) the number of such blocks,

$$\binom{2m}{m}$$

where $2m$ is the block length, becomes large (e.g., $\binom{10}{5} = 252$), which makes the technique rather unwieldy. Blocks of length six and, occasionally, eight are useful as we will see in the next subsection.

Although we have introduced RPBs for trials with just two treatments, RPBs can be used for any number of treatments. For example, for three treatments all blocks of length six comprising two As, two Bs, and two Cs could be written down and indexed by the first $M$ positive integers, where in this case, $M = 90$. Random numbers can be chosen with equal probability from $\{1, 2, ..., M\}$ and this sequence can be changed into a sequence of As, Bs, and Cs in an analogous manner to the two-treatment case.

## Example 4.2: Preparing a List of Treatment Allocations Using RPBs with Block Length Four

1. Generate a list of random numbers, each equally likely to take one of the values in $\{1, 2, 3, 4, 5, 6\}$. Suppose this results in the following: 5, 1, 1, 3, ....

2. In the enumeration of all blocks of length 4 comprising two As and two Bs, 5 corresponds to the block BAAB, 1 to AABB, and 3 to ABAB.

3. Replacing 5,1,1,3 by the preceding blocks gives the treatment allocation sequence B A A B A A B B A A B B A B A B, ...

4. Patients entering the study are then allocated in turn to the treatments indicated by this list, so the first patient gets B, the second A, the third A, and so on.

There is, however, a potentially serious drawback to the way of implementing RPBs, which has just been described. This occurs if the trial is organized in such a way that the doctors involved in the study know which treatments patients already in the study have received. In some trials, e.g., those that compare different types of surgical operations, or which compare surgical vs. nonsurgical treatments, it is almost inevitable that those admitting patients to the trial will know what past patients have received. As the numbers receiving each treatment must be equal every fourth patient, then after 3 (modulo 4) patients have been admitted (i.e., after 3, 7, 11, 15, etc., patients) knowledge of previous treatments and of the block length allows the next treatment to be predicted with certainty. For example, with blocks of length four, if three patients have been allocated to surgery and four to the nonsurgical alternative, then the next patient will receive surgery. In some circumstances, the allocation of the next two patients can be predicted with certainty.

This means that selection bias may once again become a problem. It is not as bad as with some nonrandom methods of allocation, e.g., alternation, in which the fate of every patient can be predicted with certainty. With blocks of length 4, the fate of the $n$th patient can never be predicted with certainty if $n = 1$ or 2 modulo 4. Nevertheless, the allocation of over 25% of patients in the trial could be known in advance of their allocation, and this is more than sufficient to permit an unacceptable level of selection bias.

### 4.2.2 RPBs with Random Block Length

There are several ways to modify the way RPBs are implemented in order to avoid the potential for selection bias inherent in the use of RPBs with fixed block length. The methods are all similar and a simple version is described in the following text.

The 20 blocks of length 6 comprising 3 As and 3 Bs are enumerated as follows.

| | | | | | | | | | | | | | | | | | | | | | | |
|---|---|---|---|---|---|---|---|---|---|---|---|---|---|---|---|---|---|---|---|---|---|---|
| 1. | A | A | A | B | B | B | 2. | A | A | B | A | B | B | 3. | A | A | B | B | A | B |
| 4. | A | A | B | B | B | A | 5. | A | B | A | A | B | B | 6. | A | B | A | B | A | B |
| 7. | A | B | A | B | B | A | 8. | A | B | B | A | A | B | 9. | A | B | B | A | B | A |
| 10. | A | B | B | B | A | A | | | | | | | | | | | | | | |
| 11. | B | B | B | A | A | A | 12. | B | B | A | B | A | A | 13. | B | B | A | A | B | A |
| 14. | B | B | A | A | A | B | 15. | B | A | B | B | A | A | 16. | B | A | B | A | B | A |
| 17. | B | A | B | A | A | B | 18. | B | A | A | B | B | A | 19. | B | A | A | B | A | B |
| 20. | B | A | A | A | B | B | | | | | | | | | | | | | | |

One method to produce a list of treatment allocations using RPBs with random block length is as follows:

1. Set a counter $i$ equal to 1.

2. Generate a random number $X$ from the set $\{4, 6\}$, where $\Pr(X = 4) = \frac{1}{2}$.

3. If $X = 4$ then generate a random number $Y$ from the set $\{1, 2,..., 6\}$ (each number equally likely) and set $S_i$ to be the block of length 4 corresponding to $Y$ in the enumeration in Subsection 4.2.1 of this chapter.

4. If $X = 6$ then generate a random number $Y$ from the set $\{1, 2,..., 20\}$ (each number equally likely) and set $S_i$ to be the block of length 6 corresponding to $Y$ in the preceding enumeration.

5. If you have allocated all patients then stop; otherwise, increment $i$ by 1 and go to step 2.

The sequence $S_1, S_2,..., S_k,...$ is then a sequence of As and Bs that have been produced using RPBs with random block length. This sequence has the following properties.

1. Each patient is equally likely to receive A or B.

2. The number of patients allocated to the two groups can never differ by more than three.

3. The possibility of selection bias is negligible.

Selection bias is greatly reduced because the doctor will never know the length of the current block. The only time when it will be possible to predict accurately is when the numbers in the two treatment groups differ by three. As this is only possible with blocks of length 6 and only then with blocks 1 and 11, the chance of this happening is small. Any doctor trying to predict the next allocation will soon stop because failure will be so frequent.

## 4.3 Biased Coin Designs and Urn Schemes

Random permuted blocks are an effective and easily understood method for ensuring that more or less equal numbers of patients are allocated to all treatments in the trial. However, the use of RPBs has the drawback of potentially being predictable at certain stages of the allocation procedure, although the size of this effect can be reduced by the use of several randomly chosen block lengths. More subtle ways of achieving balance are available, and although these are attractive, they are not yet as widely used as RPBs. The methods are all essentially stochastic and as such eliminate the problem of occasional allocations being predictable. They work by adjusting the probability of treatment allocation as the trial proceeds in such as way that the probability of assignment to overrepresented treatments is reduced. There are many variants of these methods, and two approaches will be outlined in the following text.

### 4.3.1 Biased Coin Designs

In a trial to compare treatments A and B, suppose that after $n$ patients have entered the study, the number allocated to treatment A is $N_A(n)$ and to B is $N_B(n)$. Write the imbalance in treatment numbers as $D(n) = N_A(n) - N_B(n) = 2N_A(n) - n$. The biased coin design was introduced by Efron (1971) and changed the allocation probability according to the value of $D(n)$ as follows:

If $D(n) = 0$, allocate patient $n+1$ to A with probability $1/2$.

If $D(n) < 0$, allocate patient $n+1$ to A with probability $P$.

If $D(n) > 0$, allocate patient $n+1$ to A with probability $1 - P$.

where $P$ is some probability $1/2 < P \le 1$. If $D(n)$ is negative, then this means that there are more patients allocated to B than to A, so allocating to A with a probability greater than $1/2$ will tend to bring the allocation back into balance. Clearly, the situation with $D(n)$ positive is analogous.

If at any stage of the trial the absolute imbalance, $|D(n)|$, is $j$ ($> 0$) then the imbalance after the next patient is allocated, $|D(n + 1)|$, must be either $j + 1$ or $j - 1$. As the scheme works to reduce the imbalance, the probability of the former is $1 - P$ and of the latter is $P$. If the trial is ever in exact balance, $|D(n)| = 0$, then after the next allocation we must have $|D(n)| = 1$. The degree of imbalance $|D(n + 1)|$ depends, in a stochastic fashion, only on the previous imbalance, $|D(n)|$: indeed the imbalances form a simple random walk on the nonnegative integers with a reflecting barrier at 0 and transition probabilities:

$$\Pr \left( |D(n + 1)| = 1 \mid |D(n)| = 0 \right) = 1$$

$$\Pr\left(\,|D(n+1)|\,=j+1\ |\ |D(n)|\,=j\right)=1-P$$

$$\Pr\left(\,|D(n+1)|\,=j-1\ |\ |D(n)|\,=j\right)=P$$

A consequence of this observation is that some pertinent properties of this method of allocation can be discerned from known properties of random walks (Rosenberger and Lachin, 2002, p. 43). One such result, which has some bearing on the choice of $P$, is that, in the long run, the probability of exact balance after the allocation of $2n$ patients is approximately $2 - P^{-1}$. (Exact balance is clearly impossible after an odd number of patients, which is why we only consider $D(.)$ with an even argument.) When $P = 1$ exact balance is assured, but in this case the biased coin design is a deterministic sequence of alternating treatments. An intermediate value, such as $P = 2/3$ gives the probability of exact balance $1/2$ and $P = 3/4$ increases the chance of balance to $2/3$.

This method of allocation reduces the chances of imbalance and gives more balanced allocations than complete randomization. However, the method does use the same probability $P$ to attempt to restore balance, whatever the degree of imbalance. A possible modification is a scheme in which the probability of allocation to the underrepresented treatment increases as the imbalance increases. Methods of this kind will be described in the following subsection.

### 4.3.2 Urn Models

The allocation methods referred to as *urn methods* are based the classic probabilist's device of an urn or urns containing balls of different colors, or in this application, bearing different treatment labels. Patients are allocated by randomly choosing a ball from the urn and assigning the patient to the treatment written on the selected ball. The urn initially contains two balls, one labeled "treatment A" and the other 'treatment B'. The first patient is allocated by randomly choosing one of these balls. The selected ball is returned to the urn and a further ball, labeled with the letter of the treatment which was not chosen, is added to the urn. The procedure for allocating a patient is repeated. However, there is now a 2:1 chance that the trial will be balanced after the second allocation. If this happens, then adding a ball labeled with the treatment not chosen will result in the urn containing two balls labeled A and two labeled B, so the next patient is equally likely to receive either treatment. On the other hand, if the second patient received the same allocation as the first, then the urn will contain four balls, three labeled with the so-far unallocated treatment, thus increasing further the chance that the next patient receives the unallocated treatment. As the trial proceeds the method naturally and stochastically limits the chance of a severe imbalance.

The scheme outlined in the preceding paragraph was first proposed by Wei (1977, 1978) and could be referred to as a UD(1,1) allocation, as the urn

starts with one ball for each treatment and one ball is added at each allocation. A more general scheme is the UD($r$,$s$) allocation in which the urn
initially contains $r$ balls of each kind and at each allocation $s$ balls of the type
not just allocated are added. The method extends naturally to trials with $K$
($>2$) treatments: the urn starts with $r$ balls of each kind and at each allocation
$s$ balls corresponding to each of the unallocated treatments are added, i.e.,
a total of $s(K - 1)$ balls are added.

Put crudely, the method weights allocation quite substantially toward
achieving balance in the early stages of a trial but is likely to be close to
simple randomization once the trial has been running for a reasonable
period. The transition probabilities for the imbalance $|D(n)|$ can be found
by counting the allocations made among the first $n$ patients. Suppose that $n$
patients have been allocated and $N_A(n)$ of these have received treatment A,
so $D(n) = N_A(n) - N_B(n) = 2N_A(n) - n$. If the allocation uses a UD($r$, $s$) scheme
then there will be $2r + ns$ balls in the urn — $2r$ initially with $s$ added after
each of the $n$ allocations. Of these, there will be $r + N_A(n)s$ balls labeled B —
$r$ initially and $s$ balls of type B are added after each allocation to treatment
A. If we require the transition probabilities for $|D(n)|$ rather than $D(n)$ we
need to be slightly careful about signs. Suppose that $j > 0$, then

$$\Pr(D(n+1) = j - 1 | D(n) = j, D(n) > 0) =$$

$$\Pr(|D(n+1)| = j - 1 \,\|\, D(n) | = j, D(n) > 0)$$

is the probability that the trial, which currently has an excess of patients on
treatment A, becomes less imbalanced at the next allocation. This will happen
if we allocate the next patient to B, an event which will have probability:

$$\Pr(|D(n+1)| = j - 1 | D(n) > 0, \ |D(n)| = j) =$$

$$\frac{r + N_A(n)s}{2r + ns} = \frac{r + \frac{1}{2}(n + D(n))s}{2r + ns} = \frac{1}{2} + \frac{D(n)s}{2(2r + ns)} \tag{4.1}$$

On the other hand, if the trial currently has an excess of patients receiving
treatment B, then for $j$ still positive, the probability the trial becomes less
imbalanced at the next stage is

$$\Pr(D(n+1) = -j + 1 | D(n) = -j, D(n) < 0) = \Pr(|D(n+1)| =$$

$$j - 1 \,\|\, D(n) | = j, D(n) < 0)$$

As this is the probability that treatment A is allocated next it is

$$\Pr(\,|D(n+1)|=j-1\,|D(n)<0,|D(n)|=j) =$$

$$\frac{r+N_B(n)s}{2r+ns} = \frac{r+\frac{1}{2}(n-D(n))s}{2r+ns} = \frac{1}{2} - \frac{D(n)s}{2(2r+ns)} \qquad (4.2)$$

By the symmetry of the process, an imbalance of a given magnitude is equally likely to be in either direction, so $\Pr(D(n)>0\,||D(n)|=j>0) = \Pr(D(n)<0\,||D(n)|=j>0) = \frac{1}{2}$. Using this expression to combine Equation 4.1 and Equation 4.2 using the law of total probability we get

$$\Pr(\,|D(n+1)|=j-1\,|\,|D(n)|=j) = \frac{1}{2} + \frac{|D(n)|s}{2(2r+ns)} \qquad (4.3)$$

A similar argument considering the probability of increasing the imbalance at the $n$th allocation gives

$$\Pr(\,|D(n+1)|=j+1\,|\,|D(n)|=j) = \frac{1}{2} - \frac{|D(n)|s}{2(2r+ns)} \qquad (4.4)$$

When supplemented by the equation for the case $j = 0$, namely $\Pr(\,|D(n+1)|=1\,|\,|D(n)|=0) = 1$, Equation 4.3 and Equation 4.4 govern the evolution of the allocation. Equation 4.3 and Equation 4.4 show that when imbalance is present, the probabilities that the next allocation reduces or increases the imbalance are adjusted up and down from $1/2$ by an amount proportional to the degree of imbalance. The presence of $n$ in the denominator of these adjustments means that the size of the adjustment will tend to decrease as the trial progresses. As stated before, in the long run, the allocation scheme tends to simple randomization, although this is certainly not the case in the short term.

The investigator will need to choose values for $r$ and $s$. If $r$ is large compared with $s$ then the initial allocations will be quite similar to complete randomization, because they will be dominated by the balls originally in the urn rather than by those added subsequently. Tighter initial control over the degree of imbalance is achieved by ensuring that $s$ is large relative to $r$. In fact, a degree of simplicity is achieved by using the special case with $r = 0$, with the convention that the first patient is equally likely to be allocated to A or B. The UD(0,1) scheme is suitable for many applications.

Urn schemes are attractive and probably underused. They ensure closer balance than simple randomization without the problems of selection bias which may accompany random permuted blocks. Other urn schemes are possible: the Ehrenfest urn scheme uses two urns, one labeled A and the other B. Initially each urn contains $w$ balls: one of these is chosen and, if it is in urn A, then treatment A is allocated and the ball is replaced in urn B.

Probabilistically, balance is achieved because at the next allocation there are more balls in urn B than urn A, so allocation to the underrepresented treatment is higher than to the overrepresented treatment. Unlike Wei's urn design the number of balls stays constant. The interested reader should consult Rosenberger and Lachin (2002, Chapter 3) for more details of this and many of the other issues discussed in this section.

The allocations made under biased coin and urn schemes depend on the previous allocations but not, of course, on the outcomes of the patients treated. As such, there is no difficulty in using these methods to prepare allocation lists before the trial starts. Designs in which the allocation depends on the outcomes of previously treated patients, so-called response-adaptive designs do exist but are beyond the scope of this book. For those interested in this topic, a good place to start is Chapter 10 of Rosenberger and Lachin (2002).

## 4.4   Unequal Randomization

Suppose we are designing a study to compare a new inhaled steroid for the treatment of asthma with the existing preparation. The outcome variable is the forced expiratory volume in 1 sec (*FEV1*) in liters, a measure of lung function. It is decided that the trial should have 90% power to detect, at the 5% level, a change in FEV1 of 0.25 l and the standard deviation of FEV1 is known to be 0.5 l, so $\tau_M/\sigma = \frac{1}{2}$. Using Equation 3.3 we obtain $\lambda = 0.154$. If the two groups are of equal size, the number in each group, $n$, is given by:

$$n = 2\lambda^{-2} = 84$$

Thus if we run an RCT in which 168 patients are allocated equally between the two groups then we will have power of 90% to detect a difference of 0.25 l.

However, suppose the patients are not allocated equally but the number in one group is $\theta$ times the number in the other group. It follows that the groups have sizes $168/(1+\theta)$ and $168\theta/(1+\theta)$ and hence the power becomes:

$$\Phi\left(\frac{\sqrt{42\theta}}{1+\theta} - 1.96\right)$$

In Figure 4.2 this is plotted against $\theta$. As expected the power declines as $\theta$ increases, but the decline is not rapid. When $\theta = 2$ the power has only declined to 86% and when $\theta = 3$ the power is 80%. However at $\theta = 4$ it is 74% and by $\theta = 8$ the power is only 53%. It is unlikely that we would tolerate a drop in power from 90% to 74% but this only occurs when one group is

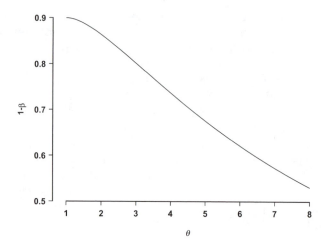

**FIGURE 4.2**
Power plotted against ratio of group sizes θ.

four times the size of the other, i.e., the groups have markedly different sizes. The loss in power that occurs when one group is twice the size of the other, relative to the power for groups of equal size, is from 90% to 86%, a difference that is unlikely to be important. However, if the group receiving the new treatment is twice the size of the other, then valuable extra experience in the use of the treatment might be obtained.

Unequal allocation can be very useful and is probably underused in practice: it can provide investigators with greater experience of a new treatment and may even encourage recruitment in certain trials. Although it inevitably entails some loss of power, provided the imbalance is no greater than 2:1, the loss is unlikely to be noticed. RPBs could easily be adapted to provide a means of ensuring an imbalance close to 2:1. Treatment allocation sequences could be built by randomly selecting from the 15 blocks of length 6, comprising 4 As and 2 Bs.

## 4.5   Stratification

### 4.5.1   The Problem of Allocation Bias

If the only use of RPBs was to ensure balance of group sizes across the whole trial, then it is unlikely that they would be used very much. Imbalance in group sizes sufficient to cause an appreciable loss of power is very unlikely. However, RPBs are widely used in practice, usually in combination with a technique known as *stratification*. Stratification is used to control the imbalance between the groups, not with respect to their size but with respect to their composition. Although randomization will, in principle, produce groups that are balanced with respect to any prognostic factor, in practice, treatments groups that are not alike with respect to important prognostic factors can and do occur. This problem, and its consequences, are made explicit in Example 4.3.

## Example 4.3: Imbalance with Respect to Prognostic Factors

Suppose we wish to compare a new method of treatment ($D$) with the existing method ($U$) to see if it improves the glycemic (i.e., blood sugar) control of patients under 16 years of age who suffer from type I diabetes mellitus. The outcome is a normally distributed variable known as HbA1c, which is the percentage of hemoglobin that has formed a complex with blood sugar. A higher value represents poorer control.

Suppose the RCT will recruit $2n$ patients and, within the patient population being recruited to the trial, a proportion $\theta$ are children (defined as patients under 12 years of age); the remaining patients, namely those over 12 years are referred to as adolescents.

Suppose we form two treatment groups each containing $n$ patients (perhaps by using RPBs). Then the number of children in the group receiving $D$, $M_D$ will have the binomial distribution Bi($n$, $\theta$). The number of children in the group receiving $U$, $M_U$ has the same distribution as $M_D$ and is independent of it. Thus, on average, we expect $\theta n$ children in each group. This is essentially what we mean when we say that, in principle, randomization will produce balanced groups: on average the groups will be balanced, but in any given trial, the actual numbers could be out of balance by an amount governed, in this example, by the two independent Bi($n$, $\theta$) distributions. (In practice, one would expect a value of $\theta$ between about 0.4 and 0.6, although the precise value of $\theta$ will not affect the following analysis.)

What you eat is a very important factor in achieving good glycemic control. Parents of children with diabetes know about this and, as they largely control the diet of their children, can impose an appropriate diet. Parents have conspicuously less control over what adolescents eat. It is widely accepted by doctors that there is a deterioration in glycemic control as patients pass through adolescence, although this is not wholly due to dietary factors.

Suppose that the treatment has no effect. Suppose also that the expected value of HbA1c is $\mu_C$ for children and $\mu_A$ for adolescents: it is expected that $\mu_A > \mu_C$ (typical values might be 6.5 to 9% for children and 7 to 11% for adolescents).

The mean HbA1c in the group receiving $D$ is then

$$\frac{\sum_{i=1}^{M_D} X_i + \sum_{i=M_D+1}^{n} X_i}{n}$$

where $X_1, \ldots, X_{M_D}$ are the HbA1c values for the children in the group and the other $X$s refer to adolescents. The expected value of this (over the distribution of HbA1c) is

$$\frac{M_D \mu_C + (n - M_D)\mu_A}{n}$$

The corresponding quantity in group $U$ is, of course,

$$\frac{M_U \mu_C + (n - M_U)\mu_A}{n}$$

The expected difference in treatments would then be the difference of these quantities, namely

$$\frac{(M_D - M_U)}{n}(\mu_C - \mu_A)$$

Because we have assumed the treatment has no effect this should be zero. However, because we are confident that $\mu_A > \mu_C$, this will only be true if $M_D$ equals $M_U$. Although this is true on average, it is certainly not guaranteed to be the case in any given trial in which we have only one realization for each of the random variables $M_D$ and $M_U$.

Example 4.3 shows that an imbalance between the treatment groups in prognostically different types of patients leads to a biased trial. This type of bias, known as *allocation bias*, was described informally in Subsection 2.2.2.

Example 4.3 is a very simple instance of allocation bias. In all trials there are likely to be several important prognostic factors which, if allocated unevenly between the treatment groups, could undermine the validity of the whole study. In Example 4.3, it would be relatively easy to argue that an additional important prognostic factor would be the length of time a patient has had diabetes.

Randomization will, in principle, allocate all prognostic factors, including ones whose importance is unsuspected by the investigators, evenly between the treatment groups. However, in practice, this may not be the case, especially with small studies, and we need to intervene in the randomization in order to ensure that specific factors are evenly spread across the treatment groups. Obviously we can only do this for factors we know are prognostically important: we must continue to rely on the good average properties of randomization to achieve balance with respect to unknown prognostic factors.

### 4.5.2 Using Stratification

Stratification is the simplest solution to the problem of allocation bias. Rather than allocate all patients in one process, we allocate patients of different types separately. So, for the case illustrated in Example 4.3 we would prepare, using RPBs, not one allocation list but two. One would be used for children and the other for adolescents. As we allocated children to the two treatments using RPBs, the number of children receiving each treatment will be very similar (differing by no more than half the maximum block length). The same holds good for adolescents, thereby producing a trial that is balanced with respect to this prognostic factor.

It is essential to realize that the allocation within each stratum must use some form of restricted randomization. If simple randomization is used, then within each stratum the numbers of patients in each treatment group may not be close, so the proportions of each type of patient in each treatment group may be quite different. Another way to think of this is that if allocation is by simple randomization, then each patient is allocated independently of all others, so the allocation is unaffected by whether or not patients are grouped into strata. With restricted randomization, this independence is lost and the stratification has an effect. Methods for achieving balanced allocations other than RPBs, such as those outlined in Section 4.3 of this chapter, can be used; it is just simple randomization that must be avoided.

In practice, when admitted to the study, the patient would have to be identified as a child (under 12) or adolescent (12 or over). If it had been decided to take account of the length of time the patient had diabetes, for example, by stratifying patients into those who were or were not diagnosed within the previous year, then this fact would also have to be known. In this case, you would need to prepare four allocation lists: one for children diagnosed within the last year, one for children who have had the disease for more than a year, and two more lists for the recently and not-so-recently diagnosed adolescents.

Of course, prognostic factors do not need to have just two levels. For patients who have had their diabetes for $t$ years, you could have three categories: e.g., $t < 1$, $1 \leq t < 5$ and $t \geq 5$. Had this been the case then six, not four allocation lists would have been needed. If there are $K$ prognostic factors, with levels $\ell_1, \ell_2, \ldots, \ell_K$, then the number of allocation lists needed would be $\Pi_{k=1}^{K} \ell_k$. This can easily become so large that the method becomes too unwieldy to be practicable (allocation lists are often held as sets of sealed envelopes in busy ward offices: for a trial with 3 prognostic factors at 2, 3, and 4 levels you need 24 such sets and keeping track of these in this environment for the duration of, say, a 2-year trial, is beyond the current capabilities of medical science).

## 4.6   Minimization

For one or two prognostic factors, each at two levels, using RPB within strata is probably the simplest method for avoiding allocation bias. However, for more complicated trials an alternative method has been available since the mid-1970s and is becoming more popular amongst investigators. This method, known as *minimization*, eliminates the awkwardness of using RPBs within strata by noting that RPBs within strata actually attempts to achieve more balance than is likely to be necessary. The drawback of the method is that it is only implemented conveniently using a computer. Until relatively recently, this was a major drawback and the recent proliferation of suitable computers in wards and hospital offices probably goes a long way to explain its recent increase in popularity.

It must be conceded that a good deal of the unmanageability of RPBs within strata would be eliminated if it were implemented on a computer. However, as the following subsection will explain, the method does have further difficulties.

### 4.6.1   Minimization for Two-Treatment Trials

Suppose there are four prognostic factors, with $I$, $J$, $K$, and $L$ levels, respectively. Altman (1991, Subsection 15.2.3) gives an example of such a trial in the treatment of patients with breast cancer. The prognostic factors are age, dichotomized as $\leq 50$ or $> 50$; stage of disease (I or II vs. III or IV); period between diagnosis of cancer and of effusion, $\leq 30$ months or $> 30$ months; and whether the patient was pre- or postmenopausal. So $I = J = K = L = 2$.

At some stage of the trial, suppose $n_{ijkl}$ patients who have these prognostic factors at levels $i, j, k,$ and $l$, respectively, have been recruited. Let the number of patients in this category, who have been allocated to treatment A or B, be denoted by $n^A_{ijkl}$ and $n^B_{ijkl}$, respectively, so $n_{ijkl} = n^A_{ijkl} + n^B_{ijkl}$.

RPB within strata would ensure that $\left| n^A_{ijkl} - n^B_{ijkl} \right| \leq \frac{1}{2} b$ for each quadruplet $(i,j,k,l)$, where $b$ is the maximum block size used in the RPBs. The impracticality of the method arises because there are so many quadruplets. However, this is an excessive aim: we generally do not want to know that we have balance in the numbers of patients under 50, have disease stage I or II, have been more than 30 months between diagnoses, and are postmenopausal. Indeed, many such subgroups will contain few patients, perhaps of the same order as the block length in the RPBs. In these circumstances, RPBs can fail to provide adequate balance.

Generally speaking, we are concerned that the groups are balanced with respect to age, disease status, interval, and menopausal status individually. This follows because we usually believe that outcomes (survival time, suppose) might be longer in younger patients, but we usually do not have reason to believe that this difference changes systematically depending on whether the patient also has stage I or II disease, is postmenopausal, etc.

It follows that it is sufficient to ensure that each of the following is small:

$$\left| n^A_{i+++} - n^B_{i+++} \right|, \text{ each } i = 1,\dots,I \; ; \; \left| n^A_{+j++} - n^B_{+j++} \right|, \text{ each } j = 1,\dots,J \; ;$$

$$\left| n^A_{++k+} - n^B_{++k+} \right|, \text{ each } k = 1,\dots,K \; ; \; \left| n^A_{+++l} - n^B_{+++l} \right|, \text{ each } l = 1,\dots,L$$

where a + sign denotes summation over that subscript, so, e.g., $n^A_{+j++} = \Sigma_{i,k,l} n^A_{ijkl}$.

Thus, $I + J + K + L$ conditions, rather than $IJKL$ conditions, are imposed; in the example, 8 conditions rather than 16 are imposed.

The method of minimization is implemented as follows.

1. The first patient is allocated by simple randomization.
2. Suppose that at some stage of the trial the number of patients with prognostic factors $i, j, k, l$ allocated to treatment A is $n^A_{ijkl}$, and similarly for $n^B_{ijkl}$.
3. A new patient is entered to the trial who has prognostic factors at levels $w, x, y, z$.
4. Form the sum

$$\left( n^A_{w+++} - n^B_{w+++} \right) + \left( n^A_{+x++} - n^B_{+x++} \right) + \left( n^A_{++y+} - n^B_{++y+} \right) + \left( n^A_{+++z} - n^B_{+++z} \right)$$

5. If the sum is negative (i.e., allocation to B has predominated thus far) then the new patient is allocated to A with probability $P$. If the sum is positive, she is allocated to B with probability $P$. If the sum is zero she is allocated to A with probability $1/2$.

Some statisticians would be happy to use a value of 1 for $P$, whereas others would prefer to keep an element of randomness in the allocation procedure and simply take a large value for $P$, such as 0.8. The use of $P < 1$ could be defended on the grounds that it amounts to a final protection against selection bias. Although knowledge of the current values of $n^A_{i+++}$ etc., would allow the next allocation to be predicted if $P = 1$, in practice it is extremely unlikely that a doctor would recall such details and would have to deliberately seek to subvert the trial in order to predict the next allocation. The relative complexity of the method is likely to be a sufficient protection against selection bias. However, nothing is lost and a little is gained by using $P < 1$, and this is becoming the accepted approach.

## Example 4.4: Application of Minimization (Altman, (1991, Subsection 15.2.3), citing LS Fentiman et al., 1983)

A trial was conducted in which breast cancer patients were randomized to receive Talc or Mustine as treatment for pleural effusions (fluid between the walls of the lung). The four prognostic factors are: age, stage of disease, time in months between diagnosis of breast cancer and diagnosis of pleural effusions, and menopausal status.

The application of minimization to this trial can be exemplified by supposing that 29 patients have already been allocated. The disposition of these patients among the prognostic factors and treatment groups is given in the following table:

| | | | General Case | | Example after 29 Patients | |
| --- | --- | --- | --- | --- | --- | --- |
| | | | Mustine (A) | Talc (B) | Mustine (A) | Talc (B) |
| Age | 1. ≤50 | | $n^A_{1+++}$ | $n^B_{1+++}$ | 7 | 6 |
| | 2. >50 | | $n^A_{2+++}$ | $n^B_{2+++}$ | 8 | 8 |
| Stage | 1. I or II | | $n^A_{+1++}$ | $n^B_{+1++}$ | 11 | 11 |
| | 2. III or IV | | $n^A_{+2++}$ | $n^B_{+2++}$ | 4 | 3 |
| Time interval | 1. ≤30 months | | $n^A_{++1+}$ | $n^B_{++1+}$ | 6 | 4 |
| | 2. >30 months | | $n^A_{++2+}$ | $n^B_{++2+}$ | 9 | 10 |
| Menopausal status | 1. Pre | | $n^A_{+++1}$ | $n^B_{+++1}$ | 7 | 5 |
| | 2. Post | | $n^A_{+++2}$ | $n^B_{+++2}$ | 8 | 9 |

Suppose the next patient is a postmenopausal woman aged 55 with stage III disease whose pleural effusions were diagnosed 20 months after her diagnosis of breast cancer. The relevant sum from step 4 of the preceding algorithm is

$$(n^A_{2+++} - n^B_{2+++}) + (n^A_{+2++} - n^B_{+2++}) + (n^A_{++1+} - n^B_{++1+}) + (n^A_{+++2} - n^B_{+++2})$$

$$= (8-8) + (4-3) + (6-4) + (8-9) = 2$$

The sum is positive so this patient is allocated to B (Talc) with probability 0.8 and the preceding table is updated.

---

Minimization does not, of course, have to use four prognostic factors and it is straightforward to see how the methods would have to be modified to accommodate a different number. It is also possible to allow judgments about differences in the relative importance of the prognostic factors to be incorporated into the allocation: this can be done by changing the sum in step 4 to a weighted sum. The technique can also be used to allocate more than two treatments: the extension required for this is not so transparent but, as it involves no essentially new ideas, it will not be covered in this book.

## Exercises

1. Suppose an RCT is conducted in which patients are randomly allocated with probability $1/2$ to one of two treatment groups: $N_1$ and $N_2$ patients are allocated to each group and the total number of patients $N = N_1 + N_2$ is fixed. What is the distribution of $N_1$? Recall that

$$\lambda(m, n) = \sqrt{\frac{1}{m} + \frac{1}{n}}$$

By writing $X = N_1 - \frac{1}{2}N$ and using a suitable normal approximation (or otherwise), show that $N - 4\lambda(N_1, N_2)^{-2}$ has a $\chi^2$ distribution with one degree of freedom. Hence, find $L$ (in terms of $N$) such that $\Pr(\lambda < L) = 0.95$. Comment on the implication for RCTs.

2. A trial in which the total number of patients $N$ is fixed allocates randomly to two groups, each with probability $1/2$, the random variables representing the numbers in the two groups are $N_1, N_2$. Show that the minimum value of $\lambda$, $\lambda_{min}$, occurs when $N_1 = N_2$ (you may assume $N$ is even). Show also that, approximately,

$$\left( \frac{\lambda}{\lambda_{min}} \right)^{-2} = 1 - \frac{Z^2}{N}$$

where $Z$ is a random variable with a standard normal distribution. Find the value of $n$ such that

$$\Pr(\lambda / \lambda_{min} > 1.5) = 0.05 : \text{find } N \text{ such that } \Pr(\lambda / \lambda_{min} > 1.1) = 0.05.$$

3. An RCT is being conducted to compare treatments A and B. The allocation is being performed using random permuted blocks (RPBs) of two lengths, namely four and six. Ten blocks are generated for the trial, the length of each block being chosen with probability $1/2$ and then for a given length, each possible block of equal numbers of As and Bs is chosen with equal probability. What is the probability that at some stage of the trial the number of patients allocated to treatment A exceeds the number allocated to B by 4? What is the probability that the number of patients on one treatment never exceeds the number on the other by more than two?

4. When allocating patients to two treatments using RPBs of length four, the allocations for the next two patients can sometimes be predicted with certainty. What are these circumstances? What is the probability of this?

5. Suppose that in Minitab you store $4N$ values in columns C1, C2, and C3 as follows:

| C1-T | C2 | C3 |
|------|----|-----|
| A | 1 | 0.199694 |
| B | 1 | 0.795802 |
| A | 1 | 0.660433 |
| B | 1 | 0.969484 |
| A | 2 | 0.231470 |
| B | 2 | 0.834883 |
| A | 2 | 0.279835 |
| B | 2 | 0.403979 |
| : | : | : |

Column C1 comprises As and Bs alternating; column C2 comprises blocks of four 1s, four 2s, etc., ending with four Ns; column C3 contains $4N$ random numbers from a uniform distribution on $(0,1)$.

Define C4 by the command `Let C4=C2+C3`. An allocation list that is essentially constructed by RPB can be formed in C5 by entering the command

```
sort C1 C5;
by C4.
```

This stores in C5 the result of applying to C1 the permutation that sorts C4 into ascending order. Explain why.

6. When $n$ patients have been allocated to a trial comparing treatments A and B, the number of patients allocated to A (B) is $N_A(n)$ ($N_B(n)$) and $D(n) = |N_A(n) - N_B(n)|$. If the allocation uses a biased coin design that allocates to treatment A with probability $P$ ($1/2 < P < 1$) when there is an excess of patients on B, it can be shown that the long-run (stationary) probability of imbalance $2k$ is

$$\lim_{n \to \infty} \Pr(D(2n) = 2k) = \frac{r-1}{r} \quad k = 0$$

$$= \frac{(r^2 - 1)}{r^{2k+1}} \quad k > 0$$

(Efron, 1971), where $r = P/(1 - P)$. Show that this is a probability distribution and find its mean. Comment on the relation of the mean to the value of $P$.

7. A trial uses an urn scheme UD($r,s$) to allocate patients to one of two treatments, A and B. Show that at the outset the probability of allocation to A for any patient entering the trial is $1/2$.

8. Suppose the imbalance between the numbers of patients in each of the two treatment groups of a trial is $D(n)$, when a total of $n$ patients have been allocated. It can be shown that when allocation follows a UD($r,s$) scheme then for large $n$

$$\Pr(|D(n)| > r) \cong 2\left[1 - \Phi\left(r\sqrt{\frac{3}{n}}\right)\right]$$

where $\Phi$ is the standard normal distribution function. Find the corresponding approximation when allocation is by simple randomization. Plot the two against a range of values of $n$ when $r = n/10$, i.e., what is the chance of an imbalance greater than 10% of the total trial size? Relate this to possible loss in power.

9. In an RCT, the minimal clinically important difference one standard deviation and we wish to detect this at the 5% significance level. If patients are to be allocated equally to the two groups, how many are needed in total to achieve 90% power? To achieve 80% power? If these numbers of patients were allocated unequally, with the ratio of the size of the larger group to the smaller being $\theta$, what would now be the values for the preceding powers for $\theta = 2$ or $\theta = 3$?

10. There are two prognostic factors, disease stage $i$ (classified into $I$ categories) and age $j$ (classified into $J$ categories) that affect the outcome, $X$, of an RCT. The outcome for a patient in categories $i$ and $j$ has expectation $\delta_i + \alpha_j + \tau_A$ if the patient received treatment A and $\delta_i + \alpha_j + \tau_B$ if treatment B was given. Suppose $n_{ijA}$ of the patients in categories $i$ and $j$ are allocated to treatment A and the remaining $n_{ijB}$ are allocated to B. The mean outcome of all the patients in the group receiving treatment A is $\overline{X}_A$ and the corresponding quantity in group B is $\overline{X}_B$. What is the expectation of $\overline{X}_A - \overline{X}_B$? Show that the bias is eliminated if our allocation procedure ensures that for each $i$ and $j$:

$$\sum_i n_{ijA} = \sum_i n_{ijB} \quad \text{and} \quad \sum_j n_{ijA} = \sum_j n_{ijB} \quad (*)$$

Show that this is satisfied if $n_{ijA} = n_{ijB}$ for all pairs $(i,j)$. By means of a simple example show that conditions (*) are less restrictive than requiring $n_{ijA} = n_{ijB}$ for all pairs $(i,j)$. How does this relate to allocation by RPB within strata and minimization?

# 5

## Assessment, Blinding, and Placebos

## 5.1  Double and Single Blindness

### 5.1.1  General Principles

A potentially important source of bias in a trial arises when either the patient or the doctor knows which treatment the patient is receiving. Many involved in trials are hopeful that the new treatment will turn out to be an improvement on the standard treatment. If an outcome measure has any element of subjectivity whatsoever and the investigator assessing the outcome is aware of which treatment the patient received, then two problems arise:

1. The investigator may err in favor of the new treatment.
2. Even if 1 does not occur, the inability to exclude that it might have happened will seriously weaken the credibility of the study.

Similar problems can arise if the patient knows which treatment they are receiving. This can be an important problem for outcomes that relate to a patient's quality of life, levels of pain, etc.

For this reason, many trials are run as single- or double-blind trials. In a single-blind study, the patient is unaware of the treatment being given. In a double-blind study, neither doctor nor patient knows what treatment is being given.

Various comments are appropriate at this point.

1. The importance of making a trial blind depends on the objectivity of the outcomes of the trial. If the outcome is whether or not the patient is alive at the end of the study, then it is difficult to see that knowing the treatment gives rise to any error in the assessment of the variable "alive/dead." However, unless you are only interested in "death from any cause," problems remain. Deciding whether a death was due to a particular cause, such as a tumor, can be surprisingly difficult, and one which can call upon a pathologist to make a judgment that has a subjective component.

2. The safety of the patient is of paramount importance, and in any study in which the doctors treating the patient do not know what treatment is being given, there must be some provision, should an emergency arise, for them to find out.

3. Some studies simply cannot be blind. Obvious examples are trials comparing surgical with nonsurgical treatment for some condition.

If a trial is run double-blind, then the assessment of outcome is no less subjective, but equally, there is no possibility of the assessor tending to make slightly higher blood pressure readings (for example) on the patients getting the new treatment, simply because the assessor does not know who is getting the new treatment. Some assessments will be a little too high, some a little too low, but this cannot happen systematically with treatment — the subjectivity might increase the standard deviation but cannot change the mean.

A very useful way of running a trial double-blind is to have the assessment of outcome made by someone outside the treatment team, usually another doctor in the relevant specialty who is not otherwise involved with these patients. In this way, the doctors responsible for the clinical management of the case are fully aware of the treatment being given to the patient but are unable to influence the data collected for the RCT. If the trial is not single-blind, then you need to be careful to ensure that the patient does not "break the blind" for the assessing doctor ("The blue tablets were very awkward to swallow, doctor").

## Example 5.1: Example of Blinding Using an Independent Assessor

Two possible treatments for coronary artery disease, in which the artery has become blocked by fatty deposits, are coronary artery bypass graft or balloon angioplasty. The former is an operation that replaces diseased coronary arteries using veins from the leg. It involves opening the chest and leaves a large and obvious scar down the chest. The latter involves passing a tube through an artery in the arm or leg and into the diseased artery and then widening it by inflating the balloon that is built into the walls of the tube. This leaves little or no scarring.

An outcome measure may well be ECG changes while walking on a treadmill. Problems of subjectivity arise because the interpretation of the ECG trace by the cardiologist will, to some extent, be a matter of judgment. Patients need to have electrodes attached to their chest for the ECG, so need to reveal their scar, thereby giving away which treatment they received. However, a technician will probably obtain the trace and if this is passed to a cardiologist unconnected with the treatment of the patient, then a blinded assessment is possible.

In some trials the analysis is also carried out blind. Obviously, the statistician needs to know, for example, that patients 1, 2, 6, 7, 10, ..., all received the same treatment, say treatment A, and that patients 3, 4, 5, 8, 9, …, all received B, but there is no need for the statistician to know any more. In particular, which of A or B is the new treatment and which is the standard need not be revealed. At first, this may seem strange, as there is little the statistician can do to bias things, is there? In fact, a statistical analysis involves many elements of judgment: should I transform this variable by taking logs, should I assess the difference using proportions or odds, or do I need to include this variable as a covariate? Each of these decisions may result in an analysis that changes the evidence presented concerning the new treatment. If you are working for a drug company whose future depends on whether the drug is approved for use by doctors, your judgments must be above suspicion and seen to be so. An unequivocal way to do this is to perform the analysis without knowing the identity of the treatment. Even if your interest in the success of the treatment is less direct than in this example, it does no harm to be able to claim that your analysis was carried out without this possibility of bias.

In summary, it should be noted that blindness is used to exclude assessment bias and to exclude the suspicion of assessment bias. For the latter reason it should be used even in cases in which you might think the outcome had so little by way of a subjective component that blindness was unnecessary.

## 5.2   Placebos

Placebos are treatments that look similar to the real thing but contain no active ingredient. Clearly, there are no such things as placebo operations (although trials using "sham" surgery have been reported). Placebo injections are sometimes given. The major use of placebos is in trials in which the treatment is an orally administered preparation, usually a tablet or capsule. Placebos must look, smell, feel, and taste the same as their active counterparts.

Placebos have essentially two roles, one is to take account of the placebo effect, whereas the other is to achieve blindness in certain types of RCT.

### 5.2.1   The Placebo Effect

In many conditions no standard therapy either is available or routinely used. Investigators contemplating an RCT to assess a new treatment in these circumstances have to decide how to handle the control group. The absence of any standard therapy means that it would be justifiable simply to carry on as before with the control group and give them no treatment at all. However, a problem arises because of what is known as the *placebo effect*. This is when a patient exhibits a response to being given a treatment, even though the treatment has no active component and cannot be having a direct

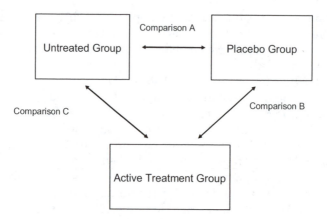

**FIGURE 5.1**
Possible comparisons in a trial with untreated and placebo groups.

effect on the condition being treated. This can arise simply because the patient reacts positively to "something being done" about their condition. This effect can be marked in minor psychiatric disorders and can extend to things such as hypertension (raised blood pressure). Moreover the effect might be quite genuine — a patient with hypertension may be reassured by being treated, thereby reducing the anxiety that was partially responsible for the raised blood pressure.

If a trial is such that an active treatment group could be compared with a control group that is either given a placebo or completely untreated, then the possible comparisons are shown in Figure 5.1.

1. Comparison B would give a measure of the effect of the active component of the drug, because the only difference between the groups is the active component. Both groups would be subject to any placebo effect, so this would cancel out in the comparison.

2. Active treatment or no treatment at all are the only options that are likely to be countenanced for future practice: doctors are seldom prepared to use placebos outside a trial as it could be construed to amount to deception. Because of this, comparison C is the comparison with greatest clinical relevance, as it compares the only groups that might be used in practice. However, a trial that only made comparison C would not be able to tell whether any effect observed was due to the active component or the placebo effect. Few doctors would be happy in using a treatment when they are unsure if the source the efficacy is the active component. For this reason some trials include both untreated and placebo control groups.

3. If both types of control are present, then it becomes possible to make comparison A, which is a direct measure of the placebo effect.

## 5.2.2 The Role of Placebos in Blinding

A slightly different role for placebos is their use to achieve blindness. If one treatment group receives no treatment at all and the other group receives something, then it is clearly impossible to make the trial either double-blind or, given the need to explain to the patient about all treatments in the trial, to make it single-blind. If you give patients in the control group a placebo that looks identical to the active treatment then you can readily achieve blindness. Of course, the comparison being made changes in the manner demonstrated in the explanation to Figure 5.1. Comparison C would be lost, but if assessment bias was a major problem, then sacrificing a biased comparison C for an unbiased comparison B may be necessary.

Placebos can also be used in trials that compare two active treatments using what is called a *double-dummy technique*. Suppose you wish to compare two treatments one given as a blue tablet, the other as a red tablet, so blindness cannot be achieved.

| Group A: | ⟵———⟶ | Group B: |
|---|---|---|
| blue active tablet | Comparison not blind: one group gets red, the other blue | red active tablet |

Most pharmaceutical companies will supply placebo versions of their products. You could then obtain placebo red and blue tablets and give group A placebo red tablets in addition to the active blue tablets, and group B placebo blue tablets in addition to the active red ones.

| Group A: | ⟵———⟶ | Group B: |
|---|---|---|
| blue active tablet red placebo | Comparison blind: both groups get red and blue | red active tablet blue placebo |

The resulting trial is then blind, with the only difference between the groups being the difference in the active components of the red and blue tablets.

## Example 5.2: Example of Using a Placebo to Achieve Blindness and Exclude a Placebo Effect

When a kidney is transplanted into the recipient, an undesirable feature is that the kidney does not pass urine from the ureter more or less as soon as the kidney has been grafted into place — this is referred to as *delayed graft function (DGF)*. An RCT was proposed to assess whether flushing the kidney prior to implantation with a special chemical would reduce the incidence of DGF. However two problems arose:

1. In the middle of an operation, there are numerous fluids flowing around the implantation site, and it would be difficult for the surgeon to be certain that a drop of fluid really was urine emerging from the ureter. The surgeon has to make this judgment but, if he or she knows that the chemical has just been flushed through the kidney, then his judgment may err in the direction of claiming that urine had been seen when the chemical was used.

2. If flushing the kidney with the new chemical reduces DGF, is it the new chemical or the flushing that has made the difference?

Both these difficulties can be overcome if a control group is used in which kidneys are flushed with saline. The patient has been randomized to one or other group by pharmacy and allotted a trial number. The anesthetist draws up a liquid from a bottle, labeled only with the trial number, into a syringe and passes it to the surgeon. The surgeon now is blind to the treatment difference, so problem 1 cannot cause a bias, and the only difference between the groups is the chemical.

## 5.3    Practical Considerations

We have defined blindness as being unaware of the treatment being given, but in practice several degrees of this are possible.

Perhaps the most satisfactory way to run a double-blind trial is for the randomization to be handled by the pharmacy. When a patient has been entered to the trial, the doctor sends the patient to pharmacy with a note which says that they have entered the trial. The pharmacist will have set up a numbered randomization list:

| Patient | Allocation |
|---------|------------|
| 1 | diuretic |
| 2 | diuretic |
| 3 | beta-blocker |
| 4 | diuretic |
| . | |
| . | |
| 10 | beta-blocker |

The first patient receives the drug against their number (in this case diuretic), the second patient the drug against number 2, etc. The patient will receive a bottle of pills (or possibly two bottles if a double-dummy technique is being used), each labeled with only the trial number. Hospital pharmacies usually have 24-h contact numbers, so the blind can be broken at any time that an emergency might arise.

This system is far preferable to one in which patients are given bottles labeled A or B. Even if the doctor does not know which is which of A or B, it is likely he or she will soon find out. If a single case of a side-effect or adverse reaction that only happens with one of the drugs occurs, then the blind will be broken for all patients.

Other methods of randomization involve placing a predetermined sequence of random allocations into sealed envelopes. Alternatively, telephoning to a central randomization center is possible.

## Exercises

1. Explain what is meant by a single-blind trial and a double-blind trial? What are the important features of an outcome variable when deciding whether or not to make a trial double-blind?

2. In a randomized controlled clinical trial, one treatment is a tablet that must be given twice a day, morning and evening, whereas the other treatment must be given three times, morning, evening, and midday. Can you make the trial double-blind? If so, how?

# 6

## Analysis of Results

### 6.1 Example

Throughout this chapter it will be convenient to use data from a real trial to illustrate the application of certain techniques and how they are interpreted.

One of the long-term complications of diabetes is kidney disease or nephropathy. One of the problems that can exacerbate this condition is raised blood pressure, and therefore there is some purpose to seeing if medication can reduce blood pressure in this group of patients. An RCT was reported by Hommel et al. (1986) in which insulin-dependent patients with diabetic nephropathy were randomized to receive either Captopril, a drug intended to reduce blood pressure, or a placebo (reduction of blood pressure is not quite the whole story: Captopril is one of a class of drugs that will reduce blood pressure, but it also has other actions that are thought to be of specific benefit in diabetic nephropathy). The systolic blood pressure was measured before randomization, giving a baseline value and then again after one week on treatment. The data are given in Table 6.1 with all blood pressures in mmHg.

The trial is quite small and in this respect is not wholly typical (it appeared to recruit all eligible, consenting patients attending the investigators' clinic in 1984). However, in other respects its structure is similar to many trials.

### 6.2 Use of Confidence Intervals

The randomization should have produced groups that are comparable, so the primary comparison is between the outcomes $X$ in the two groups. The summary statistics for the two groups can easily be computed as

|           | Sample Size | Mean (mmHg) | SD (mmHg) | SE (mmHg) |
|-----------|-------------|-------------|-----------|-----------|
| Captopril | 9           | 135.33      | 8.43      | 2.8       |
| Placebo   | 7           | 141.86      | 6.94      | 2.6       |

**TABLE 6.1**

Data from Trial by Hommel et al. (1986)

| | Captopril | | | Placebo | |
|---|---|---|---|---|---|
| Patient | Baseline (B) | Outcome at 1 Week (X) | Patient | Baseline (B) | Outcome at 1 Week (X) |
| 1 | 147 | 137 | 1 | 133 | 139 |
| 2 | 129 | 120 | 2 | 129 | 134 |
| 3 | 158 | 141 | 3 | 152 | 136 |
| 4 | 164 | 137 | 4 | 161 | 151 |
| 5 | 134 | 140 | 5 | 154 | 147 |
| 6 | 155 | 144 | 6 | 141 | 137 |
| 7 | 151 | 134 | 7 | 156 | 149 |
| 8 | 141 | 123 | | | |
| 9 | 153 | 142 | | | |

*Source:* From Hommel, E. et al. (1986), Effect of Captopril on kidney function in insulin-dependent diabetic patients with nephropathy, *British Medical Journal*, 293, 467–470.

The difference in sample mean systolic blood pressure is 141.86 – 135.33 = 6.53 mmHg. Is this evidence that blood pressure has been reduced in the group taking Captopril? The first step is to exclude the possibility the difference has arisen by chance, so a hypothesis test is performed.

The assumption of equal variances in the two groups seems reasonable, so the pooled estimate of standard deviation is

$$\sqrt{\frac{8 \times 8.43^2 + 6 \times 6.94^2}{8+6}} = 7.82 \text{ mmHg}$$

The $t$ statistic is then:

$$t = \frac{6.53}{7.82\sqrt{\frac{1}{7} + \frac{1}{9}}} = 1.65$$

Under the null hypothesis that the mean systolic blood pressure at the end of the week of treatment is the same in the two treatment groups, this statistic will have a $t$-distribution with 14 degrees of freedom. From this we obtain $P = 0.12$.

As discussed in Section 3.2, this does not provide strong evidence against the null hypothesis, so we cannot assert that treatment with Captopril has had any effect on blood pressure. However, neither can we assert that Captopril has had no effect.

When planning the study, we hope to avoid this kind of outcome by ensuring that a "nonsignificant" result is unlikely if the true difference between the groups is above a minimal, clinically important threshold. However, even if carefully planned, obtaining a nonsignificant *P*-value does not mean that the true difference between the groups is necessarily less than the clinically important minimum. Among the reasons for this are

1. If, for example, the trial has been planned to have a power of 80% to detect a difference of 8 mmHg, then we still have a 1 in 5 chance of failing to detect a clinically important difference.

2. Sample size estimates are sensitive to the values chosen for the parameters on which they are based, and an unfortunate choice of these may have led to us underestimating the number of patients that were really needed to have 80% power.

3. Practicalities may mean that we simply failed to recruit the number of patients we said we needed.

In addition to these difficulties, there may be interest in a difference between treatments even if it is less than that previously specified to represent the threshold of clinical importance.

We are left with a test result that is compatible with a true treatment effect of zero, $\tau = 0$, but which is also compatible with other true treatment effects $\tau \neq 0$. Here compatible means that the data are unable to reject the null hypothesis that the treatment difference is $\tau$ at the 5% level. We want to know what values of $\tau$ are compatible with the data. That is, we wish to determine the set:

$$\left\{ \tau \, \middle| \, \frac{|6.53 - \tau|}{7.82\sqrt{\frac{1}{7} + \frac{1}{9}}} \leq t_{14;0.975} = 2.145 \right\} \tag{6.1}$$

where $t_{14;0.975}$ is the value that cuts off the top 2.5% of the *t*-distribution with 14 degrees of freedom. Performing the arithmetic gives the result $\{\tau \, | -1.9 \leq \tau \leq 15.0\}$: note that 0 is in this set, as it must be because we have already found that a zero treatment difference is compatible with the data.

Rewriting this for the general case, the analogue of Equation 6.1 is

$$\left\{ \tau \, \middle| \, \frac{|\bar{x}_1 - \bar{x}_2 - \tau|}{s\sqrt{n_1^{-1} + n_2^{-1}}} \leq t_{n_1+n_2-2;0.975} \right\}$$

which can be written as

$$\left\{ \tau \, \middle| \, \bar{x}_1 - \bar{x}_2 - t_{n_1+n_2-2;0.975} s\sqrt{n_1^{-1} + n_2^{-1}} \leq \tau \leq \bar{x}_1 - \bar{x}_2 + t_{n_1+n_2-2;0.975} s\sqrt{n_1^{-1} + n_2^{-1}} \right\}$$

Of course, this is simply the 95% confidence interval for the treatment effect. One of the definitions of a $100\alpha\%$ confidence interval is as the set of values of a parameter that cannot be rejected by a significance test performed at the $100(1 - \alpha)\%$ level.

It follows that we can be 95% sure that the change in mean blood pressure effected by Captopril is somewhere between a reduction of 15 mmHg and an increase of about 2 mmHg. It may be that this is adequate for clinical purposes: a change in mean blood pressure of 2 mmHg is probably of no clinical importance, so we have excluded the possibility that Captopril may increase blood pressure by a clinically important amount. However, Captopril is a powerful drug with potent side effects and few doctors would be happy to prescribe it without good evidence that it did some good, as opposed to evidence that its main effect will not do harm and then rely on the vague hope that it might do some good.

This example illustrates how much more informative it is to present a confidence interval than simply to give the result of a significance test. Confidence intervals should be used to present the results of all RCTs, whether or not the hypothesis test of no treatment difference is significant. Appropriate confidence intervals should also be used when the outcome is not normal, e.g., when it is binary. There is nothing unusual about the application or interpretation of confidence intervals when they are applied to RCTs, it is simply that they are especially informative in this context.

Confidence (about the location of the treatment effect) is the concept that should be used once data have been collected: it is the analogue of power at the planning stage. Some trials attempt to calculate the power they have achieved once the trial has been concluded. This might be possible by computing $\psi(\bar{x}_1 - \bar{x}_2)$, where $\psi$ is the power function defined in Section 3.2. This is inappropriate because $\psi$ is a function of the parameter and not the sample. It is unclear what is achieved by computing $\psi$ at $\bar{x}_1 - \bar{x}_2$. Computing $\psi(\bar{x}_1 - \bar{x}_2)$ - because it is the best estimate of power at the true treatment difference not only ignores the sampling variation in $\bar{x}_1 - \bar{x}_2$ but also the fact that power at the true difference is not usually of interest, it is the power at clinically important thresholds that usually demands attention. Attempts to compute post hoc power are unhelpful and should be eschewed in favor of confidence intervals.

## 6.3   Baselines: Uses and Abuses

In Section 6.1 of this chapter, values of blood pressure were also recorded before the patients were randomized: such measurements are often called *baseline measurements*. Could these values be usefully incorporated into the analysis? The answer is yes. Although there are several ways to do this, only the best one will be described in Section 6.4. Other methods, some of which are mistaken, are described below.

### 6.3.1 Comparison of Baseline Values

Randomization ensures that the baseline values (which cannot be affected by any difference in treatments) in the treatment groups are all samples from the same population. So, on average, they will be balanced between treatment groups. However, as with any prognostic factor, imbalances may occur in any particular trial (cf. Section 4.5). The extent of any imbalance could be assessed by looking at the baseline data from the trial. For the example this gives the following results.

|  | Baseline Mean (mmHg) | Baseline SD (mmHg) |
|---|---|---|
| Captopril | 148.0 | 11.4 |
| Placebo | 146.6 | 12.3 |

These look reassuringly balanced, but why not do things properly and compare these data using a hypothesis test? Performing a $t$-test gives $P = .81$.

Informally assessing the difference between baseline values by computing means and standard deviations may offer some reassurance about balance and is quite acceptable, but the final step is logically flawed. A hypothesis test is used to see if the difference between two groups could be due to chance. In an RCT, the groups are formed by randomization, so the difference between baselines must, by construction, be due to chance. Comparing baselines using significance tests is only appropriate if you suspect that the randomization is flawed for some reason.

### 6.3.2 Analyzing Change from Baseline

The drug is intended to reduce blood pressure. If it does so by similar amounts in each person, then the values after one week will still exhibit marked variation because everyone started from a different value. A way around this would be to analyze the change in blood pressure over the week. The same analysis as shown in Section 6.2 of this chapter would be presented, but instead of using the values in columns 3 and 6 of Table 6.1, we would use the difference between columns 3 and 2 and compare it with the difference between columns 6 and 5. If this is done we obtain:

|  | Sample Size | Mean Change (mmHg) | SD of Change (mmHg) | SE of Change (mmHg) |
|---|---|---|---|---|
| Captopril | 9 | 12.67 | 8.99 | 3.00 |
| Placebo | 7 | 4.71 | 7.91 | 2.99 |

The difference in mean changes shows that Captopril reduces blood pressure by nearly 8 mmHg more than placebo. A two-sample $t$-test gives $P = 0.086$ with a 95% confidence interval for the difference in changes of $(1.3, 17.2)$.

The *P*-value is a little smaller, the treatment effect is still in favor of Captopril and has similar magnitude to that obtained previously, the confidence interval is also of similar width to that obtained before. It is reassuring that the two analyses do not point to conclusions that are qualitatively at odds with one another. However, the analyses are different — so is one analysis better than the other? To answer this, it is helpful to develop some theory.

Suppose a baseline measurement from group 1 (placebo) is represented by the random variable $B_1$ and the corresponding outcome is $X_1$, with $B_2, X_2$ similarly defined for group 2 (Captopril). Suppose:

$$E(X_1) = \mu$$

$$E(X_2) = \mu + \tau$$

$$E(B_1) = E(B_2) = \mu_B$$

The randomization entitles us to assume the two baselines have a common mean. It is convenient (and often reasonable in practice) to assume:

$$\text{var}(X_1) = \text{var}(X_2) = \text{var}(B_1) = \text{var}(B_2) = \sigma^2$$

The sample mean of the *X*s in group 1 will have expectation $\mu$ and in group 2 it will be $\mu + \tau$, so the difference in means will have expectation $\tau$, as required. If we analyze not the outcomes *X* but the differences *X-B*, then the analogous quantity has expectation:

$$E(X_2 - B_2) - E(X_1 - B_1) = (\mu + \tau - \mu_B) - (\mu - \mu_B) = \tau$$

So the analysis based on changes is also unbiased. The analysis ignoring baselines is based on data with variance $\sigma^2$, whereas that based on change uses

$$\text{var}(X_2 - B_2) = \text{var}(X_2) + \text{var}(B_2) - 2\,\text{cov}(X_2, B_2)$$

$$= \sigma^2 + \sigma^2 - 2\rho\sigma^2 = 2\sigma^2(1 - \rho)$$

where $\rho$ is the true correlation between *X* and *B*, which is assumed to be the same for both groups. There is an identical expression for $\text{var}(X_1 - B_1)$. It follows that the analysis of changes from baseline uses variables with a different variance and, if $\rho > \frac{1}{2}$, it will be a smaller variance. This makes sense: if there is marked positive correlation between baseline and outcome such that higher outcomes go with higher baselines, etc., then some of the variability between patients will be reduced if we remove some of the variability by studying changes from baseline. Thus, if the baselines have a correlation with outcome that exceeds $1/2$, we should obtain narrower confidence intervals and more powerful tests by studying changes rather than raw outcomes. If the correlation is below $1/2$, then using change from baseline is essentially just introducing unhelpful noise into the analysis.

More will be said about the use of baselines in Section 6.4.

### 6.3.3 An Erroneous Analysis Based on Change from Baseline

Another way to use baselines that is too often encountered is to assess changes separately within each treatment group and then make some informal comparison of the results. An application to the present example will make this clearer.

Within each group, perform a paired $t$-test on the difference between baseline and outcome, giving

|  | $t$ Statistic (Degrees of Freedom) | $P$-Value |
|---|---|---|
| Captopril | 4.23 (8) | .003 |
| Placebo | 1.58 (6) | .17 |

There appears to be strong evidence that Captopril effects a change in blood pressure, whereas there is no such evidence for placebo. As there is a change in blood pressure for Captopril but not for the placebo, a difference between the treatments has been established.

This analysis is flawed. There are two criticisms:

1. Having conducted an RCT, in which the primary aim is to compare two groups, it is an odd approach to make this comparison so indirectly, namely through $P$-values.

2. A more direct problem is that the logic is flawed. The $P$-value of 0.17 in the placebo group does not show that there is no effect in the placebo group — it demonstrates that we cannot reject the null hypothesis, and not that the null hypothesis is true. Consequently, there may well be a difference in the placebo group, perhaps comparable to that in the Captopril group, so from the comparison of $P$-values we certainly cannot conclude that there is a difference between treatments.

The proper analysis is, as always with RCTs, to compare directly the differences in the treatment groups, i.e., as in Subsection 6.3.2.

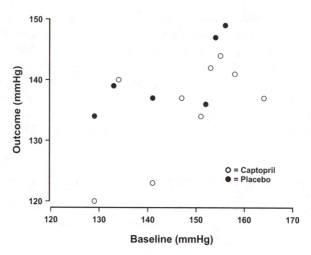

**FIGURE 6.1**
Plot of final blood pressure against baseline, distinguishing the treatments.

## 6.4  Analysis of Covariance

### 6.4.1  Baseline Bias Leads to Outcome Bias

Consider the following observations.

1. It is common to find that outcome measurements are related to the corresponding baseline measurement — often quite strongly related. In the example in this chapter, it would not be surprising if the patients who started with the higher blood pressures finished with the higher blood pressures, notwithstanding the effect of the treatment. This is indeed the case and is demonstrated in Figure 6.1.

2. Although randomization ensures that, on average, the baseline measurements will be balanced between the treatment groups, it does not follow that in a given trial the baseline values in the two groups will be identical.

If the outcome is positively related to the baseline, and if in a given trial the baseline is higher in one group than the other, would we not expect the outcome also to be higher in that group, even in the absence of a treatment effect? If this is the case, how could we then decide if a difference in outcomes was related to a difference in treatments or is simply the difference we would expect given that the baselines were different? To be more specific, in the example the baseline mean blood pressure in the Captopril group was 148.0 mmHg, whereas in the placebo group it was 146.6 mmHg; so if Captopril and the placebo had the same effect, should we not expect the Captopril group to have slightly higher mean blood pressure at the end of the study? (Clinically, the difference of 1.4 mmHg is unimportant and the randomization has performed well in this instance, but the difference illustrates the general point and, in any case, it might have been greater.)

This problem is indeed genuine. Randomization is worthwhile not only because of its desirable average properties but because its use means that, by and large, differences between treatment groups are not large. However, for variables that are strongly associated with the outcome, it is often fruitful to use a method of analysis that makes allowance for the imbalances that remain despite randomization. This method is the *analysis of covariance* (ANCOVA). It has several advantages and can be introduced in several ways: the following introduction is framed around its use in RCTs.

The ideas behind the rest of this section apply to all manner of outcomes, but we will restrict our attention to the case when the baseline and outcome have a normal distribution. We will also need some results for jointly distributed normal variables and these will now be derived.

### 6.4.2 Interlude: Bivariate Normal Variables

Suppose $X$ and $Y$ are two random variables that are jointly normally distributed. For our purposes, this essentially means that $X$ and $Y$ each have a normal distribution with means and variances $\mu_X, \sigma_X^2$ and $\mu_Y, \sigma_Y^2$, respectively, and the correlation between $X$ and $Y$ is $\rho$.

By this definition

$$E(Y) = \mu_Y$$

However, suppose we know that $X$ has the value $x$, what is now the expected value of the corresponding $Y$? If $\rho > 0$ then higher values of $X$ are associated with higher values of $Y$, so if, for example, $x$ is from the upper part of the $X$ distribution, the distribution $Y$ conditional on this value of $X$ is not the same as the unconditional distribution of $Y$. Consequently, the expectation of $Y$ conditional on $X = x$, written $E(Y \mid X = x)$, is not the same as $E(Y)$.

This is illustrated in Figure 6.2, which shows a typical elliptical contour of the joint density function. The distribution of the $Y$s associated with $X = 1$ is clearly shifted up relative to the unconditional distribution of $Y$.

However, if $W$ is another random variable that is independent of $Y$, then specifying a value for $W$ does not affect the distribution of $Y$, so:

$$E(Y \mid W = w) = E(Y)$$

Also, if two normal variables are uncorrelated, they are independent. We can use these two observations to calculate $E(Y \mid X = x)$.

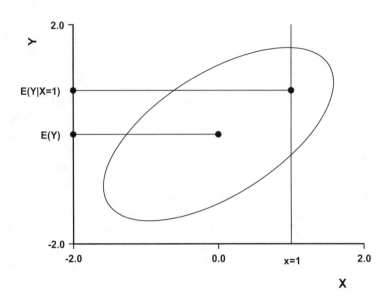

**FIGURE 6.2**
A contour of the bivariate normal distribution.

The first step is to compute the covariance of $X$ and $Y - kX$ for any constant $k$. This is straightforward, as

$$cov(X, Y - kX) = E[(X - \mu_X)(Y - kX - \mu_Y + k\mu_X)]$$

$$= E[(X - \mu_X)(Y - \mu_Y) - k(X - \mu_X)^2]$$

$$= \rho\sigma_X\sigma_Y - k\sigma_X^2$$

This is zero if $k = \rho\sigma_Y / \sigma_X = \beta$, say. Therefore, as $Y - kX$ is also normally distributed, $X$ and $Y - \beta X$ are independent, hence:

$$E(Y - \beta X \mid X = x) = E(Y - \beta X) = \mu_Y - \beta\mu_X$$

However, conditioning on $X = x$ means we take $X$ to be fixed at this value, so $E(\beta X \mid X = x) = \beta x$, and so we obtain the result we want:

$$E(Y \mid X = x) = \mu_Y + \beta(x - \mu_X)$$

We can use the same general approach to obtain $var(Y \mid X = x)$. The definition of this quantity is

$$var(Y \mid X = x) = E[(Y - E(Y \mid X = x))^2 \mid X = x] = E(Y^2 \mid X = x) - [E(Y \mid X = x)]^2$$

In order to evaluate this we need an expression for $E(Y^2 \mid X = x)$. To obtain this, we use the same device as before and note that $X$ and $(Y - \beta X)^2$ are independent. Consequently, we obtain:

$$E[(Y - \beta X)^2 \mid X = x] = E[(Y - \beta X)^2] = S^2 + (\mu_Y - \beta \mu_X)^2$$

where $S^2 = \sigma_Y^2 + \beta^2 \sigma_X^2 - 2\beta\rho\sigma_Y\sigma_X = \sigma_Y^2(1 - \rho^2)$ (substituting for $\beta$).

Expanding the left-hand side we find that this expression is equal to:

$$E[Y^2 \mid X = x] - 2\beta x E(Y \mid X = x) + \beta^2 x^2 = E[Y^2 \mid X = x] - 2\beta x(\mu_Y - \beta\mu_X) - \beta^2 x^2$$

Equating the two expressions and rearranging we obtain:

$$E[Y^2 \mid X = x] = S^2 + (\mu_Y - \beta\mu_X)^2 + 2\beta x(\mu_Y - \beta\mu_X) + \beta^2 x^2$$

Expanding the square of $E(Y \mid X = x) = \mu_Y + \beta(x - \mu_X) = (\mu_Y - \beta\mu_X) + \beta x$ we obtain:

$$[E(Y \mid X = x)]^2 = (\mu_Y - \beta\mu_X)^2 + 2\beta x(\mu_Y - \beta\mu_X) + \beta^2 x^2$$

and subtracting these expressions we find:

$$\text{var}(Y \mid X = x) = S^2 = \sigma_Y^2(1 - \rho^2)$$

Note that the conditional variance of $Y$ does not depend on $x$. Note also that the conditional variance of $Y$ never exceeds the unconditional variance and is only equal to it when the variables are uncorrelated.

### 6.4.3 Allowing for Baseline Imbalance: The Theory

Suppose that the outcome measurement from a clinical trial is a random variable $X$, which has mean $\mu$ in the control group (C) and mean $\mu + \tau$ in the new treatment group (T), so the aim of the RCT is to obtain an estimate of $\tau$, the treatment effect. Suppose also that the standard deviation of $X$ is $\sigma$ in both groups. Suppose further that the measurement of the same quantity at the start of the trial, the baseline, is a random variable $B$. By randomization, this will have the same true mean $\mu_B$ and standard deviation in both groups; it is convenient and not all that unrealistic to assume that this standard deviation is the same as that for $X$, i.e., $\sigma$. The true correlation between $B$ and $X$ is $\rho$, again assumed to be the same in both groups. It is also convenient to assume that the RCT comprises groups of equal size $N$.

If we observe baseline values $b_1$, $b_2$, ..., $b_{2N}$, then, given these values, we find:

$$E(X_i \mid b_i) = \mu + \rho(b_i - \mu_B) \quad \text{Group C}$$
$$E(X_i \mid b_i) = \mu + \tau + \rho(b_i - \mu_B) \quad \text{Group T} \tag{6.2}$$

Denote the mean of the Xs by $\bar{X}_C$ in group C and $\bar{X}_T$ in group T, with the mean of the observed baselines in the two groups being $\bar{b}_C$ and $\bar{b}_T$. From this we obtain:

$$E(\bar{X}_T - \bar{X}_C \mid \bar{b}_T, \bar{b}_C) = \tau + \rho(\bar{b}_T - \bar{b}_C) \tag{6.3}$$

So, if we start from the observation that in our particular trial there is an imbalance in the baseline values, $\bar{X}_T - \bar{X}_C$ is not unbiased. There is an extra term in Equation 6.3 that allows for the difference you would expect in outcome because of the difference in baselines. Even if there is no treatment effect, $\bar{X}_T - \bar{X}_C$ will not have zero expectation; put more loosely, if you do not start with groups that are quite alike, you should not expect to end up with groups that are alike. The exception is if $\rho = 0$, i.e., if baselines and outcomes are unrelated, then imbalance in baselines has no effect on the outcome. However, this situation rarely occurs in practice.

The problem cannot be solved by analyzing changes from baseline, that is if we use $(\bar{X}_T - \bar{b}_T) - (\bar{X}_C - \bar{b}_C)$ to estimate $\tau$. This is because it follows from Equation 6.3 that

$$E[(\bar{X}_T - \bar{b}_T) - (\bar{X}_C - \bar{b}_C) \mid \bar{b}_T, \bar{b}_C] = \tau + (\rho - 1)(\bar{b}_T - \bar{b}_C)$$

and in practice $\rho$ will never be 1; so using change from baseline does not provide an unbiased estimate.

Of course, if we adjust for baseline imbalance by using $(\bar{X}_T - \bar{X}_C) - \rho(\bar{b}_T - \bar{b}_C)$, then this quantity will have expectation $\tau$ as we require. Moreover, as the correlation between $\bar{X}_T - \bar{X}_C$ and $\bar{B}_T - \bar{B}_C$ is $\rho$, the result in the previous subsection shows that

$$\text{var}[(\bar{X}_T - \bar{X}_C) - \rho(\bar{b}_T - \bar{b}_C)] = \text{var}[\bar{X}_T - \bar{X}_C](1 - \rho^2)$$
$$= \frac{2\sigma^2(1 - \rho^2)}{N}$$

Thus, by taking account of the baseline values in the manner described, we have not only obtained a more accurate estimate of $\tau$, we have one which has a smaller variance.

### 6.4.4　Allowing for Baseline Imbalance: The Practice

The previous subsection outlines how we ought to go about taking account of baseline information, but it is not a practical proposition as it stands. An obvious problem is that the proposed estimator $(\bar{X}_T - \bar{X}_C) - \rho(\bar{b}_T - \bar{b}_C)$ depends on the unknown parameter $\rho$. The second problem is that, in practice, we would not wish to impose the constraints that the variance of the baseline should equal to the variance of the outcome nor that the treatment groups have equal size.

The solution is to analyze the data using a statistical model in which the expectation of the outcome includes a linear term in the observed baseline. Thus we fit the model:

$$x_i = \mu + \gamma b_i + \varepsilon_i \qquad \text{in group C}$$

$$x_i = \mu + \tau + \gamma b_i + \varepsilon_i \qquad \text{in group T}$$

where $\varepsilon_i s$ are independent, normally distributed errors, with mean 0 and variance $\sigma^2$. The observed outcomes are $x_1, x_2, \ldots, x_{N_T + N_C}$ and the baselines are $b_1, b_2, \ldots, b_{N_T + N_C}$ where groups T and C have sizes $N_T, N_C$, respectively. The parameters $\mu, \tau, \gamma$ and $\sigma^2$ need to be estimated from the data and, for the first three, this is done by minimizing the sum of squares:

$$S(\mu, \tau, \gamma) = \sum_{i \text{ in } T} (x_i - \mu - \tau - \gamma b_i)^2 + \sum_{i \text{ in } C} (x_i - \mu - \gamma b_i)^2$$

If the estimates thereby obtained are denoted by $\hat{\mu}$, $\hat{\tau}$, and $\hat{\gamma}$ we estimate $\sigma^2$ by:

$$\hat{\sigma}^2 = \frac{S(\hat{\mu}, \hat{\tau}, \hat{\gamma})}{N_T + N_C - 3}$$

This technique is a well-established statistical method known as the analysis of covariance (ANCOVA) and is implemented in many statistical packages. In Minitab (version 14), you can apply this method to the data from Section 6.1 of this chapter by selecting successively the menus Stat -> ANOVA -> General Linear Model .... Three columns of data are required: the columns "Outcome" and "Baseline" are self-explanatory and the column "Treatment" is a text column whose entries are T for Captopril and C for placebo (this slightly odd coding is to conform to our notion of T = "test" and C = "control," in which placebo is naturally the control). In the dialog box that is presented following the preceding choice of menus, you enter

1. "Outcome" in the Responses box
2. "Treatment" in the Model box

You must click on the Covariates ... box and then enter "Baseline" in the Covariates box.

Under Options: ... it is convenient to put "Treatment" in the Display least squares means corresponding to the terms: box.

The output obtained (after slight editing) is as follows:

## General Linear Model: Outcome vs. Treatment

```
Analysis of Variance for Outcome using Adjusted SS for
Tests

Source      DF   Seq SS   Adj SS   Adj MS      F      P
Baseline     1   374.66   409.11   409.11   11.88  0.004
Treatment    1   202.04   202.04   202.04    5.87  0.031
Error       13   447.75   447.75    34.44
Total       15  1024.44

S = 5.86872  R-Sq = 56.29%  R-Sq(adj) = 49.57%

Term         Coef SE    Coef     T      P
Constant       71.16   19.62   3.63   0.003
Baseline      0.4578  0.1328   3.45   0.004
Treatment
C              3.589   1.482   2.42   0.031

Least Squares Means for Outcome

Treatment  Mean SE  Mean
C          142.2    2.221
T          135.0    1.958
```

The estimates of the various parameters can be found from this output as follows.

1. $\hat{\sigma}^2$ is found as the mean square (MS column) in the Error row of the Analysis of Variance table, namely 34.44 (mmHg$^2$). Its square root, S, can be found in the line below the table starting S = 5.86872.

2. $\hat{\gamma}$ is found under Coef in the table of output below the Analysis of Variance table: it is in the row corresponding to Baseline — so $\hat{\gamma} = 0.4578$. Both $\hat{\mu}$ and $\hat{\tau}$ can be found from the same table, although there is usually little interest in $\hat{\mu}$. The Treatment column is a text column with entries C and T, so internally Minitab must ascribe a numerical code for these, and it has used 1 and 1, respectively. Thus, in essence, Minitab fitted the model

$$x_i = \mu' + \tau' + \gamma b_i + \varepsilon_i \text{ in group C (Placebo)}$$

$$x_i = \mu' - \tau' + \gamma b_i + \varepsilon_i \text{ in group T (Captopril)}$$

This is easily seen to be equivalent to the preceding model, once we have made the identifications $\mu = \mu' + \tau'$, $\mu + \tau = \mu' - \tau'$. The estimates of $\mu'$ and $\tau'$ are the numbers under Coef corresponding to Constant and Treatment, respectively, i.e., 71.16 and 3.589. From the identification of the parameters in the two models, note that $\tau = -2\tau'$, giving $\tilde{\tau} = -2 \times 3.589 = -7.179$ mmHg. This shows that after adjustment for baseline blood pressure, patients treated with Captopril have a mean blood pressure 7.18 mmHg lower than those given the placebo. This adjusted value compares with a reduction of 6.53 mmHg based on an analysis of outcomes alone (cf. Section 6.2). The adjusted reduction is slightly greater than the unadjusted change, reflecting the fact that the Captopril group started with a slightly higher mean blood pressure than the placebo group.

3. Some users of clinical trial results would want adjusted (or least squares) means to be presented. These are not fundamental quantities, as they depend for their definition on certain conventions. Nevertheless they are encountered quite often. In general, if the mean response in group $i$ is $\bar{y}_i$, the mean covariate in group $i$ is $\bar{z}_i$ and the estimate of the coefficient for the covariate is $c$, then one convention for the definition of an adjusted mean for group $i$ is $\bar{y}_i - c(\bar{z}_i - \bar{z})$ where $\bar{z}$ is the mean of the covariate computed across all groups. This is the convention adopted by Minitab in the preceding output. Thus, our estimate for $\tau$, namely $(\bar{x}_T - \bar{x}_C) - \hat{\gamma}(\bar{b}_T - \bar{b}_C)$, following from Equation 6.3, can be found as the difference between the adjusted means, namely, $135.05 - 142.23 = -7.18$ mmHg, agreeing with the preceding estimate of $\tau$.

The test of the null hypothesis $\tau = 0$ is performed in the Analysis of Variance table and the $P$-value is found in the appropriate column under the row labeled Treatment, so $P = 0.031$. The $P$-value is smaller than in the earlier analyses based on outcome alone or on change. This is, at least in part, because the inclusion of the baseline information has reduced the residual variance. In the analysis of outcomes alone, the residual standard deviation was 7.82 mmHg, whereas in the present analysis it is reduced to $\sqrt{34.44} = 5.87$ mmHg.

A 95% confidence interval for the adjusted difference is found from the standard error associated with the estimate of $\tilde{\tau}$. This is found next to the estimate of 3.589 under the column SE Coef and has value 1.482. The standard error of $\hat{\tau}$ is therefore $2 \times 1.482 = 2.964$. Thus, a 95% confidence interval for the adjusted treatment effect is $7.179 \pm t_{0.975;13} \times 2.964$, where $t_{0.975;13} = 2.160$ is the two-sided 95% point of the $t$ distribution with the same degrees of freedom as for the estimate of $\sigma^2$. This gives a confidence interval of (0.78, 13.58) mmHg for the adjusted reduction in blood pressure on Captopril, relative to the placebo.

### 6.4.5   Conditional vs. Unconditional Inference

It has been asserted in various parts of this chapter that $\bar{X}_T - \bar{X}_C$ and $(\bar{X}_T - \bar{B}_T) - (\bar{X}_C - \bar{B}_C)$ are unbiased estimators of $\tau$. Then in Equation 6.3, it is shown that the expectation of $\bar{X}_T - \bar{X}_C$ is $\tau + \rho(\bar{b}_T - \bar{b}_C)$, that is we have a biased estimator, as is the estimator based on changes from baseline. This raises the question of the consistency of these assertions.

There is, in fact, no contradiction. When claiming that $\bar{X}_T - \bar{X}_C$ and $(\bar{X}_T - \bar{B}_T) - (\bar{X}_C - \bar{B}_C)$ are unbiased for $\tau$, we are taking expectations over all possible outcomes $X$ and all possible baselines $B$; we say that the expectations are unconditional. To put it more loosely, before we had any data we knew that the average of these quantities taken over hypothetical repetitions of the trial, including repetitions of the baseline values, is the required treatment effect. When claiming that the expectation of $\bar{X}_T - \bar{X}_C$ is $\tau + \rho(\bar{b}_T - \bar{b}_C)$, we are taking the baseline values to be fixed at the values we actually observed. The average of $\bar{X}_T - \bar{X}_C$ over hypothetical repeated trials that had the same baseline difference as that we actually observed would not give $\tau$ but the biased $\tau + \rho(\bar{b}_T - \bar{b}_C)$. We say the expectation is conditional. Conditional and unconditional expectations are not necessarily equal, as Figure 6.2 illustrates.

However, this explanation raises the next question: why do we treat the baselines as if they were fixed at the observed value and are we entitled to do so? Why do we not also take the outcomes to be fixed?

Taking the outcomes to be fixed would destroy our ability to make any statistical inferences, so this is clearly an unhelpful approach. We are not solely interested in the estimates of the treatment effect in this trial, but we want to know what can be said about what treatment effects might have been found if we had repeated the trial. However, it is the treatment effect that is the focus of our attention and the baseline values, being taken before treatments are administered, cannot contain direct information on the effect of the treatment. So we are not concerned about how baselines vary across repeated trials. If the outcomes vary less in the conditional distribution than in the unconditional one, we may be able to make more precise inferences if we work with this conditional distribution rather than the unconditional one.

This is a heuristic explanation of the deep statistical property of ancillarity. Ancillary statistics contain no direct information on the parameters of interest, and the principle of ancillarity asserts that inferences will be improved if they are made conditional on the observed values of the ancillary statistics. It also demonstrates the important point that the argument does not work if the baseline values do contain direct information about the treatment effect. It is of the utmost importance that baselines are taken before any administration of treatment to ensure they cannot be affected by it.

### 6.4.6 Some General Remarks on Covariates

#### 6.4.6.1 Choice of Analysis

In this chapter, three analyses of the introduced data in the first section, differing in the way they make use of baseline data, have been presented. The first analysis ignored baselines, the second considered changes from baseline, and the third included the baseline as the covariate in an analysis of covariance. Three different sets of results were obtained, and the most important aspects of these are summarized in the following table.

|  | $\hat{\tau}$ | 95% Confidence Interval | *P*-Value |
|---|---|---|---|
| Ignoring baseline | 6.5 mmHg | 1.9, 15.0 mmHg | 0.12 |
| Change from baseline | 8.0 mmHg | 1.3, 17.2 mmHg | 0.086 |
| Baseline as covariate | 7.2 mmHg | 0.8, 13.6 mmHg | 0.031 |

The results are broadly the same but there are differences and, in particular, the *P*-values change noticeably. An investigator eager to obtain $P < .05$ might be more easily persuaded of the value of using the baseline as a covariate after seeing this table. This raises an important point about choosing analyses. With a choice between a range of legitimate analyses, there is the danger of choosing one because it gives more appealing results; this is discussed further in Chapter 9.

#### 6.4.6.2 Other Types of Covariate

The second analysis in the preceding table, namely the change from baseline, is only possible if we can subtract the baseline from the outcome, and this is only possible if they measure the same variable. The presence of a coefficient $\gamma$ in the adjustment by ANCOVA, namely $(\bar{x}_T - \bar{x}_C) - \hat{\gamma}(\bar{b}_T - \bar{b}_C)$, means that the baseline does not have to be the same variable, nor even have the same units, as the outcome when adjustments are made this way. Although the pre-randomization value of the outcome variable is often an important baseline, it is not the only possibility. As long as the values were obtained before randomization, and so cannot be affected by the treatment, considering other baseline variables is a legitimate and possibly desirable approach.

#### 6.4.6.3 Which Covariates Should Be Used?

The observation that ANCOVA allows a wide range of variables measured at baseline to be used to adjust the treatment effect opens up an important but complicated area. In most trials, many variables are recorded at baseline and using them all is not a practical or desirable proposition. However, some of the variables could profitably be used in this way, so how do we choose which variables to use?

An analysis of a trial with a normal outcome using ANCOVA does two things that are potentially beneficial. First, it allows for chance imbalances that have occurred in a variable despite randomization. Second, it gives a more precise estimate of the treatment effect, because some of the variation in the outcome can be ascribed to concomitant variation in the covariate. If the covariate is not related to the outcome, then the second advantage does not hold good, and adjustment for imbalances in variables that are unrelated to the outcome does not have value. It is therefore important that only baseline variables that are related to the outcome variable, the so-called prognostic variables, be contemplated as possible covariates in an ANCOVA.

One approach to selecting covariates is to choose those baseline variables that are imbalanced, perhaps by looking for variables that exhibit a statistically significant difference at baseline. The practice of performing significance tests on baseline variables to obtain reassurance regarding the balance of the treatment groups has been criticized in Subsection 6.3.1. The use of significance testing just proposed is slightly different. If a large number of variables are observed at baseline, then a few will be not be balanced just by chance, and the proposed approach could be seen as identifying which ones exhibit chance imbalance and thus should be used to adjust the estimate of the treatment effect. Unfortunately, this method is not helpful for two reasons. First, there is no guarantee that the variables found to be imbalanced are prognostic, so the imbalance may be immaterial. Second, if a variable is closely related to the outcome, then an imbalance that fails to reach conventional levels of statistical significance may still have a marked effect on the estimate of the treatment effect and some adjuctment should be used.

The safest approach to selecting the variables that are to be used in adjusting the treatment effect using ANCOVA is to decide which variables should have this role in the primary analysis before the trial commences. These will usually comprise important prognostic variables. If after the trial is run, a prognostic variable was overlooked, or a variable is unexpectedly found to be related to the outcome, then these variables could be included in a secondary analysis in order to check the sensitivity of the estimate found in the primary analysis.

There is a special place in this approach for variables used to stratify the allocation of patients. Only prognostic variables will be used to stratify the allocation, so these variables should always be included as covariates in the ANCOVA. This applies whichever technique, e.g., RPB within strata or minimization, has been used to balance the allocation. There should be little imbalance between the treatment groups with respect to variables that have been used to stratify the allocation, so the ANCOVA is likely to have little to achieve by way of adjusting for baseline imbalances in these variables. However the prognostic nature of the stratifying variables means that including them in the analysis will give a more precise estimate of the treatment effect. This advantage can only be realized by including the variables in the ANCOVA.

A further and more subtle way ANCOVA can be used to extract information from baseline covariates is to investigate whether the treatment effect differs between different types of patient. To do this, the ANCOVA needs to include a term for a treatment by covariate interaction, with the covariate in question defining the types of patient. This amounts to looking for subgroup effects, which is a delicate matter that will be discussed in detail in Chapter 9.

## Exercises

1. Suppose that the outcome measurement from a clinical trial is a random variable $X$, which has mean $\mu$ in the control group (C) and mean $\mu + \tau$ in the new treatment group (T), and standard deviation $\sigma_X$ in both groups. Suppose further that the measurement of the same quantity at the start of the trial, the baseline, is a random variable $B$, which by randomization will have the same mean $\mu_B$ and standard deviation $\sigma_B$ in both groups. The correlation between $B$ and $X$ is $\rho$, assumed to be the same in both groups.

   If we observe baseline values $b_1$, $b_2$, ..., $b_{N+M}$ then, given these values, show that the expected difference in the means in the two groups, $\bar{X}_T, \bar{X}_C$, is

   $$E(\bar{X}_T - \bar{X}_C \mid \bar{b}_T, \bar{b}_C) = \tau + \rho \frac{\sigma_X}{\sigma_B}(\bar{b}_T - \bar{b}_C)$$

2. An RCT is conducted to compare a control group C (with $N_C$ patients) with a treated group T (with $N_T$ patients) in which the outcome, $x_i$, and baseline, $b_i$, are assumed to be related by the following model ($\varepsilon_i$s are independent normal errors with zero mean and common variance)

   $$x_i = \mu + \gamma b_i + \varepsilon_i \qquad \text{in group C}$$
   $$x_i = \mu + \tau + \gamma b_i + \varepsilon_i \qquad \text{in group T}$$

   The estimators of the parameters $\mu, \tau, \gamma$, namely $\hat{\mu}, \hat{\tau}, \hat{\gamma}$, are the values of the parameters that minimize:

   $$S(\mu, \tau, \gamma) = \sum_{i \text{ in T}} (x_i - \mu - \tau - \gamma b_i)^2 + \sum_{i \text{ in C}} (x_i - \mu - \gamma b_i)^2$$

   (a) By differentiation, show that the estimators satisfy the following:

$$\begin{pmatrix} N & N_T & N\bar{b} \\ N_T & N_T & N_T\bar{b}_T \\ N\bar{b} & N_T\bar{b}_T & S^0_{bb} \end{pmatrix} \begin{pmatrix} \hat{\mu} \\ \hat{\tau} \\ \hat{\gamma} \end{pmatrix} = \begin{pmatrix} N\bar{x} \\ N_T\bar{x}_T \\ S^0_{bx} \end{pmatrix},$$

where $N = N_T + N_C$, $\bar{b}, \bar{b}_T$ are the means of the $b_i$ over both groups or in group T, respectively, with similar definitions for $\bar{x}, \bar{x}_T$. Also,

$$S^0_{bb} = \sum b^2_i, \quad S^0_{bx} = \sum x_i b_i$$

with both summations taken over all patients in the study.

(b) Show that for any value of $\hat{\gamma}$, the first two rows of the preceding matrix equation are satisfied by $\hat{\mu} = \bar{x}_C - \hat{\gamma}\bar{b}_C$, $\hat{\tau} = (\bar{x}_T - \bar{x}_C) - \hat{\gamma}(\bar{b}_T - \bar{b}_C)$, with the obvious definitions for $\bar{x}_C, \bar{b}_C$.

(c) Hence show that

$$\hat{\gamma} = \frac{\sum\limits_{i \text{ in T}} (x_i - \bar{x}_T)(b_i - \bar{b}_T) + \sum\limits_{i \text{ in C}} (x_i - \bar{x}_C)(b_i - \bar{b}_C)}{\sum\limits_{i \text{ in T}} (b_i - \bar{b}_T)^2 + \sum\limits_{i \text{ in C}} (b_i - \bar{b}_C)^2}$$

(d) Explain, in qualitative terms, how the estimator in (c) is the sample analogue of the population quantity shown in question 1.

3. Note that the answer to question 2 (c) can be written as

$$\hat{\gamma} = \frac{\sum\limits_{i \text{ in T}} x_i(b_i - \bar{b}_T) + \sum\limits_{i \text{ in C}} x_i(b_i - \bar{b}_C)}{\sum\limits_{i \text{ in T}} (b_i - \bar{b}_T)^2 + \sum\limits_{i \text{ in C}} (b_i - \bar{b}_C)^2}$$

(a) Show that in any random sample, the covariance between $\bar{x}$ and $\Sigma\lambda_i x_i$, where the $\lambda_i$s are constants such that $\Sigma\lambda_i = 0$, is zero.

(b) Use this result to show that, in the notation of question 2, $\text{cov}(\bar{x}_T - \bar{x}_C, \hat{\gamma}) = 0$.

(c) Hence find an expression for the variance of $\hat{\tau}$ in terms of $\text{var}(\hat{\gamma})$ and other relevant quantities.

(d) By substituting for the $x_i$ from the underlying model, find an expression for the variance of $\hat{\gamma}$.

4. The following data are from a small trial in which patients with familial adenomatous polyposis (FAP) were treated with Sulindac

(S) or placebo (P). FAP is a condition in which the patient is predis-
posed to the formation of polyps (small growths) in the colon which,
although not serious in themselves, may turn into colon cancer. The
number of polyps in the colon were counted before randomization
and after 12 months of treatment with P or S. The data in the following table are the logs (to base 10) of the numbers of polyps (data
from Giardiello et al., 1993, cited in Piantadosi [2005, p. 425] renum-
bering patients and omitting cases with missing data at 12 months).

| Patient | Log (Base 10) Number of Polyps at Baseline | Log (Base 10) Number of Polyps at 12 Months | Treatment (1 = Sulindac) |
|---|---|---|---|
| 1 | 0.84510 | 0.60206 | 1 |
| 2 | 0.69897 | 1.41497 | 0 |
| 3 | 1.36173 | 1.20412 | 1 |
| 4 | 1.54407 | 1.60206 | 0 |
| 5 | 1.04139 | 1.14613 | 1 |
| 6 | 1.07918 | 1.20412 | 0 |
| 7 | 0.84510 | 1.04139 | 0 |
| 8 | 2.50243 | 2.63749 | 0 |
| 9 | 2.20412 | 1.41497 | 1 |
| 10 | 0.90309 | 0.84510 | 1 |
| 11 | 1.30103 | 1.65321 | 0 |
| 12 | 1.04139 | 1.50515 | 0 |
| 13 | 1.38021 | 1.90309 | 0 |
| 14 | 1.53148 | 1.53148 | 1 |
| 15 | 1.73239 | 1.57978 | 0 |
| 16 | 1.47712 | 1.75587 | 0 |
| 17 | 1.00000 | 0.84510 | 1 |
| 18 | 1.30103 | 0.00000 | 1 |
| 19 | 1.07918 | 0.90309 | 1 |

Ignoring the baseline information, test the null hypothesis that the
treatment has had no effect on the log of the number of polyps.
Estimate the difference in the effects of the two treatments. Between
what limits would you expect this difference to lie?

5. Reanalyze the data in question 4, but this time, do not ignore
baseline information. Use analysis of covariance in Minitab (or any
other suitable package) to compare treatments with baseline value
as the covariate. What is now the $P$-value for the comparison of
the treatments? What is the difference in the adjusted treatment
means? (Remember to use Options to display means corresponding
to the treatment term, and Graphs can be useful to check whether
the assumption of normal residuals is reasonable.) Repeat the analysis, still using baseline as a covariate but with outcome equal to
the difference between the value at 12 months and baseline. Comment on the differences and similarities between the analyses. (In
Minitab 14, you will need to use the general linear model option
under ANOVA.)

# 7

## Further Analysis: Binary and Survival Data

In Chapter 6, some of the key ideas behind the analysis of data from randomized trials were introduced. The development was entirely in terms of a normally distributed outcome. This was because: (1) the methods used, such as $t$-tests, were likely to be widely familiar, (2) the effect to be estimated is unambiguous, namely, the difference in means, and (3) the theory behind certain aspects, such as the way baseline information is taken into account, is relatively accessible. In this chapter, some further aspects of the analysis of data from RCTs will be considered.

The first issue that will be addressed is that the outcome variable in many trials is not normally distributed. A lack of space does not permit a comprehensive review of all kinds of outcomes, and our attention will be focused on two types — binary data and survival data, with greater emphasis being given to the former. Both of these types of outcomes will, to a certain extent, require the fitting of a statistical model and, in general, the issue of how well the model fits the data needs to be considered. The second issue is that a powerful alternative approach to the analysis of all kinds of data from an RCT exists, which is based directly on the way patients are randomized. This will be introduced briefly in the final section of this chapter.

### 7.1   Binary Data: An Example and a Statistical Model

Gordon et al. (1999) reported a trial comparing two treatments for psoriasis. This is a scaly, itchy skin condition that can be treated by exposing the affected area to ultraviolet (UV) light. However, as is now widely known through campaigns warning of the dangers of sunbathing, there are risks associated with exposing the skin to too much UV radiation. Therefore, dermatologists try to refine the use of this treatment so as to minimize the toxic effects of the treatment while maintaining its efficacy. UV light can be classified into shorter wavelength radiation (UVB) and longer wavelength (UVA). Giving patients a drug, methoxsalen, followed by exposure to UVA, is an established treatment for psoriasis, often referred to as PUVA therapy (the "P" comes from Psoralen, the proprietary name for methoxsalen). Shorter wavelength UVB is not, in general, as effective as PUVA, but is likely to be less toxic. A new lamp, known as the TL-01 lamp, that focused the radiation into a narrow band of the UVB spectrum was developed, which was thought to be highly effective in treating psoriasis. Gordon et al. (1999) reported a comparison of PUVA with TL-01.

The principal outcome is whether or not the patient was clear of psoriasis at or before the end of the course of treatment. This was a judgment made on the basis of clinical observation by a dermatologist who was unaware of which treatment the patient had received (cf. Chapter 5). For each patient, this outcome takes one of two possible outcomes, namely, clear or not clear. As discussed in Subsection 3.4.1, the natural way to model this kind of response is using the binomial distribution. The number of patients clearing on PUVA, $R_P$, will have a binomial distribution $Bi(n_P, \pi_P)$, where $n_P$ patients have received PUVA, and $\pi_P$ is the probability a patient treated with PUVA clears in the defined period. A similar distribution, $Bi(n_T, \pi_T)$, applies to the number of patients who clear when allocated to TL-01.

The aim of the analysis is to make inferences about $\pi_P$ and $\pi_T$. Point estimates of these quantities and point and interval estimates for some measure of discrepancy between these parameters will all be needed. In addition, ways to test the null hypothesis that $\pi_P = \pi_T$ will be required.

## 7.2   Point Estimates and Hypothesis Tests

### 7.2.1   Methods Based on Informal Derivations

Suppose that the data observed in a trial of PUVA vs. TL-01 are written with the notation in Table 7.1. The actual values obtained in the trial reported by Gordon et al. (1999) are shown in Table 7.2.

The parameter $\pi_P$, the proportion of patients who clear when treated with PUVA, can be estimated by the corresponding sample proportion, $p_P = r_P/n_P$, where $r_P$ is the realization. The mean and variance of the binomial distribution show that the expectation of this estimator is $\pi_P$ and its variance is

**TABLE 7.1**

General Notation for Outcomes from a Trial
with Binary Outcome

|  | Cleared | Did Not Clear | Total |
|---|---|---|---|
| TL-01 | $r_T$ | $n_T - r_T$ | $n_T$ |
| PUVA | $r_P$ | $n_P - r_P$ | $n_P$ |
| Total | $r$ | $N - r$ | $n$ |

**TABLE 7.2**

Principal Outcomes from the PUVA vs. TL-01 Trial

|  | Cleared | Did Not Clear | Total |
|---|---|---|---|
| TL-01 | 32 | 19 | 51 |
| PUVA | 41 | 8 | 49 |
| Total | 73 | 27 | 100 |

*Source:* Reported in Gordon, P.M. et al. (1999), A randomized comparison of narrow-band TL-01 phototherapy and PUVA photochemotherapy for psoriasis, *Journal of the American Academy of Dermatology*, 41, 728–732.

$\pi_P(1 - \pi_P)/n_P$. If we write $y_{iP}$ for the variable, which is 1 if the *i*th patient receiving PUVA clears and 0 otherwise, then

$$r_P = \sum_{i=1}^{n_P} y_{iP}$$

and, therefore, the central limit theorem suggests that the sampling distribution of $p_P$ can be approximated under many circumstances by a normal distribution. Consequently, we could test the null hypothesis that $\pi_P = \pi_T$ by referring $(p_P - p_T)$ to a normal distribution with mean 0 and a suitable variance. The variance is

$$\frac{\pi_P(1 - \pi_P)}{n_P} + \frac{\pi_T(1 - \pi_T)}{n_T} \tag{7.1}$$

and this could be estimated by replacing $\pi_P$ and $\pi_T$ with $p_P$ and $p_T$, respectively. However, as the test statistic is calculated assuming that $\pi_P = \pi_T = \pi$, say, then it may be better to use

$$\pi(1 - \pi)\left(\frac{1}{n_P} + \frac{1}{n_T}\right) \tag{7.2}$$

as the variance of $(p_P - p_T)$ under the null hypothesis. In calculations $\pi$ would be replaced with $p$, an estimate of the common probability of clearance under the null hypothesis. As the null hypothesis essentially says that the distributions under the two treatments are the same, the data from them can be pooled, giving an estimate of the probability of clearance from all the patients of $p = (r_P + r_T)/(n_P + n_T)$. Therefore, a test of the null hypothesis can be found by computing

$$Z = \frac{(p_P - p_T)}{\sqrt{p(1-p)\left(\dfrac{1}{n_P} + \dfrac{1}{n_T}\right)}}$$
(7.3)

The test is completed by referring this statistic to a standard normal distribution.

Implementing these methods for the trial of Gordon et al. (1999) gives the following:

The proportion of patients clearing on PUVA is estimated to be
$p_P = 41/49 = 0.84$.

The proportion of patients clearing on TL-01 is estimated to be
$p_T = 32/51 = 0.63$.

These point estimates summarize what is perhaps the simplest, most easily understood, and most important aspect of the study, namely, the proportion clearing on each treatment.

A test of the null hypothesis $\pi_P = \pi_T$ requires an estimate of the common proportion clearing, assuming the null hypothesis is true, namely $p = (41 + 32)/(49 + 51) = 0.73$. Using this value, the statistic in Equation 7.3 can be found as

$$Z = \frac{0.8367 - 0.6275}{\sqrt{0.73 \times 0.27 \times \left(\frac{1}{49} + \frac{1}{51}\right)}} = 2.357$$

(Note the use of extra precision in the calculation.) The probability that a standard normal variable exceeds this value is $1 - \Phi(2.357) = 0.0092$. For a two-sided hypothesis test (see Subsection 3.2.3, of Chapter 3), this needs to be doubled, giving $P = 0.018$. This provides good evidence that there is a difference between the probabilities of clearance with the two treatments.

Another way of testing the same hypothesis is the widely used $\chi^2$ test, which is actually equivalent to the test just described. The test proceeds by working out the version of Table 7.2 that would be "expected" if the null hypothesis were true. The expected table is found by noting that under the null hypothesis, the probability of clearance is $73/100$ and, therefore, the number of patients receiving PUVA who would be expected to clear is $(73/100) \times 49 = 35.77$. Similar arguments lead to the other entries in the expected table and these are given in Table 7.3.

The next stage is to compute a statistic, $X^2$, which measures, in some sense, the distance between the expected table and the table that was actually observed. If this statistic is large, then this furnishes evidence against the null hypothesis. If the elements of the observed and expected tables are $o_i$ and $e_i$, $i = 1, \ldots, 4$, then the so-called $\chi^2$ statistic is defined as

**TABLE 7.3**

Table of Expected Values from Table 7.2

|  | Cleared | Did Not Clear | Total |
|---|---|---|---|
| TL-01 | 37.23 | 13.77 | 51 |
| PUVA | 35.77 | 13.23 | 49 |
| Total | 73 | 27 | 100 |

$$X^2 = \sum_{i=1}^{4} \frac{(o_i - e_i)^2}{e_i} \tag{7.4}$$

If the null hypothesis is true, then $X^2$ has a $\chi^2$ distribution with one degree of freedom. For observed and expected values in Table 7.2 and Table 7.3, respectively, $X^2$ has the value

$$\frac{(32 - 37.23)^2}{37.23} + \frac{(19 - 13.77)^2}{13.77} + \frac{(41 - 35.77)^2}{35.77} + \frac{(8 - 13.23)^2}{13.23} = 5.553$$

This gives $P = 0.018$, which is the same as derived using the statistic in Equation 7.3. In fact, it should be noted that the test statistic just derived, 5.553, is the square of that derived before, 2.357. In fact, it is generally true that $X^2 = Z^2$, so the tests are almost wholly equivalent. The only distinction between them is that with the approach based on Equation 7.3, it is possible to conduct a one-sided test, whereas this is not possible with the $\chi^2$ test.

## 7.2.2 Methods Based on More Formal Derivations

Although the informal methods are readily understood and adequate in straightforward circumstances, they do not lay a useful foundation for more complicated analyses. These can be derived using more formal methods, such as maximum likelihood. Before embarking on more complicated methods, it is useful to see how the formal approach would work in the simpler cases.

Using the definition of $y_{iP}$ adopted earlier, the contribution to the likelihood from the $i$th patient allocated to PUVA is $\pi_P^{y_{iP}}(1 - \pi_P)^{1-y_{iP}}$, and a similar expression is obtained for patients allocated to TL-01. Combining these into the complete likelihood $L(\pi_P, \pi_T \mid \{y_{iP}\}, \{y_{iT}\})$ and gathering like factors together gives

$$L(\pi_P, \pi_T \mid \{y_{iP}\}, \{y_{iT}\}) = L(\pi_P, \pi_T \mid n_P, n_T, r_P, r_T) = \pi_P^{r_P}(1 - \pi_P)^{n_P - r_P} \pi_T^{r_T}(1 - \pi_T)^{n_T - r_T}$$

and the corresponding log likelihood is

$$\ell(\pi_P, \pi_T \mid n_P, n_T, r_P, r_T) = r_P \log \pi_P + (n_P - r_P) \log(1 - \pi_P)$$

$$+ r_T \log \pi_T + (n_T - r_T) \log(1 - \pi_T)$$

Here, and throughout this chapter, all logarithms are to base $e$. Differentiating the log likelihood with respect to $\pi_P$ and $\pi_T$ and setting equal to zero shows that the maximum likelihood estimators are $\hat{\pi}_P = r_P/n_P = p_P$ and $\hat{\pi}_T = r_T/n_T = p_T$, respectively. It is comforting to observe that the estimators based on a sound theoretical method coincide with the intuitively based ones used previously. If we assume that the probability of clearance is the same for both treatments, $\pi$, then the maximum likelihood estimator of the common probability of clearance is found by maximizing $\ell(\pi, \pi \mid n_P, n_T, r_P, r_T)$ with respect to $\pi$, and this also yields the same estimator as that obtained earlier when the null hypothesis $\pi_P = \pi_T$ was assumed, namely, $\hat{\pi} = P$.

The likelihood ratio test of the null hypothesis $\pi_P = \pi_T$ is formed by considering the difference between the value of the log likelihood maximized over both parameters and the corresponding value under the null hypothesis, i.e., when the two parameters are constrained to have a common value, $\pi$. If the null hypothesis is true then, for sufficiently large $n_P$ and $n_T$, $G^2 = 2\{\ell(\hat{\pi}_P, \hat{\pi}_T \mid n_P, n_T, r_P, r_T) - \ell(\hat{\pi}, \hat{\pi} \mid n_P, n_T, r_P, r_T)\}$ will follow a $\chi^2$ distribution with one degree of freedom (because there is one more parameter under the alternative hypothesis than under the null). Evaluating this expression gives the following test statistic:

$$G^2 = 2\left\{ \begin{aligned} & r_P \log(\frac{r_P}{n_P}) + (n_P - r_P) \log(\frac{n_P - r_P}{n_P}) + r_T \log(\frac{r_T}{n_T}) + (n_T - r_T) \log(\frac{n_T - r_T}{n_T}) \\ & -(r_P + r_T) \log(p) - (n_P - r_P + n_T - r_T) \log(1 - p) \end{aligned} \right\}$$

$$= 2\left\{ \begin{aligned} & r_P \log(\frac{r_P}{n_P p}) + (n_P - r_P) \log(\frac{n_P - r_P}{n_P(1 - p)}) + r_T \log(\frac{r_T}{n_T p}) \\ & + (n_T - r_T) \log(\frac{n_T - r_T}{n_T(1 - p)}) \end{aligned} \right\}$$

This second form can be rewritten in a simple manner in terms of the elements of the observed and expected tables (Table 7.2 and Table 7.3, respectively), namely

$$G^2 = 2 \sum_{i=1}^{4} o_i \log\left(\frac{o_i}{e_i}\right) \tag{7.5}$$

and this has value 5.687 for the data from the PUVA vs. TL-01 trial, giving $P = 0.017$. Although the formula looks quite different, the value is similar to that obtained from Equation 7.4. In fact, under the null hypothesis, $G^2$ and $X^2$ are asymptotically equivalent.

---

## 7.3   Interval Estimates for the Binary Case

### 7.3.1   Different Measures of Difference between Treatments

Unlike hypothesis tests, interval estimates or confidence intervals attempt to measure the size of the difference between the effects of a treatment, rather than simply focus on whether or not there is a difference. When the outcome is continuous, the difference is almost always summarized by the difference in treatment means, $\mu_1 - \mu_2$. Occasionally, the ratio of means, $\mu_1/\mu_2$, is considered, although this is often done when the outcome variable has a skewed distribution and then the $\mu$s will be geometric means. Even if the ratio is chosen to summarize the discrepancy between treatments, the analysis is broadly the same as for the difference; the data are usually transformed using logs before a conventional analysis is applied. A feature of summarizing treatment differences when the outcome is binary is that there are several commonly used ways of measuring the difference between two proportions $\pi_P, \pi_T$. The various measures of difference require rather different approaches.

For binary data, the difference, $\pi_P - \pi_T$, often referred to as the *absolute risk difference* (ARD), is certainly used. However, the risk ratio (RR), $\pi_P/\pi_T$, the odds ratio (OR), $\{\pi_P/(1 - \pi_P)\}/\{\pi_T/(1 - \pi_T)\}$, and the number needed to treat (NNT), $1/(\pi_P - \pi_T)$, are also encountered quite frequently. The ARD is a natural way of measuring the treatment difference. If the outcome is "cured" or "not cured," then $N \times$ ARD is the number of extra patients you would expect to cure if you treated $N$ patients with P rather than T.

The NNT has its origins in clinical trials with binary outcomes. It is motivated by being the value of $N$ such that $N \times$ ARD $= 1$, that is, it is the number of patients you would have to treat before you would bring benefit to one extra patient if you used the better treatment. For example, if $\pi_P = 0.25$ and $\pi_T = 0.2$, then ARD $= 0.05$ and NNT $= 20$, so after treating 20 patients with P, you would expect to have cured 5 patients, whereas with T you would have expected to cure only 4. If the proportions are small, say 0.02 and 0.01, then NNT $= 100$, so a clinician might feel that the difference is not sufficiently large for a change of practice to be worthwhile, especially if aspects such as cost and safety are not in favor of P. The fact that ARD and NNT are reciprocals of each other means that many statisticians are not wholly persuaded of the need for both measures. However, it must be conceded that many clinicians find NNT easier to interpret than ARD. Nevertheless, NNT has some awkward statistical properties, as will be seen when interval estimates of NNT are discussed in the following text, and its use must be approached with care.

The other measures, RR and OR, are more often found in epidemiology, but they do appear quite frequently in the reporting of trials (especially ORs). Apparently, quite impressive differences can be reported with these measures: for example, if $\pi_P = 0.003$ and $\pi_T = 0.001$ then RR = 3, so a patient would be expected to be three times more likely to be cured using P than T. However, in this case NNT = 500, which gives a less impressive view of the difference between the treatments. These measures arise more naturally when the issue of baseline adjustment is considered. This will be covered in Section 7.4, essentially, the key technique is logistic regression and, as will be seen in that section, the OR is a natural measure of difference when logistic regression is used.

Substituting estimates of $\pi_P$ and $\pi_T$ in the formulae for RR, OR, and NNT gives straightforward estimates of each of the measures of difference. The only complications are if one or possibly both of the estimates is 0 (OR and RR) or 1 (OR) or if the estimates coincide (NNT). Methods for obtaining interval estimates will be explained in the next subsection.

### 7.3.2   Interval Estimates or Confidence Intervals

#### 7.3.2.1   *Interval Estimates for ARD and NNT*

A very widely used and easily implemented method for finding a confidence interval for the ARD is to note that the distribution of $(p_P - p_T) - (\pi_P - \pi_T)$ is approximately normal with mean 0 and variance that can be estimated by $p_P(1 - p_P)/n_P + p_T(1 - p_T)/n_T$. Consequently, a $100(1 - \alpha)\%$ confidence interval is given by

$$p_P - p_T - z_{\frac{1}{2}\alpha}\sqrt{\frac{p_P(1-p_P)}{n_P} + \frac{p_T(1-p_T)}{n_T}},$$

$$p_P - p_T + z_{\frac{1}{2}\alpha}\sqrt{\frac{p_P(1-p_P)}{n_P} + \frac{p_T(1-p_T)}{n_T}}$$

(7.6)

where the probability that a standard normal variate falls between $\pm z_{\frac{1}{2}\alpha}$ is $1 - \alpha$. It is convenient to recall that for a 95% confidence interval, $\alpha = 0.05$ and $z_{\frac{1}{2}\alpha} = 1.96$.

Applied to the PUVA vs. TL-01 trial, we obtain ARD = 0.836 − 0.627 = 0.209, with 95% confidence interval (0.041, 0.378). Thus, there is evidence that the proportion of patients who clear is higher if PUVA is used rather than TL-01, although the lower limit of the confidence interval shows that the difference may not be that marked.

Taking the reciprocal of the ARD gives an estimate of the NNT of 1/0.209 = 4.78. Thus you need to treat nearly five patients before one more patient is cleared if you use PUVA than if you use TL-01. Taking reciprocals of the limits of the interval estimate for ARD gives the 95% confidence interval for NNT as 2.65, 24.39. The NNT is the reciprocal of a quantity that is approximately normally distributed and therefore has a distribution with long tails, as exemplified by the wide interval estimate for NNT.

To see what complications arise when the difference is not significant, it is useful to consider a smaller trial. Suppose, for illustration only, that the trial had only been about half the size reported in Table 7.2. To be specific, suppose 25 patients had been treated in each group and 16 had cleared with TL-01 and 20 with PUVA. Then the ARD would have been 0.16, with 95% confidence interval (−0.085, 0.405). The smaller sample size has led to a confidence interval spanning 0; on the basis of the reduced trial, PUVA could be superior to TL-01 but the superiority of TL-01 has by no means been ruled out. As before, the NNT can be estimated as the reciprocal of the ARD, i.e., $1/0.16 = 6.25$. However, because the confidence interval spans 0, trying to construct a confidence interval from the reciprocals of the limits of the interval for ARD, namely, 2.470 and 11.775, needs great care.

There are several difficulties. The first is that if $\pi_P - \pi_T = 0$, then the treatments have the same effect, and you would not expect to cure more patients on one treatment rather than the other, no matter how many you treated. Therefore, it is quite reasonable that in this case the NNT is infinite. However, if an interval estimate for ARD includes 0, then in some way, an interval estimate for NNT must include infinity. The second problem is that in defining NNT, we have been rather cavalier about the consequences of different signs for the ARD. When only point estimates are considered, any difficulties can be avoided. Negative ARDs, which would correspond to negative NNTs, can be avoided by taking the difference in the other direction. This approach can be used to form confidence intervals when, as in the real PUVA vs. TL-01 trial, both limits are positive (possibly after adjusting the direction of the difference). However, this casual approach cannot be sustained when the limits of the confidence interval for ARD do not have the same sign.

Part of the problem is, as Altman (1998) pointed out, that the terminology is not sufficiently specific. A positive NNT can be thought of as the number of patients you need to treat before one additional patient benefits from the better treatment, which Altman suggested might be called the NNTB, the "number needed to benefit one extra patient." Although a negative NNT can be interpreted (after removal of the negative sign) as the NNTB by using the "other" treatment, it could also be interpreted, without this reversal in the order the treatments are compared, as the "number needed to harm one extra patient" (NNTH) on the inferior treatment. Being able to interpret both positive and negative NNTs allows interval estimates for NNTs to be framed corresponding to intervals for ARD that span 0. Suppose the confidence interval for $\pi_P - \pi_T$ is $(-L, U)$, with $L, U > 0$. As the value of $\pi_P - \pi_T$ decreases from $U$ to 0, the corresponding NNT, actually the NNTB, increases from $1/U$ without limit as 0 is approached. As $\pi_P - \pi_T$ decreases from 0 toward $-L$, NNT increases from $-\infty$ to its lower limit, $-1/L$. The interval

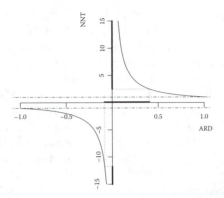

**FIGURE 7.1**
The interval estimate for NNT when the confidence interval for ARD spans 0. The interval for
ARD is the bold horizontal line and the corresponding interval for NNT is the union of the
emboldened parts of the vertical axis (extended to infinity in both directions).

estimate for NNT is therefore the union of $(-\infty, -1/L)$ and $(1/U, \infty)$; thus, the
negative interval corresponding to an interval $(1/L, \infty)$ for the NNTH and
the positive part being an interval for the NNTB. The situation is illustrated
in Figure 7.1. Note that if $x \in [-1,1]$ then $1/x$ cannot lie in $(-1,1)$, thus,
provided the confidence interval for ARD is proper, in the sense that it lies
wholly within $[-1,1]$, then no part of the interval for NNT can lie within
$(-1,1)$. The interval unavailable to NNT is shown as that between the dot-
ted/dashed tramlines in Figure 7.1.

For the confidence interval for ARD for the preceding artificially reduced
trial, namely, $(-0.085, 0.405)$, the 95% confidence is that, for PUVA more
beneficial than TL-01, more than 2.47 patients need to be treated with PUVA
for one more patient to clear and, when TL-01 is more beneficial, more than
11.78 patients need to be treated with PUVA to have one fewer patient clear.
Although Altman (1998) has tried hard to present confidence intervals for
NNTs in a convincing way, there is no doubt that NNT is at its least compelling when this must be derived from a confidence interval from an interval for ARD, which spans zero.

### 7.3.2.2   Problems with the Confidence Interval for ARD and a Simple Solution

The confidence interval in Equation 7.6 is easy to compute and is very widely
used. It is also widely implemented in statistical software. Nevertheless, it
has a number of flaws and was the worst-performing method of the 11
scrutinized by Newcombe (1998). If the denominators of the proportions are
not too small and the probabilities are not too close to 0 or 1, then the
problems are not too great. However, the method has coverage probability
much lower than its nominal value. The putative 95% interval is closer to a

90% or even 85% interval. Another difficulty is that the limits of Equation 7.6 are not guaranteed to lie within [–1,1].

Newcombe (1998) considered several methods, including profile likelihood methods, most of which were computationally awkward. For a single proportion, an interval derived from score statistics* is relatively easily implemented. Newcombe described an *ad hoc* adaptation of this methodology to the case of two independent samples, which is also easy to implement. This method has good coverage properties and gives limits that must lie within [–1,1]. The rationale for the method is described briefly here. The derivation has three parts.

1. An alternative interval estimate is found for the case of a single proportion.

2. It is noted that the interval estimate for the difference in Equation 7.6 has a width that is the square root of the sum of squares of the widths for the confidence intervals of the individual proportions making up the difference.

3. The new interval estimate argues by analogy with 2 using widths derived in 1. Some slight adaptations are needed because the intervals in 1 are not symmetric about the point estimate of the parameter.

The first point proceeds by noting that a $100(1 - \alpha)\%$ confidence interval for a single proportion $\pi$, estimated by $p$ with denominator $n$ could be found as

$$\left\{ \pi \;\middle|\; \frac{|p - \pi|}{\sqrt{\pi(1 - \pi)/n}} \leq z_{\frac{1}{2}\alpha} \right\} = \left\{ \pi \;\middle|\; (p - \pi)^2 \leq z_{\frac{1}{2}\alpha}^2 \pi(1 - \pi)/n \right\}$$

The analogous interval to Equation 7.6 for a single sample can be obtained by substituting $p$ for $\pi$ in the expression on the RHS of the inequality in the second version shown in the preceding text: this might be called the *elementary* method. The alternative pursued here is to solve the quadratic in $\pi$ implied by setting the inequality to equality in the aforementioned second expression: this is referred to as the *score-based* method. The required interval estimate is $(l, u)$, where $l < u$ are the solutions of the quadratic; the solutions are always distinct and in the interval $[0,1]$. The situation can be seen graphically in Figure 7.2, illustrated using the data from the PUVA group in the PUVA vs. TL-01 trial, with $p = 41/49$. Note that $p$ is not the midpoint of $l$ and $u$; this fact and the reason for it can clearly be seen in Figure 7.2.

---

* Score statistics are based on consideration of the slope of the log likelihood function, and its rate of change, near to the maximum likelihood estimate.

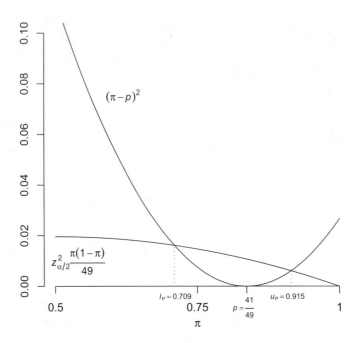

**FIGURE 7.2**
Graphical illustration of score-based interval for a single proportion, $p = 41/49 = 0.837$; 95% limits are 0.709 and 0.915; $z_{\frac{1}{2}\alpha} = 1.96$.

A formal adaptation of these arguments to the two sample case is not straightforward. However, Newcombe (1998) proceeded as follows. The interval in Equation 7.6 can be written as

$$p_P - p_T - \sqrt{w_P^2 + w_T^2}, p_P - p_T + \sqrt{w_P^2 + w_T^2}$$

where $w_P$ ($w_T$) is the width, measured from the point estimate $p_P$ ($p_T$), using the elementary method for a single sample. Newcombe's approach is to proceed analogously, but using the widths based on the score-based method.
An immediate difficulty is that for the score-based method, the widths $p_P - l_P$ and $u_P - p_P$ are unequal. Newcombe used the lower limit for $p_P$ and the upper limit for $p_T$ when constructing the lower limit for $p_P - p_T$, and vice versa for the upper limit, giving:

$$p_P - p_T - \sqrt{(p_P - l_P)^2 + (u_T - p_T)^2}, p_P - p_T + \sqrt{(p_T - l_T)^2 + (u_P - p_P)^2}$$

Although slightly intricate, all the calculations are easy to perform and no iterative methods are needed. The method has a somewhat *ad hoc* basis but its performance, as assessed in the simulation studies reported by Newcombe (1998), is impressive and far superior to that of Equation 7.6.

The interval for $\pi_P - \pi_T$ from the PUVA vs. TL-01 trial using the score-based method is 0.035, 0.367, which compares with 0.041, 0.378 for the interval based on Equation 7.6.

### 7.3.2.3   Interval Estimates for RR and OR

Before dealing with the details of interval estimates for these quantities, it is worth thinking a little more carefully about these scales for measuring the discrepancy between two proportions — they are very different to those for ARD and NNT. The first thing to note is that both RR and OR are necessarily nonnegative and, in each case, the null value, i.e., the value when the two treatments are the same is one. Thus, RR = OR = 1 if, and only if, ARD = 0; so a test of the null hypothesis that ARD = 0 is equivalent to testing RR = OR = 1. Thus, special tests for RR and OR are not needed — those described in Section 7.2 of this chapter remain appropriate. New approaches are only needed for deriving confidence intervals, which is reasonable as confidence intervals are concerned with measuring differences, and new measurement scales are being used here.

The order in which we compare two treatments in a trial is arbitrary. If we compare PUVA with TL-01 we would obtain one difference, ARD, whereas if we made the comparison in the other direction we would obtain −ARD. Moreover, confidence intervals for ARD should lie in [−1,1], and intervals for a difference computed in the opposite direction will also lie in the same interval, being the reflection of the first interval about the origin. For an RR or OR, the discrepancy between the proportions is measured by a ratio, so comparing PUVA with TL-01 would give an estimate for the RR of $p_P/p_T = (41/49)/(32/51) = 1.334$. However, a comparison the other way round would give an essentially equivalent RR of $p_T/p_P = 1.334^{-1} = 0.750$. In other words, comparing treatments the other way around on the RR scale gives values that are reciprocals of one another. The limits of an interval estimate for an RR are nonnegative and those for the same comparison, but made in the opposite directions, will be reciprocals of the original interval. For example, if the interval estimate is (10, 100) when the comparison is made in one direction, the interval becomes (0.01, 0.1) in the other direction.

These observations should focus attention on the inherent lack of symmetry in the RR scale. A very large RR (say, 1000) is in essence the same as a very small RR (say, 0.001) because the direction of the comparison is arbitrary. Therefore, there is an equivalence between the interval $[1,\infty)$ and $(0,1]$ in that any value in the former (which is of infinite width) has a natural partner in the latter (of width 1). Consequently, there is a clear sense in which the intervals $(^1/_2, 2)$, $(^1/_3, 3)$, $(^1/_4, 4)$ are all symmetric intervals — one treatment might be two, three, or four times as good as the other, or possibly the other treatment might be two, three, or four times as good. If two treatments were equivalent, then interval estimates for the RR (or OR) ought to be symmetric about 1 (the null value) in this sense. Consequently, when constructing intervals for RR, we should not expect them to follow the additively symmetric format *point estimate* $\pm z \times SE$.

However, intervals such as $(^1/_2, 2)$ and $(^1/_3, 3)$ are additively symmetric when expressed on the log scale, so if $(^1/_3, 3)$ is the interval estimate for RR, the corresponding estimate for log RR is $(\log(^1/_3), \log(3)) = (-\log(3), \log(3))$, which is symmetric in the additive sense about the null value for log RR, which is $\log(1) = 0$. Therefore, it is likely to be sensible to try to construct an interval for log RR along the customary lines of *point estimate* $\pm z \times SE$ in a way that it would not be for RR directly.

An interval estimate for log RR can be obtained by a direct approach. Define $\phi = \log(\pi_P/\pi_T)$ and consider its natural estimate $\log(p_P/p_T) = \log(p_P)$ $- \log(p_T)$. The approximate normality and independence of the estimated proportions together show that $\log(p_P/p_T)$ is approximately normal with mean $\phi$ and variance $\mathrm{var}(\log(p_P)) + \mathrm{var}(\log(p_T))$. Applying the delta method (see Subsection 3.4.2) gives:

$$\mathrm{var}(\log(p_P)) = \mathrm{var}\left(\log\left(\frac{r_P}{n_P}\right)\right) \approx \frac{\pi_P(1-\pi_P)}{n_P} \times \left(\frac{1}{\pi_P}\right)^2 = \frac{1}{n_P\pi_P} - \frac{1}{n_P}$$

so an estimate of this variance is $r_P^{-1} - n_P^{-1}$. Note that in applying the delta method, we have used the fact that the derivative of log $x$ is $x^{-1}$, so in using these results, it is essential that natural logarithms are used throughout.

From the result that $\log(p_P/p_T)$ is approximately normal with mean $\phi$ and variance $r_P^{-1} - n_P^{-1} + r_T^{-1} - n_T^{-1}$, we can derive an approximate $100(1 - \alpha)\%$ confidence interval for $\phi$ as $(l_{RR}, u_{RR})$:

$$l_{RR} = \log(p_P / p_T) - z_{1-\frac{1}{2}\alpha}\sqrt{\frac{1}{r_P} - \frac{1}{n_P} + \frac{1}{r_T} - \frac{1}{n_T}},$$

$$u_{RR} = \log(p_P / p_T) + z_{1-\frac{1}{2}\alpha}\sqrt{\frac{1}{r_P} - \frac{1}{n_P} + \frac{1}{r_T} - \frac{1}{n_T}}$$

with the corresponding interval for the RR being $(e^{l_{RR}}, e^{u_{RR}})$.

All the aforementioned remarks about the RR apply equally well to the OR. The log OR, $\psi$, namely, $\log[\{\pi_P/(1 - \pi_P)\}/\{\pi_T/(1 - \pi_T)\}]$, is naturally estimated by

$$\log\left(\frac{r_P}{n_P - r_P} \times \frac{n_T - r_T}{r_T}\right)$$

An argument analogous to that just used for RR gives a $100(1-\alpha)\%$ confidence interval for $\psi$ of $(l_{OR}, u_{OR})$, namely

$$\log\left(\frac{r_P}{n_P - r_P} \times \frac{n_T - r_T}{r_T}\right) \pm z_{\frac{1}{2}\alpha}\sqrt{\frac{1}{r_P} + \frac{1}{n_P - r_P} + \frac{1}{r_T} + \frac{1}{n_T - r_T}}$$

with the corresponding confidence interval for OR being $(e^{l_{OR}}, e^{u_{OR}})$. As with the interval for $\phi$, and for the same reason, the natural logarithm must be used in this formula.

Note that if any of the entries in Table 7.1 is zero then the above formulae will not be defined. In this case one possible solution is to add $1/2$ to each element in that table, and then to apply the preceding formulae, giving:

$$\log\left(\frac{r_P + \frac{1}{2}}{n_P - r_P + \frac{1}{2}} \times \frac{n_T - r_T + \frac{1}{2}}{r_T + \frac{1}{2}}\right) \pm z_{\frac{1}{2}\alpha}\sqrt{\frac{1}{r_P + \frac{1}{2}} + \frac{1}{n_P - r_P + \frac{1}{2}} + \frac{1}{r_T + \frac{1}{2}} + \frac{1}{n_T - r_T + \frac{1}{2}}}$$

This straightforward, seemingly rather heuristic approach is slightly less *ad hoc* than might appear at first glance. If $c$ is added to each element in Table 7.1 and the log OR calculated as before, then $c = 1/2$ minimizes the bias in the log OR.

### 7.3.2.4 Summary of Results

The results of applying each method to the PUVA vs. TL-01 trial are shown in Table 7.4. This trial shows a clear advantage for PUVA, and the intervals do not contain the null value. To illustrate the methods when the difference between the treatments is not clear-cut, the reduced, hypothetical version of the trial, introduced in the discussion of NNT, in which the clearance proportions are 20/25 (PUVA) and 16/25 (TL-01) is also presented.

The hypothesis test that there is no difference between the treatments shows clear evidence of a difference for the full trial (with $P = 0.018$) but not for the reduced trial $P = 0.208$. Consequently, the 95% confidence intervals for the full trial do not include the null value for the measure but they do

**TABLE 7.4**

Point and Interval Estimates for the Different Measures of Discrepancy for Real and Reduced PUVA vs. TL-01 Trial

| Measure of Discrepancy | Full Trial ($P = 0.018$) | | Reduced Trial ($P = 0.208$) | |
|---|---|---|---|---|
| | Point Estimate | 95% Confidence Interval | Point Estimate | 95% Confidence Interval |
| ARD (Equation 7.6) | 0.209 | 0.041, 0.378 | 0.160 | −0.085, 0.405 |
| ARD (Newcombe) | 0.209 | 0.035, 0.367 | 0.160 | −0.088, 0.384 |
| NNT | 4.78 | 2.65, 24.39 | 6.25 | $(2.47,\infty)\cup(-\infty, 11.78)$ |
| RR | 1.334 | 1.044, 1.704 | 1.25 | 0.878, 1.780 |
| OR | 3.043 | 1.181, 7.842 | 2.25 | 0.628, 8.058 |

*Note:* Treatments compared as PUVA minus or over TL-01.

for the reduced trial. For ARD the null value is 0, for the RR and OR it is 1, and for the NNT it is essentially an infinite value, the values are included in the interval estimates for the reduced version of the trial but not for the full trial. Notice also that the OR tends to give a rather more exaggerated value than the RR.

## 7.4  Adjusting Binary Outcomes for Baseline Observations

### 7.4.1  Using a Logistic Model

In Section 6.3, the role of observations taken before randomization, so-called baseline variables, was discussed. Methods based on differences were seen to have poorer properties than the method of analysis of covariance. In this technique, a linear model was used to allow estimation of treatment effects, adjusted for one or more baseline variables. In Subsection 6.4.5, the need to include any variables used in the stratification of the treatment allocation was described. If the trial compares treatments A and B, then the model used could be presented as, e.g.,

$$\text{outcome}_i = \mu + \tau I_i + \beta_1 \times \text{baseline value}_{1i} + \beta_2 \times \text{baseline value}_{2i} + \text{error}_i$$

where $I_i$ is an indicator function taking the value 1 if treatment A had been allocated and 0 if B had been allocated to patient i. When the outcome is binary, there is also a need for a method to adjust treatment effects for baseline imbalances or to allow for stratification of the allocation.

An approach that is widely used is similar to that described in Subsection 6.4.3 and 6.4.4, and uses a version of the preceding model. However, some adaptations of the model for normal outcomes are necessary to make it suitable for binary data. Adding an error term to a mean is natural for normal outcomes — an outcome will have a normal distribution if, and only if, the error term is normally distributed. If the outcome has a binomial distribution, then deviations of this variable from the mean of the binomial variable will not follow a binomial distribution. Consequently, an analysis based on a binomial likelihood, with the amended model

$$\text{mean outcome}_i = \mu + \tau I_i + \beta_1 \times \text{baseline value}_{1i} + \beta_2 \times \text{baseline value}_{2i}$$

is to be preferred. There is one further problem, namely, that the mean outcome is the probability the binary outcome has value 1. As this must be between 0 and 1, problems arise because the linear term on the right-hand side is not similarly constrained. The final amendment is to use

$$f(\text{mean outcome}_i) = \mu + \tau I_i + \beta_1 \times \text{baseline value}_{1i} + \beta_2 \times \text{baseline value}_{2i}$$

where $f(.)$ is a function that maps $(0,1)$ to the whole real line. This approach is essentially a description of a generalized linear model for a binary outcome. See McCullagh and Nelder (1989) for a full treatise on this class of models and Collett (2002) for an account focused on binary data.

The usual approach to the analysis of binary data is to use a logistic regression, which is obtained when we choose $f(\pi) = \log\{\pi/(1-\pi)\}$: this is extensively discussed in Collett (2002). This form of $f$ is known as the *logit* function and is the natural logarithm of the odds of the outcome taking the value 1.

Suppose such a model was fitted to data from a trial comparing two treatments, A and B, in which the effect of two baseline variables, say $x_1$ and $x_2$, had to be taken into account. Suppose that an outcome of 1 indicates a successful outcome and 0 a failure, then if $\pi = \Pr(\text{successful outcome})$ the model gives:

$$\text{logit}(\pi) = \log\left(\frac{\pi}{1-\pi}\right) = \log(\text{odds of success}) = \mu + \tau + \beta_1 x_1 + \beta_2 x_2$$

(treatment A)

$$\text{logit}(\pi) = \log\left(\frac{\pi}{1-\pi}\right) = \log(\text{odds of success}) = \mu + \beta_1 x_1 + \beta_2 x_2$$

(treatment B)

If a patient has given values for $x_1$ and $x_2$, then taking the difference between these expressions shows that

$$\log(\text{odds of success on treatment A}) - \log(\text{odds of success on treatment B})$$

$$= \log\left(\frac{\text{odds of success on treatment A}}{\text{odds of success on treatment B}}\right) = \log(OR) = \tau.$$

In other words, $\tau$ is the log OR, or $e^\tau$ is the OR of success on treatment A relative to treatment B, adjusted for variables $x_1$ and $x_2$. In other words, whereas changes in the values of the baseline variables $x_1$ and $x_2$ may give rise to changes in the probability of successful treatment, $\tau$ is a measure of the difference between treatments for patients with the same baseline values.

Models for adjusted ARD might have been obtained had $f(x) = x$ been used in the preceding analysis and for adjusted RR if $f(x) = \log(x)$ had been used. However, neither function maps $(0,1)$ to the whole real line, so difficulties could arise in the modeling procedure. These models can be used, but their use is a delicate matter and they are not routinely employed. When an adjusted treatment difference is required for a trial with a binary outcome, the OR is a convenient measure to use.

The preceding illustration uses two baseline variables. However, there is nothing special about two variables and more or fewer can be used as required, although as with any regression model, some judgment needs to be exercised to keep the number in check. Also, the variables can be continuous or categorical; in the latter case, a variable with $c$ levels would require $c - 1$ dummy variables to be fitted.

### 7.4.2 Fitting a Logistic Regression

The standard way to fit a logistic regression is to use maximum likelihood. To explain this analysis, a notation is needed for the variables fitted in the model, and the vector notation $x_i^T \beta$ to denote the variables fitted for the $i$th patient will be used. This is simply

$$x_i^T \beta = \sum_{j=0}^{q} x_{ij} \beta_j \ ,$$

where $x_{ij}$ is the value on the $i$th patient of the $j$th of $q + 1$ variables and $\beta_j$ are the elements of the $(q + 1)$-dimensional vector $\beta$. Usually, $x_{i0} = 1$ for all $i$, such that $\beta_0$ corresponds to $\mu$ in the notation used in the previous section, and $x_{i1} = 0$ or 1 depending on whether treatment A or B was allocated, so $\beta_1$ corresponds to $\tau$ in the previous notation.

If $\pi_i$ is the success probability for the $i$th patient ($i = 1, \ldots, n$), then the logistic model specifies these $n$ parameters in terms of the $q + 1$ parameters $\beta_j$ via the $n$ expressions $\text{logit}(\pi_i) = x_i^T \beta$. The log likelihood of the data is

$$\ell(\{\pi_i\} \,|\, \text{data}) = \sum_{i=1}^{n} [y_i \log(\pi_i) + (1 - y_i) \log(1 - \pi_i)]$$

$$= \sum_{i=1}^{n} [y_i \log(\frac{\pi_i}{1 - \pi_i}) + \log(1 - \pi_i)]$$

where $y_i$ is 1 or 0 depending on whether the $i$th patient is successfully treated or not. This can be rewritten in terms of the $\beta_j$ as

$$\ell(\{\beta_j\} \,|\, \text{data}) = \sum_{i=1}^{n} [y_i x_i^T \beta - \log(1 + e^{x_i^T \beta})]$$

The model is fitted by choosing the $\beta_j$ that maximize this expression. This can be done in a variety of ways but, in general, a numerical method is needed because no explicit solution is available. One approach is to solve the $q + 1$ normal equations $\partial \ell / \partial \beta_r = 0$ and these are

$$\sum_{i=1}^{n}(y_i - \pi_i)x_{ir} = 0, \quad r = 0, \ldots, q$$

Suppose that the maximizing values of the βs are denoted by $\{\hat{\beta}_r\}$. The general theory of maximum likelihood estimation shows that for large $n$, the covariance of the estimates $\hat{\beta}_r$ and $\hat{\beta}_s$ is given by $(r, s)^{th}$ element of the inverse of the matrix with $(r, s)^{th}$ element equal to $-E(\partial^2\ell/\partial\beta_r\partial\beta_s)$ (with variances given by the case $r = s$). These expectations are quantities given by

$$\sum_{i=1}^{n}\pi_i(1-\pi_i)x_{ir}x_{is}, \quad r,s = 0,\ldots,q \tag{7.7}$$

This matrix can be estimated by substituting $\hat{\pi}_i$ for $\pi_i$, the former being the latter evaluated at $\{\hat{\beta}_j\}$, i.e.,

$$\sum_{i=1}^{n}\hat{\pi}_i(1-\hat{\pi}_i)x_{ir}x_{is}, \quad r,s = 0,\ldots,q \tag{7.8}$$

The estimate of $\tau = \beta_1$ is the estimate of the log OR, adjusted for the variables $x_{i2},\ldots,x_{iq}$. The estimate of the standard error of $\hat{\beta}_1$, $\sqrt{\hat{v}_{11}}$, is the square root of the entry in column 1 and row 1 of the inverse of the matrix in Equation 7.8 (remembering the numbering starts at 0), and this can be used to perform a test of the null hypothesis that the adjusted log OR is zero and to form confidence intervals for the adjusted log OR and adjusted OR.

The test of the null hypothesis computes the ratio $\hat{\beta}_1/\sqrt{\hat{v}_{11}}$ ; under the null hypothesis this will approximately have a standard normal distribution. The $100(1 - \alpha)\%$ confidence interval for the adjusted log OR is $(\hat{\beta}_1 - z_{\frac{1}{2}\alpha}\sqrt{\hat{v}_{11}}, \hat{\beta}_1 + z_{\frac{1}{2}\alpha}\sqrt{\hat{v}_{11}})$ and the interval for the adjusted OR is found by exponentiating the ends of the this interval.

An alternative way to perform the hypothesis test is to evaluate the maximized log likelihood, which we could write as $\ell(\hat{\beta}_0,\hat{\beta}_1,\{\hat{\beta}_j\}_{j\geq2}\,|\,\text{data})$. Then refit the model, but with the term for the treatment effect omitted, this could be written $\ell(\hat{\beta}_0,\{\hat{\beta}_j\}_{j\geq2}\,|\,\text{data})$. General maximum likelihood theory implies that under the null hypothesis $\beta_1 = 0$, $2[\ell(\hat{\beta}_0,\hat{\beta}_1,\{\hat{\beta}_j\}_{j\geq2}\,|\,\text{data})-\ell(\hat{\beta}_0, \{\hat{\beta}_j\}_{j\geq2}\,|\,\text{data})]$ follows a $\chi^2$ distribution with 1 degree of freedom. This test, called the *likelihood ratio test*, is broadly equivalent to the one previously described for large samples but often has better properties in smaller samples. The approach can be extended to yield confidence intervals, a technique known as *profile likelihood intervals*, but this is beyond the scope of this book (but see question 6 in this chapter).

### 7.4.3   Adjusting the OR in the PUVA vs. TL-01 Trial

The first approach will use logistic regression, which can be fitted in many packages including Minitab and R; in this illustration we will use R. The variable fitted, other than the constant term and the indicator for the treatment, is the plaque size, which is a binary variable. The plaque size is a description of the nature of the psoriasis affecting the patient. In psoriasis, scaly areas arise on the skin and, in some patients, the predominant size of these scales is large, whereas in others it is small. It was believed before the trial started that it would be harder to achieve clearance in patients with predominantly large plaques. Consequently, the treatment allocation used random permuted blocks stratified according to whether the predominant plaque size was above or below 3 cm (cf. Section 4.4).

The following analysis is purely illustrative. As explained in Subsection 6.4.5, the model should include all variables used in the stratification of the allocation. This means that plaque size must be included. To maintain the simplicity of the exposition the other variable used in stratification in the real trial, skin type, is not considered here but it would have to be included in any genuine analysis.

Fitting this model in R gives the output in Table 7.5. The first thing to note is the variables used for fitting treatment have been coded as 1 for PUVA and 0 for TL-01 and the variable for plaque size has used 1 for large plaques and 0 for small plaques. Given this, we can interpret the fitted model, namely

$$\log \frac{\text{Pr(clearance)}}{1-\text{Pr(clearance)}} = 1.200 + 1.2195 I(\text{treatment} = \text{PUVA}) -$$

$$1.4352 I(\text{plaque size} = \text{large}))$$

where $I(.)$ denotes an indicator function taking values 1 and 0, according to whether or not the argument is true. The aforementioned coefficients are shown in Table 7.5, under `Coefficients` in the column headed `Estimate`. In terms of the notation of Subsection 7.4.2, the values 1.200, 1.2195, and –1.4352 are, respectively, $\hat{\beta}_0, \hat{\beta}_1, \hat{\beta}_2$. The odds of clearance can be estimated from this equation for the following four groups:

|                | TL-01                          | PUVA                                              |
| -------------- | ------------------------------ | ------------------------------------------------- |
| Small plaques  | exp(1.200) = 3.320             | exp(1.200 + 1.2195) = 11.240                       |
| Large plaques  | exp(1.200 – 1.4352) = 0.790    | exp(1.200 – 1.4352 + 1.2195) = 2.676              |

These figures illustrate the nature of the model; though the odds of clearing is lower for patients with large plaques, those patients with a given plaque

**TABLE 7.5**

R Output from Fitting a Logistic Regression to the Data from the PUVA vs. TL-01 Trial

```
Call:
glm(formula = Clear ~ Treatment + Plaque, family = binomial,
  data = gordon)

Deviance Residuals:
    Min       1Q    Median        3Q       Max
 -2.2382  -1.0793    0.4129    0.7434    1.2788

Coefficients:
              Estimate   Std. Error   z value   Pr(>|z|)
(Intercept)     1.2000       0.3994     3.005    0.00266 **
Treatment       1.2195       0.5099     2.392    0.01676 *
Plaque         -1.4352       0.4975    -2.885    0.00392 **
---
Signif. codes: 0 '***' 0.001 '**' 0.01 '*' 0.05 '.' 0.1 ' ' 1

(Dispersion parameter for binomial family taken to be 1)

   Null deviance: 116.65 on 99 degrees of freedom
Residual deviance: 102.00 on 97 degrees of freedom
AIC: 108

Number of Fisher Scoring iterations: 4
```

*Note:* Effect of treatment is adjusted for baseline plaque size.

size who were treated with PUVA have odds of clearing $\exp(1.2195) = 3.385$ times greater than similar patients treated with TL-01.

The null hypothesis that, once adjusted for the effect of plaque size, the treatment has no effect can be tested by noting that the estimated standard error of $\hat{\beta}_1$ is 0.5099, in the column headed Std. Error in Table 7.5. The ratio $\hat{\beta}_1 / \sqrt{\hat{v}_{11}} = 1.2195/0.5099$ is given in the next column of the table and the corresponding $P$-value is 0.017. The 95% confidence interval for adjusted OR can be found by first finding the interval for its logarithm, namely,

$$(\hat{\beta}_1 - z_{\frac{1}{2}\alpha} \sqrt{\hat{v}_{11}}, \hat{\beta}_1 + z_{\frac{1}{2}\alpha} \sqrt{\hat{v}_{11}}) = 1.2195 \pm 1.96 \times 0.5099 = 0.2201, 2.2189,$$ which

gives an interval for the adjusted OR of 1.246, 9.197.

The residual deviance for this model, found toward the bottom of the output in Table 7.5 is 102.00; this is essentially $-2 \times$ maximized log likelihood. The corresponding value for the model omitting the term for the treatment is 108.19. The likelihood ratio test proceeds by referring $108.19 - 102.00 = 6.19$ to a $\chi^2$ variable on 1 degree of freedom, giving $P = 0.013$. This is similar to the $P$-value obtained from the ratio $\hat{\beta}_1 / \sqrt{\hat{v}_{11}}$.

**TABLE 7.6**

R Output from Fitting a Logistic Regression to the Data from the PUVA vs. TL-01 Trial

```
Call:
glm(formula = Clear ~ Treatment, family = binomial, data = gordon)

Deviance Residuals:
     Min        1Q     Median        3Q        Max
 -1.9039   -1.4053     0.5971    0.9655     0.9655

Coefficients:
               Estimate    Std. Error    z value    Pr(>|z|)
(Intercept)      0.5213        0.2896      1.800      0.0719 .
Treatment        1.1128        0.4830      2.304      0.0212 *
---
Signif. codes:  0 `***' 0.001 `**' 0.01 `*' 0.05 `.' 0.1 ` ' 1

(Dispersion parameter for binomial family taken to be 1)

    Null deviance: 116.65 on 99 degrees of freedom
Residual deviance: 110.96 on 98 degrees of freedom
AIC: 114.96

Number of Fisher Scoring iterations: 4
```

*Note:* Effect of treatment but with no adjustment for plaque size.

In Table 7.6, the same approach is taken but with no variable included for plaque size — in other words, the analysis of the treatment effect is not adjusted for any variable. The log OR is estimated as 1.1128, with confidence interval (0.1661, 2.059), which transforms to point and interval estimates for the OR of 3.043 and (1.181, 7.842), which coincide with those from Table 7.4. Therefore, when this method is applied with no adjusting variables in the model, the results do indeed reduce to the unadjusted values found in Subsection 7.3.2. Also, the adjusted OR and confidence interval, namely, 3.385 and (1.246, 9.197) are not too far from the unadjusted values. The degree of adjustment effected by the inclusion of the plaque size variable in the analysis might be anticipated to be small because the allocation was stratified by plaque size.

The method can be used in just the same way to adjust for baseline variables that are continuous, such as age. The recommendations regarding which covariates to include are broadly similar to those outlined in Subsection 6.4.5. Although the use of logistic regression to allow for baseline variables in an RCT is desirable, the benefits obtained are not quite the same as for a normal regression and continuous outcome. The logistic regression allows for adjustment of imbalances between groups, but the position vis-à-vis improved precision is more subtle than might be imagined and is beyond the scope of this book: a fuller discussion can be found in Robinson and Jewell (1991).

It should also be noted that the logistic regression is essentially a statistical model and some consideration needs to be given to whether or not the model fits the data. Sophisticated model checks can be employed, but these are standard for models for binary data and will not be considered here: the interested reader should consult Collett (2003).

### 7.4.4 An Alternative Approach

An approach to adjusting for baseline variables, which does not use a logistic regression exists. It is somewhat less flexible, e.g., adjusting for continuous variables is not really possible. On the other hand, because the method does not require the use of a complex fitting algorithm for which a computer is essential, it is probably more transparent, and this can be advantageous when explaining the analysis to non-statisticians.

The method divides the data into strata and compares the treatments separately within each stratum and then combines the results from each stratum. As such it is an approach which fits well with stratified allocation, and will prove useful in Section 7.6 on randomization models. The ideas involved in a stratified analysis can be implemented in several ways, and the one discussed in the following text is associated with the names of Mantel and Haenszel. The method gives similar answers to the use of logistic regression. Underlying the combination of results across strata is the assumption that the difference between the treatments is the same for all strata. However, a similar assumption is made when adjustments are based on logistic regression — the model contains a term for a treatment effect and terms for the adjusting variables but no interactions between the two. The issue of differing treatment effects between different groups of patients is a delicate one that is discussed more fully in Chapter 9.

In order to understand the formulae associated with the Mantel–Haenszel (MH) procedure it is necessary to have a brief digression into slightly deeper properties of $2 \times 2$ tables, and this requires some knowledge of the hypergeometric distribution.

### 7.4.4.1 *The Hypergeometric Distribution*

Consider the key part of Table 7.1 reproduced as follows:

$$
\begin{array}{ccc}
r_T & n_T - r_T & n_T \\
r_P & n_P - r_P & n_P \\
r & n - r & n
\end{array}
$$

In the context of a clinical trial, the group sizes, $n_T$ and $n_P$, are (or should be) largely fixed before the trial starts. The total number of patients who clear, $r$, is not fixed in advance but depends on the parameters of the two binomial distributions, $\text{Bi}(n_T, \pi_T)$, $\text{Bi}(n_P, \pi_P)$. The likelihood of the data can be written as

$$\pi_P^{r_P}(1-\pi_P)^{n_P-r_P}\pi_T^{r_T}(1-\pi_T)^{n_T-r_T} = \left(\frac{\pi_P}{1-\pi_P}\right)^{r_P}\left(\frac{\pi_T}{1-\pi_T}\right)^{r_T}(1-\pi_P)^{n_P}(1-\pi_T)^{n_T}$$

The kernel of this likelihood, which is the part in which the data and parameters are inextricably linked, comprises the first two factors that involve the odds $\pi_P/(1-\pi_P)$ and $\pi_T/(1-\pi_T)$. This can be rewritten as $\phi^{r/2}\psi^{(r_P-r_T)/2}$, where $\phi$ is the product of the odds and $\psi$ is the odds ratio. The interest in the analysis is due to the discrepancy between the treatments and this is captured by $\psi$, with $\phi$ being a nuisance parameter. The expression from the likelihood also shows that $r$ is a sufficient statistic for $\phi$. Standard statistical theory indicates that we should make our inferences about $\psi$ from the distribution of the data conditional on the sufficient statistic for the nuisance parameter, because this maneuver eliminates $\phi$ from the distribution to be used for inferences about $\psi$. In other words, we base inferences on the table with not only the group sizes fixed but also $r$ is taken to be fixed.

The distribution of $(r_P, r_T)$ conditional on $r$ is, of course, essentially the same as the distribution of any one element of the $2 \times 2$ table, because with all the marginal totals fixed, knowledge of just one element within the body of the table fixes all the other values. We therefore focus on the distribution of $r_T$ conditional on $r$. This is $\Pr(R_T = a \mid R = r)$ and is the simplest form of the hypergeometric distribution; in writing this expression upper case letters are used to denote the random variables underlying the realizations written in the above table.

In computing this distribution, there are two issues that need to be addressed. The preceding expression denotes the conditional probability that the top-left cell in the $2 \times 2$ table has value $a$, and we need to think carefully what range of values are possible for $a$. The second issue is that we need to compute $\Pr(R = r)$ and, in general, this does not have a neat closed form. However, our use of the hypergeometric distribution will only extend to performing tests of the hypothesis that $\psi = 1$ and, under this hypothesis, $\Pr(R = r)$ is simply a binomial probability.

The constraints on the value of $a$ arise from the fact that none of the four values within the $2 \times 2$ table can be negative. A first attempt might set the range at $0 \le a \le \min\{r, n_T\}$. However, this range might be too extensive because $r_P = r - a \le n_P$, and this implies that $a \ge r - n_P$, so the range for $a$ is, in fact, $\max\{0, r - n_P\} \le a \le \min\{r, n_T\}$.

Now, $\Pr(R_T = a \mid R = r) = \Pr(R_T = a \text{ \& } R = r)/\Pr(R = r) = \Pr(R_T = a \text{ \& } R_P = r - a)/\Pr(R = r)$. This can be calculated under the assumption that $\psi = 1$ as

$$\frac{\binom{n_T}{a}\pi^a(1-\pi)^{n_T-a}\binom{n_P}{r-a}\pi^{r-a}(1-\pi)^{n_P-r+a}}{\binom{n}{r}\pi^r(1-\pi)^{n-r}} = \frac{\binom{n_T}{a}\binom{n_P}{r-a}}{\binom{n}{r}}$$

The use of this distribution is largely confined to its mean and variance, which can be calculated in the usual way. The mean is

$$\sum_a a\frac{\binom{n_T}{a}\binom{n_P}{r-a}}{\binom{n}{r}} = \sum_a n_T\frac{\binom{n_T-1}{a-1}\binom{n_P}{r-a}}{\binom{n}{r}} = \frac{n_T}{\binom{n}{r}}\sum_a \binom{n_T-1}{a-1}\binom{n_P}{r-a}$$

$$= \frac{n_T}{\binom{n}{r}}\binom{n-1}{r-1} = \frac{n_T r}{n}$$

where the first summation is over the range of a. The second expression comes from manipulating the binomial coefficient; if the range of summation includes $a = 0$ then this term is omitted as it does not affect the result. The third summation can be calculated by noting that it is the coefficient of $z^{r-1}$ in the expansion of $(1+z)^{n_T-1}(1+z)^{n_P} = (1+z)^{n-1}$. Observe that the answer is the expected value calculated in the *ad hoc* approach to the computation of the $\chi^2$ test outlined in Subsection 7.2.1. The variance can be found similarly and is $[n_T n_P r(n-r)]/[n^2(n-1)]$.

### 7.4.4.2 The Mantel–Haenszel Method

The concern underlying stratification in a clinical trial is that the outcome depends on the stratifying variable and this must not be imbalanced between the groups. In terms of the present example, this would mean that the probability of clearing will be different for patients with large and small plaques. However, the difference between the treatments in patients with large plaques may be the same as that for patients with small plaques.

The position is shown in Table 7.7, in which the data from the TL-01 vs. PUVA trial are shown broken down by plaque size. The proportion of patients with small plaques who clear is 84%, whereas for patients with large plaques the figure is 58%. The data in Table 7.7 are presented as two 2 × 2 tables, one for each type of patient. The difference between treatments can be described by first applying separately to each of the tables any of the measures discussed in Subsection 7.3.1 of this chapter. In this section, emphasis is placed on using the OR; an analogous method using ARD can be found

**TABLE 7.7**

Data from the Tl-01 vs. PUVA Trial, Shown Separately for Patients with Small and Large Plaques

| | Small Plaques | | | Large Plaques | | |
|---|---|---|---|---|---|---|
| | Cleared | Not Cleared | Total | Cleared | Not Cleared | Total |
| TL-01 | 23 | 6 | 29 | 9 | 13 | 22 |
| PUVA | 25 | 3 | 28 | 16 | 5 | 21 |
| Total | 48 | 9 | 57 | 25 | 18 | 43 |
| | OR = 2.17 | | | OR = 4.62 | | |

in Section 15.6 of Armitage, Berry, and Matthews (2002). The differences obtained in this way are then combined appropriately.

A test that the two treatments have the same effect can be constructed by considering in turn the $2 \times 2$ tables for patients with small and large plaques. If the subscript $k$ refers to the plaque size ($k = 1$ or 2 according to whether the plaques size is small or large, respectively) then $r_{Pk}$ denotes the number of patients with plaque of size $k$ who cleared when given PUVA. A similar modification to the notation will apply to the other symbols in Table 7.1, with $n$ remaining as the total number of patients and $n_k$ ($r_k$) being the total number (number clearing) with plaque size $k$. If the treatments do have the same effect then, taking the group sizes within each type of patient and the $r_k$ to be fixed then $r_{P1}$ and $r_{P2}$ have independent hypergeometric distributions. From the preceding calculations, the means and variances of these distributions are seen to be

$$e_{Pk} = \frac{r_k n_{Pk}}{n_k} \text{ and } v_{Pk} = \frac{n_{Pk} n_{Tk} r_k (n_k - r_k)}{n_k^2 (n_k - 1)}, k = 1, 2$$

Consequently, $(r_{P1} - e_{P1}) + (r_{P2} - e_{P2})$ has mean zero and variance $v_{P1} + v_{P2}$. Approximating this quantity by a normal distribution (the $r$ quantities are sums, so a central limit theorem argument gives a basis for this), the Mantel–Haenszel test refers

$$MH = \frac{\left[ (r_{P1} - e_{P1}) + (r_{P2} - e_{P2}) \right]^2}{v_{P1} + v_{P2}}$$

to a $\chi^2$ distribution on one degree of freedom.

For the data from the TL01 vs. PUVA, the following values are obtained

| | $r$ | $e$ | $v$ |
|---|---|---|---|
| Small plaques ($k = 1$) | 25 | 28×48/57 = 23.579 | 29×28×48×9/(57²×56) = 1.928 |
| Large plaques ($k = 2$) | 16 | 21×25/43 = 12.209 | 22×21×25×18/(43²×42) = 2.677 |

Consequently, the Mantel–Haenszel statistic is

$$MH = \frac{\left[(25 - 23.579) + (16 - 12.209)\right]^2}{1.928 + 2.677} = 5.899$$

which gives $P = 0.015$. The square root of $MH$ is 2.43, which is close to the $z$ value for the treatment effect adjusted for plaque size obtained using the logistic regression reported in Table 7.5.

The estimate of the OR separately for plaque size is

$$\frac{r_{Pk}(n_{Tk} - r_{Tk})}{r_{Tk}(n_{Pk} - r_{Pk})}, \quad k = 1, 2$$

The combined estimate of the OR proposed by Mantel and Haenszel (1959) is

$$\frac{\sum_k r_{Pk}(n_{Tk} - r_{Tk}) / n_k}{\sum_k r_{Tk}(n_{Pk} - r_{Pk}) / n_k}$$

For the TL-01 vs. PUVA trial this estimator has value

$$\frac{(25 \times 6) / 57 + (16 \times 13) / 43}{(23 \times 3) / 57 + (9 \times 5) / 43} = 3.309$$

A 95% confidence interval can be computed using the method given by Robins, Breslow, and Greenland (1986). The formula for this method is straightforward to compute if somewhat intricate to present: a description can be found in the cited paper or in Section 19.5 of Armitage, Berry, and Matthews (2002). Applying this method gives the interval estimate to be (1.234, 8.860). These values are close to the values found for the OR (3.385) and its 95% confidence interval (1.246, 9.197) found earlier using logistic regression.

Although the Mantel–Haenszel method may have some advantages in terms of the transparency of the method, the widespread availability of appropriate software makes logistic regression almost the universal choice for analysts. However, the Mantel–Haenszel has attractive features, both conceptual and practical, when a randomization model is used. This method will be described briefly in Section 7.6.

Two comments are pertinent here. First, the approach of measuring the difference between the treatments and then combining these is necessary. A simpler alternative which might be thought to be adequate would be to combine the data and then measure the treatment difference. Adding the two tables together (thereby recovering Table 7.2) and then computing the OR, or some other measure, will often give broadly similar results. However, if the variable distinguishing the tables is associated with the outcome, and the treatment groups are imbalanced with respect to this variable then combining the tables before analysis leaves the analysis open to Simpson's paradox.

A full description of this phenomenon is in Section 15.6 of Armitage, Berry, and Matthews (2002) but a brief illustration in general terms is in Figure 7.3. The outcome scale could be quite general, but for definiteness, it can be thought of as the proportion cured. The figure supposes that a trial compares treatments A and B and that patients are of one or two types. For each type of patient, treatment B gives a higher outcome than treatment A. The outcome for all the patients receiving a given treatment is a weighted combination of the outcome for each type of patient and therefore lies between the outcomes for each type taken individually. In the figure, the open circles, denoting the combined outcome, must lie between the closed circles. How close the outcome for the treatment group as whole is to the outcome of one or other type of patient depends on the make-up of the treatment group in terms of patient type. If the make-up of patient type is different between the treatment groups, then the position of the overall outcome for each can be located differently relative to the outcomes for each patient type for the treatments. In extreme cases, this can lead to the situation illustrated in Figure 7.3, in which the outcome for the combined treatment groups is actually lower for treatment B.

For stratified random allocations, this difference in make-up of the treatment groups should not occur. This is why analysis of Table 7.2 is valid, even if an analysis respecting the stratification is preferable. The approach parallels the use of the logistic regression. Analyzing the 2 × 2 tables for each plaque size and then combining the results is analogous to fitting the model with a term for plaque size and a term for treatment effect used in Subsection 7.4.3.

A second point is that the approach of combining estimates of treatment effect from patients of different types assumes that the true measure of difference between the treatments is the same in each such group. For example, the difference observed in OR for the patients with small and large plaques, 2.17 and 4.62, is taken to reflect sampling variation. Of course, the possibility exists that the treatment effect may actually be different for the two types of patient. Methods derived in a similar manner to the Mantel–Haenszel procedure are available to address this issue but are not considered here. The same issue arises when using a logistic model — the treatment effect is estimated without checking if a term for the interaction between the effect of treatment and the plaque size is significant. However, this is a more complicated issue than it may at first appear because of matters related to how models to be fitted or tests to be performed are chosen. This is essentially a matter of looking for subgroup effects — a subtle and surprisingly troublesome aspect of the analysis of clinical trials — which is mentioned in Chapter 9.

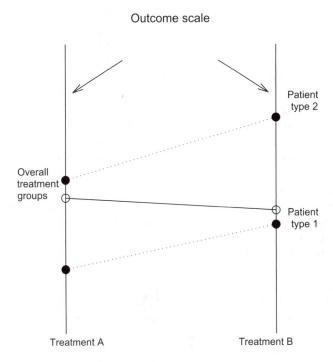

**FIGURE 7.3**
Simpson's paradox; the outcome (solid circles) is higher for treatment B than treatment A for patients in both group 1 and group 2; for the combined groups, the outcome (open circles) is higher for treatment A than B.

## 7.5 Survival Analysis

A common form of data that arise in clinical trials is survival data (or lifetime data). Data of this form are usually times until some event. Much of the motivation behind the development of this branch of statistics came from the rise in the number of trials in the treatment of cancer that occurred in the 1960s and 1970s. In these cases, the event concerned was often death or the metastatic spread, i.e., the spread of cancer to parts of the body remote from the site of the original tumor. Other examples of events might be a disease being cured or time to death from a specific cause. Occasionally, survival data may not involve time explicitly — it may refer to the number of visits a patient makes to the hospital before a cure is effected.

There are two aspects of survival data which mean that the methods considered so far in this book are inadequate for this kind of data. Although survival data are essentially continuous, they are often quite noticeably skewed, so methods based on the normal distribution are not generally encountered in this area of statistics.

The second aspect is that the survival times are not always fully observed. For some patients in a sample, the event in question will be observed and so too will the time to that event. However, for other patients the event will not be observed. Examples of why this might happen may be because the study closes before the event has occurred to some of the patients, or because the patient leaves the study. For such patients, the survival time cannot be observed. However, for these patients a time $t$, say, will be observed at which they were last seen free of the event in question. Although the survival time is unknown, we do know something about it — it must exceed $t$. These partially observed survival times are known as *censored* times.

An analysis that treated censored times as if they were fully observed would clearly be unsatisfactory and biased; it would report survival experiences that were systematically shorter than appropriate. An analysis that ignored censored times would also be inadequate, as it would waste information and potentially be biased. For example, if half of a sample of patients died quickly but the other half lived for a long period, then many studies would close before the latter group of patients died and the survival times on these patients is likely to be censored. Consequently, an analysis that ignored the survivors would inevitably underestimate the survival time of the underlying population. An important component of the analysis of survival data is to ensure that censored times are incorporated into the analysis appropriately.

Survival data analysis is a newer branch of statistics than the analysis of normally distributed or binary data. Moreover the demands of accommodating censored observations and the skewed shape of the usual survival distribution make this a more challenging branch of the subject. It is also one in which pitfalls abound and Altman (1991, Section 13.5) outlines some of these. In this section, only a very superficial presentation will be attempted; a good introduction to more thorough treatments can be found in Collett (2003). In this section, ways of describing the survival experience of samples of patients will be considered together with ways of assessing whether this differs between groups and how to adjust for baseline values.

### 7.5.1 The Hazard Function, the Survival Curve, and Some Estimators

In the analysis of normally or binomially distributed data, attention is naturally focused on the parameters of the distributions, as other aspects of these distributions, such as their shape, are well understood. In a survival analysis, it is common to find that more attention is paid to the shape of the whole distribution, perhaps because no one distribution has a role analogous to that which the normal distribution has in the analysis of continuous data. The most easily understood quantity is the survival function, $S(t)$, which is the probability that an individual survives more than time $t$.

The survival curve is the plot of $S(t)$ (vertical axis) against $t$ (horizontal axis). The definition has two general consequences: first, as an individual is

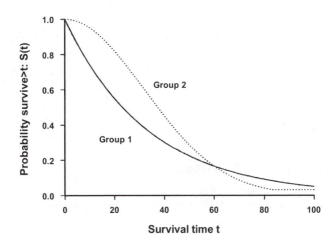

**FIGURE 7.4**
Example of two survival curves.

certain to survive more than zero time, $S(0) = 1$; second, as it is impossible for an individual to survive more than time $t_2$ without surviving all times $t_1 < t_2$, $S(t)$ cannot increase $t$ gets bigger. Figure 7.4 shows two examples of survival curves.

A second and somewhat less accessible quantity that is nonetheless important in survival analysis is the hazard function $h(t)$. This is the probability that an individual who has survived up to time $t$ fails just after time $t$ — a measure of the instantaneous failure probability at time $t$. If $T$ denotes the random variable for the survival time then the definitions of $S(t)$ and $h(t)$ are

$$S(t) = \Pr(T > t) \quad \text{and} \quad h(t) = \lim_{s \to 0+} \frac{\Pr(t < T < t+s \mid T > t)}{s}$$

The definition of conditional probability allows the second expression to be written as $h(t) = f(t)/S(t) = -S'(t)/S(t)$ where $f(.)$ is the probability density of $T$. Unlike the survival function, which must lie between 0 and 1, the hazard function can take any positive value. The log of the hazard function is thus useful in the modeling of survival data in a way that is analogous to the logit of the probability of success in logistic regression.

Estimates of these functions can be obtained in two ways. One way is to assume that the functions arise from some underlying distribution for $T$ which has a form known up to the value of some parameters — the parametric approach. The other approach is to try to make progress without making any assumptions about the distribution of $T$ — a nonparametric approach. The two approaches are available for continuous data, but the second method is not widely adopted in statistical circles, partly because methods based on the normal distribution have been found to be so widely applicable. The lack of any obvious counterpart to the normal distribution for survival data has meant that nonparametric (and as will be encountered later, semi-parametric) methods are widely used in survival analyses. Nevertheless, both methods have their virtues and some attention will be paid to both approaches.

In the descriptions that follow, the terminology usually adopted is that death is taken as the "event," but it should be kept in mind that this is merely a convenience that fits with the general survival terminology, and the event in question could have many other interpretations.

### 7.5.1.1    The Kaplan–Meier Estimator

The idea behind this nonparametric estimator is that $S(t)$ is calculated by first dividing the interval $[0,t]$ into many short, contiguous intervals, so

$$[0,t] = \bigcup_{k=0}^{K} [s_k, s_{k+1}]$$

where $s_k < s_{k+1}$ with $s_0 = 0$ and $s_{K+1} = t$. The probability of surviving beyond time $t$ is then calculated as the product of the probabilities of surviving each of the successive intervals $[s_k, s_{k+1}]$. As the Kaplan–Meier estimator is non-parametric, no distributional form is assumed and the probability of surviving $[s_k, s_{k+1}]$ is simply estimated as $1 - Q$, where $Q$ is the number who die in the interval divided by the number at risk of death in that interval. A consequence is that the estimate of $S(t)$ only changes at those values of $t$ at which a death occurs, so the plot of $S(t)$ against $t$ will be a series of horizontal lines, with steps down at the times at which deaths occur. To be more precise, suppose that deaths are observed at times $t_1 < t_2 < \ldots < t_n$ and that the number dying at time $t_j$ is $d_j$ out of a number at risk at that time of $n_j$. Then if $t$ is in the interval $[t_j, t_{j+1})$ then $S(t)$ is estimated by

$$\hat{S}(t) = \prod_{j=0}^{J} \frac{(n_j - d_j)}{n_j}$$

Note that the number at risk at $t_{j+1}$ will be the number at risk at $t_j$ less the number dying at $t_j$ less the number with survival times censored at values in the interval $[t_j, t_{j+1})$. In this way, the calculation incorporates information from individuals with censored survival times for as long as they were observed and only excludes them after this time.

### 7.5.1.2    Parametric Estimators

This approach assumes that the distribution of $T$ follows some particular form, specified up to unknown parameters, and then these are estimated from the data. A particularly simple distribution is the exponential distribution, with density $f(t) = \lambda \exp(-\lambda t)$, survival function $S(t) = \exp(-\lambda t)$ and mean survival time equal to $1/\lambda$. This distribution is not particularly flexible and often does not fit survival data well. A related, more useful distribution is the Weibull distribution that has an additional parameter, $\gamma$, known as the *shape parameter*. For this distribution, $S(t) = \exp(-\lambda t^\gamma)$, so the exponential distribution is the special case when $\gamma = 1$. For the Weibull and the exponential distributions, the unknown parameters are estimated by maximum likelihood. The important ideas are the same for both distributions, so although the Weibull distribution is of more use in practice, it is technically more awkward, and the exponential distribution will suffice for the following discussion.

Suppose that the sample comprises $n$ times $t_1$, $t_2$, ..., $t_n$ with $m$ of them fully observed and the remaining $n - m$ are censored. Let $\delta_1$, $\delta_2$, ..., $\delta_n$ be a series of indicators, with $\delta_i = 1$ if the $i$th observation is fully observed and $\delta_i = 0$ if it is censored. The likelihood would usually be computed as the product of the density functions evaluated at the values in the sample. However, for the censored times the densities would not be the correct probability to use because for cases with $\delta_i = 0$ we only know that the survival time exceeds $t_i$. For such observations, the survival function gives the correct contribution to the likelihood. Consequently, the required likelihood, $L$, can be written as

$$L = \prod_{i=1}^{n} f(t_i)^{\delta_i} S(t_i)^{1-\delta_i}$$

The log likelihood for an exponential distribution is therefore found as

$$\ell = \sum_{i=1}^{n} \delta_i (\log \lambda - \lambda t_i) - \sum_{i=1}^{n} (1 - \delta_i) \lambda t_i = m \log \lambda - \lambda \sum_{i=1}^{n} t_i = m \log \lambda - \lambda t_+ \text{, say.} (7.9)$$

Note that the sum of the $\delta_i$s is simply the number of fully observed times, $m$. The maximum likelihood estimator, $\hat{\lambda}$, is therefore $m/t_+$ and the expected information is $m/\lambda^2$. Consequently, the variance of $\hat{\lambda}$ is approximately $\lambda^2/m$, which can be estimated as $m/t_+^2$. Notice that the denominator in the expression of the variance of $\hat{\lambda}$ is not the sample size, $n$, but the number of fully observed times, $m$. Censored times need to be incorporated into the analysis to make full use of the data and to avoid bias, but if the aim is to learn about the distribution of survival times, there is a limit to what can be learnt from incompletely observed times. Thus, it is important that trials in which the outcome is a survival time should follow the patients for long enough that a sufficient number of events is observed.

The dependence of the standard error on $m$ rather than $n$ has important consequences for the calculation of sample sizes for trials in which the primary outcome requires a survival analysis. The power may first be expressed in terms of $m$, the number of fully observed times. An essentially separate calculation is then needed to determine the number of patients who need to be recruited and for how long they need to be followed in order that the analysis be based on a sufficient number of fully observed times. This important issue is not pursued here; interested readers can consult Chapter 9 of Machin et al. (1997).

The estimated survival curve for the analysis based on the exponential distribution is the plot of $t$ vs. $e^{-\hat{\lambda}t}$, which is the analogue of the Kaplan–Meier plot from the nonparametric analysis. A single number summary could be the estimated mean survival time, $\hat{\lambda}^{-1}$, or the estimated median survival time, $\hat{\lambda}^{-1}\log 2$. The analogue of the mean is not readily obtained from the Kaplan–Meier plot, but the median time can be readily found as the value on the time axis corresponding to $^1/_2$ on the vertical axis.

## Example 7.1: (Part I) Survival Analysis of the PUVA vs. TL-01 Trial

The trial comparing two treatments for psoriasis introduced previously (Gordon et al. 1999) as an example of a trial with a binary outcome admits a second analysis using methods from survival analysis. Each patient has to attend the phototherapy clinic on several occasions. The number of visits each patient had to make before their psoriasis cleared was recorded, and there is interest in which treatment required fewer visits. If a treatment requires fewer visits to achieve clearance, then this may be preferable as it may reduce toxicity and patient inconvenience, enhance compliance, and reduce waiting times for new patients. The data on the number of attendances are shown in Table 7.8. The number of visits until clearance was not observed for patients who did not clear, and the observations for these patients are considered to be censored for the purposes of analysis.

In the first analysis of these data the information on plaque size will not be used.

**TABLE 7.8**

Data on Number of Visits to Clearance in the PUVA vs. TL-01 Trial

| PUVA | Small Plaques | 2, 3*, 6*, 6, 7, 7, 8, 8, 9, 9, 9, 10, 10, 11, 11, 13, 13*, 15, 15, 16, 16, 16, 16, 17, 22, 27, 28, 30 |
|------|---------------|----|
|      | Large Plaques | 2*, 7, 9, 11, 12, 13, 14*, 16, 16, 16, 18, 19, 20, 21, 22, 25, 26*, 29, 32*, 32*, 34 |
| TL-01 | Small Plaques | 10, 11, 12, 13, 13, 14*, 15, 16, 16*, 16, 17, 17, 17, 19, 19*, 21, 21, 23, 24, 24, 24, 24*, 26, 29, 30, 32, 33*, 35*, 36 |
|      | Large Plaques | 7*, 11, 14, 17*, 19*, 21, 23*, 24*, 24*, 24, 24, 26, 26*, 27*, 31*, 31*, 31, 32*, 32*, 33, 34*, 36 |

*Note:* Asterisks denote censored observations.

**TABLE 7.9**

Calculations for the Kaplan–Meier Estimator
of the Survival Curve for the TL-01 Group

| $t_j$ | $n_j$ | $d_j$ | $(n_j - d_j)/n_j$ | $\hat{S}(t_j)$ |
|---|---|---|---|---|
| 0 | 51 | 0 | 1 | 1 |
| 10 | 50 | 1 | 0.980 | 0.980 |
| 11 | 49 | 2 | 0.959 | 0.940 |
| 12 | 47 | 1 | 0.979 | 0.920 |
| 13 | 46 | 2 | 0.957 | 0.880 |
| 14 | 44 | 1 | 0.977 | 0.860 |
| 15 | 42 | 1 | 0.976 | 0.840 |
| 16 | 41 | 2 | 0.951 | 0.799 |
| 17 | 38 | 3 | 0.921 | 0.736 |
| 19 | 34 | 1 | 0.971 | 0.714 |
| 21 | 31 | 3 | 0.903 | 0.645 |
| 23 | 28 | 1 | 0.964 | 0.622 |
| 24 | 26 | 5 | 0.808 | 0.502 |
| 26 | 18 | 2 | 0.889 | 0.446 |
| 29 | 14 | 1 | 0.929 | 0.415 |
| 30 | 13 | 1 | 0.923 | 0.383 |
| 31 | 12 | 1 | 0.917 | 0.351 |
| 32 | 9 | 1 | 0.889 | 0.312 |
| 33 | 6 | 1 | 0.833 | 0.260 |
| 36 | 2 | 2 | 0.000 | 0.000 |

Assuming an exponential distribution for the number of visits, the estimated parameter for the patients treated with PUVA is $\hat{\lambda}_p = 41/754 = 0.0544$ because, from Table 7.8, the sum of the number of visits is $2 + 3 + 6 + \ldots + 32 + 34 = 754$, and the number of patients on PUVA who cleared is 41. The corresponding quantities for TL-01 are 1154 and 32, giving $\hat{\lambda}_T = 0.0277$.

The Kaplan–Meier estimator cannot be shown so succinctly; the calculations for the the TL-01 group are set out in Table 7.9. The number at risk at time 0 is the sample size, namely 51. At the time of the first clearance, i.e., at 10 visits, the number at risk is only 50 because of the censored observation at 7 visits. The number at risk at each of the subsequent few times is the number at risk at the previous time less the number clearing at the previous time. However, this fails going from visit 14 to visit 15: the number at risk at visit 15 is 42, which is not $44 - 1$ because there is a censored observation at visit 14. The construction of the table proceeds in this way: the entries in the final column, i.e., the estimated survival probabilities, are found as the partial products of the previous column. The estimator for the PUVA group is found in the same way.

Figure 7.5 shows the Kaplan–Meier plots and the estimated survival curves assuming an exponential distribution.

Note that in Figure 7.5, there are occasional small vertical lines on the Kaplan–Meier estimates. These indicate the visit numbers at which censored values have been observed — there are fewer of these than censored obser-

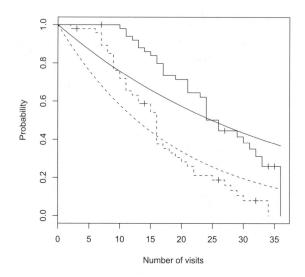

**FIGURE 7.5**
Kaplan–Meier plots and exponential survival curves for the PUVA (dashed lines) and TL-01 (solid lines) treatment groups. Probability of non-clearance plotted against the number of visits.

vations because they are not plotted when censored observations occur at a visit number at which a clearance also occurs.

## 7.5.2    Comparing Survival Curves

As with all clinical trials, comparison of the treatment groups is of paramount importance. Therefore, a means of testing a suitable null hypothesis and deriving appropriate confidence intervals is needed. The usual null hypothesis is that the survival curves under the different treatments are the same. A confidence interval is usually presented in terms of a suitable numerical summary, and the one that will be mentioned briefly in the following is the hazard ratio.

For a parametric analysis, the null hypothesis that the survival curves are the same reduces to assessing the equality of the parameters defining the distributions. Standard likelihood methods, such as the likelihood ratio test, can be used for this.

If no distributional form is assumed, then various tests are possible, perhaps the most widely used of which is the log-rank test. This is computed by forming a series of $2 \times 2$ tables and then combining information across these tables in a way which is essentially the same as for the Mantel–Haenszel method described in Subsection 7.4.4. The method constructs a $2 \times 2$ table at each time at which an event is observed in either group. Suppose events are observed at times $t_j$ and at this time $n_j$ patients are "at risk" of the event and $d_j$ events are observed. Suppose also that the groups are labeled

1 and 2 and in the following subscripts 1 and 2 refer to these groups, so the table at time $t_j$ is

| Group | Number "Surviving" | Number "Failing" | Number "at Risk" |
|-------|--------------------|-----------------| -----------------|
| 1 | $n_{1j} - d_{1j}$ | $d_{1j}$ | $n_{1j}$ |
| 2 | $n_{2j} - d_{2j}$ | $d_{2j}$ | $n_{2j}$ |
| Total | $n_j - d_j$ | $d_j$ | $n_j$ |

If the null hypothesis is true, i.e., if the survival curves are the same, then the number of failures would be expected to be distributed *pro rata* between the groups, with the expected number in group $k$ being $e_{kj} = n_{kj} \times (d_j/n_j)$. Of course, $e_{1j} + e_{2j} = d_{1j} + d_{2j}$. From the discussion of the Mantel–Haenszel test in Subsection 7.4.4, it follows that if the margins of this table are taken to be fixed, then $d_{1j}$ has a hypergeometric distribution with mean $e_{1j}$ and variance $v_j$, where

$$v_j = \frac{n_{1j} n_{2j} d_j (n_j - d_j)}{n_j^2 (n_j - 1)}$$

As the numbers failing at successive times are independent, under the null hypothesis, $U = \Sigma_j (d_{1j} - e_{1j})$ will have asymptotically a normal distribution with mean 0 and variance $V = \Sigma_j v_j$. The log-rank test is obtained by referring $U^2/V$ to a $\chi^2$ distribution on one degree of freedom.

In fact, several variants of the log-rank test are available. A commonly used version notes that under the null hypothesis, the expected number of events in group $k$ is $E_k = \Sigma_j e_{kj}$ and the observed number is $O_k = \Sigma_j d_{kj}$. The standard formula for $\chi^2$ is applied and the alternative test statistic is

$$\frac{\left(O_1 - E_1\right)^2}{E_1} + \frac{\left(O_2 - E_2\right)^2}{E_2} \tag{7.10}$$

It can be shown (see question 7 in this chapter) that this is always less than $U^2/V$ so always provides a slightly conservative test (i.e., larger $P$-value).

In terms of estimating a difference between the groups, a quantity that is widely used is the hazard ratio, which is

$$h = \frac{O_1/E_1}{O_2/E_2}$$

As with the odds ratio, a confidence interval for $h$ first requires that a confidence interval for $\log(h)$ be found. Again, as with the odds ratio, the base of the logarithms must be $e$. The formula for the variance of $\log(h)$ is

$$\mathrm{var}(h) = \sqrt{\frac{1}{E_1} + \frac{1}{E_2}}$$

There are alternative formulae and which is preferable and when is discussed in Section 17.6 of Armitage, Berry, and Matthews (2002).

## Example 7.1: (Part II) Comparing Survival Curves in the PUVA vs. TL-01 Trial

If an exponential distribution is assumed for the time to clearance and if $\ell_P(\hat{\lambda}_P)$ denotes the maximized log likelihood for the group given PUVA, with $\ell_T(\hat{\lambda}_T)$ being the corresponding quantity in the TL-01 group, then the log likelihood for the two groups is simply the sum of these, because the groups are independent. Substituting the expression for the maximum likelihood estimator into Equation 7.9 gives the following expression for the maximized log likelihood,

$$m_P \log(m_P / t_{+P}) - m_P + m_T \log(m_T / t_{+T}) - m_T$$

where $m$ is the number of fully observed times and $t_+$ is the sum of all times and, as usual, subscripts $P$ and $T$ refer to the PUVA and TL-01 groups, respectively. The null hypothesis is that $\lambda_P = \lambda_T$ and, under this hypothesis, the maximized log likelihood is

$$m \log(m / t_+) - m$$

where the quantities have the same meanings as before and the absence of subscripts indicates that they refer to the combined groups. Therefore, the likelihood ratio test of the equality of the distribution to clearance in the two groups is found by referring

$$2\{m_P \log(m_P / t_{+P}) + m_T \log(m_T / t_{+T}) - m \log(m / t_+)\}$$

to a $\chi^2$ distribution on one degree of freedom. The confidence interval for the difference between $\lambda_P$ and $\lambda_T$ can be found by computing the asymptotic variances of the estimate of each parameter, namely $\lambda_P^2 / m_P$ and $\lambda_T^2 / m_T$. Therefore, a 95% confidence interval can be estimated as

$$\frac{m_P}{t_{+P}} - \frac{m_T}{t_{+T}} \pm 1.96 \sqrt{\frac{m_P}{t_{+P}^2} + \frac{m_T}{t_{+T}^2}}$$

For the PUVA vs. TL-01 trial, the pertinent values for PUVA are $m_P = 41$ and $t_{+P} = 754$, and for TL-01 $m_T = 32$ and $t_{+T} = 1154$; so $m = 73$ and $t_+ = 1908$. This gives a likelihood ratio test statistic of 8.22 and thus $P = 0.004$. The estimated difference in the parameters is 0.0266 and the associated 95% confidence interval is (0.0074, 0.0459). In fact, the parameters are hazard rates and a more usual way to estimate their difference is through the hazard ratio (see question 6 in this chapter).

The calculations for the log-rank test are rather less succinct. Rather than write down the $2 \times 2$ table at each appropriate time, the key quantities should be tabulated. These are $n_{Pj}$ and $d_{Pj}$, and the corresponding values for the TL-01 group, and the other quantities required can easily be calculated from these. These values, together with some other useful quantities are shown in Table 7.10.

The observed and expected numbers of events in the PUVA group are, respectively, 41 and 24.242. Note that in this group, more events have been observed than would have been expected under the null hypothesis, as in this example, an event is a good outcome (clearance of psoriasis), in keeping with the emerging picture that PUVA is the superior treatment. This is in distinction to many survival analyses in which the outcome is bad (death or relapse). The corresponding values for TL-01 are 32 and 48.758. The value of $V$ is not shown in the table but is 14.797. So the log-rank statistic can be calculated as $(41 - 24.242)^2 / 14.797 = 18.98$, $P < 0.001$. The alternative expression for the log-rank statistics gives

$$\frac{(41\text{-}24.242)^2}{24.242} + \frac{(32\text{-}48.758)^2}{48.758} = 17.34$$

which also yields $P < 0.001$

The value of $O_P / E_P$ is $41/24.242 = 1.691$ and for $O_T / E_T$ it is $32/48.758 = 0.656$, so the hazard ratio $h$ is $1.691/0.656 = 2.578$. The log of $h$ is 0.947 and the standard error of this quantity is the square root of $24.242^{-1} + 48.758^{-1}$, which is 0.2485. The 95% confidence interval for $\log(h)$ is (0.4595, 1.4337), so the confidence interval for $h$ is (1.583, 4.194).

Therefore, there is clear evidence that a patient will clear after fewer visits on PUVA than on TL-01. The chance of clearing on PUVA is over twice as large as on TL-01 as measured by the hazard ratio with a lower limit to the confidence interval of about 1.5.

### 7.5.3 Adjusting Survival Analyses for Baseline Values

As in clinical trials with continuous and binary outcomes, it is often the case that the analyst would wish to adjust analyses of survival outcomes for baseline observations. This is possible and can be done in an analogous way, i.e., by fitting a model that involves not only a term indicating the treatment

**TABLE 7.10**

Calculations for the Log-Rank Test Comparing the Survival Curves of the PUVA and TL-01 Groups

| | PUVA | | | TL-01 | | | | |
|---|---|---|---|---|---|---|---|---|
| $t_j$ | $n_{Pj}$ | $d_{Pj}$ | $e_{Pj}$ | $n_{Tj}$ | $d_{Tj}$ | $e_{Tj}$ | $n_j = n_P + n_{Tj}$ | $d_j = d_{Tj} + d_{Tj}$ |
| 2 | 49 | 1 | 0.49 | 51 | 0 | 0.51 | 100 | 1 |
| 6 | 46 | 1 | 0.474 | 51 | 0 | 0.526 | 97 | 1 |
| 7 | 44 | 3 | 1.389 | 51 | 0 | 1.611 | 95 | 3 |
| 8 | 41 | 2 | 0.901 | 50 | 0 | 1.099 | 91 | 2 |
| 9 | 39 | 4 | 1.753 | 50 | 0 | 2.247 | 89 | 4 |
| 10 | 35 | 2 | 1.235 | 50 | 1 | 1.765 | 85 | 3 |
| 11 | 33 | 3 | 2.012 | 49 | 2 | 2.988 | 82 | 5 |
| 12 | 30 | 1 | 0.779 | 47 | 1 | 1.221 | 77 | 2 |
| 13 | 29 | 2 | 1.547 | 46 | 2 | 2.453 | 75 | 4 |
| 14 | 26 | 0 | 0.371 | 44 | 1 | 0.629 | 70 | 1 |
| 15 | 25 | 2 | 1.119 | 42 | 1 | 1.881 | 67 | 3 |
| 16 | 23 | 7 | 3.234 | 41 | 2 | 5.766 | 64 | 9 |
| 17 | 16 | 1 | 1.185 | 38 | 3 | 2.815 | 54 | 4 |
| 18 | 15 | 1 | 0.306 | 34 | 0 | 0.694 | 49 | 1 |
| 19 | 14 | 1 | 0.583 | 34 | 1 | 1.417 | 48 | 2 |
| 20 | 13 | 1 | 0.295 | 31 | 0 | 0.705 | 44 | 1 |
| 21 | 12 | 1 | 1.116 | 31 | 3 | 2.884 | 43 | 4 |
| 22 | 11 | 2 | 0.564 | 28 | 0 | 1.436 | 39 | 2 |
| 23 | 9 | 0 | 0.243 | 28 | 1 | 0.757 | 37 | 1 |
| 24 | 9 | 0 | 1.286 | 26 | 5 | 3.714 | 35 | 5 |
| 25 | 9 | 1 | 0.333 | 18 | 0 | 0.667 | 27 | 1 |
| 26 | 8 | 0 | 0.615 | 18 | 2 | 1.385 | 26 | 2 |
| 27 | 7 | 1 | 0.318 | 15 | 0 | 0.682 | 22 | 1 |
| 28 | 6 | 1 | 0.3 | 14 | 0 | 0.7 | 20 | 1 |
| 29 | 5 | 1 | 0.526 | 14 | 1 | 1.474 | 19 | 2 |
| 30 | 4 | 1 | 0.471 | 13 | 1 | 1.529 | 17 | 2 |
| 31 | 3 | 0 | 0.2 | 12 | 1 | 0.8 | 15 | 1 |
| 32 | 3 | 0 | 0.25 | 9 | 1 | 0.75 | 12 | 1 |
| 33 | 1 | 0 | 0.143 | 6 | 1 | 0.857 | 7 | 1 |
| 34 | 1 | 1 | 0.2 | 4 | 0 | 0.8 | 5 | 1 |
| 36 | 0 | 0 | 0 | 2 | 2 | 2 | 2 | 2 |
| Sum | | 41 | 24.242 | | 32 | 48.758 | | |

allocated but also the values of baseline observations, such as stratification variables. These are quite advanced statistical techniques, and this section will be a very superficial introduction to this area of statistics — those interested in a more thorough treatment should perhaps start with Collett's (2003) book.

The idea is to model the hazard, and this is done on the log scale. This is in part for reasons similar to those that applied to the use of the logit function in the adjustment of binary outcomes, and also because it leads naturally to an adjusted estimate of the hazard ratio. If the hazard for patient $i$ at time $t$ is written as $h_i(t \mid x_i)$ to emphasize its dependence on a vector of covariates $x_i$, then most models assume that

$$\log h_i(t \mid x_i) = \log h(t) + \sum_j \beta_j x_{ij} , \qquad (7.11)$$

where the $\beta_j$ are parameters to be estimated and $x_{i1}, x_{i2}, \ldots, x_{iq}$ are baseline observations. The function $h(t)$ is a baseline hazard function.

These models are known as *proportional hazards* models because the hazard functions for the different patients are all proportional. If you consider $h_r(t \mid x_r)/h_s(t \mid x_s)$ for patients $r$ and $s$ then the preceding model implies that this ratio does not depend on $t$. Consequently, patients may have different hazards, perhaps because they are older or had more advanced disease when they presented, but the extent of this difference is unchanged over time. When using this kind of model this is an aspect that needs to be checked.

So, for example, if $\sum_j \beta_j x_{ij} = \beta_0 x_{i0} + \beta_1 x_{i1}$ with $x_{i0} = 1$ for all patients and $x_{i1} = 1$ or 0, according to whether treatment A or B was allocated, then the difference in the log hazard for a patient on treatment A from a patient on treatment B is simply $\beta_1$; thus the hazard ratio between patients receiving treatment A relative to treatment B is $\exp(\beta_1)$. If, instead, a more complicated model with, e.g., $\sum_j \beta_j x_{i0} = \beta_0 x_{i0} + \beta_1 x_{i1} + \beta_2 x_{i2}$ with $x_{i2}$ being the age of the patient was used, then $\exp(\beta_1)$ would still be the hazard ratio between the treatments but now adjusted for age.

As with the analyses discussed in the previous subsections, an approach making a distributional assumption for the survival time can be adopted or avoided. In this context, the difference largely hinges on the extent to which the baseline hazard, $h(t)$, is specified. If the distribution of survival time is assumed to come from a family of distributions, then $h(t)$ can be derived. If the density of the survival time is $\lambda e^{-\lambda t}$ then $h(t) = \lambda$, i.e., a constant, and the model is simply a linear model for this constant hazard.

A more subtle approach, introduced by Cox (1972), is to avoid specifying the form of $h(t)$ altogether. This approach relies on a method known as *partial likelihood* to derive estimates of the $\beta$s and associated variances without specifying the distribution of the survival times any more fully than is implied by Equation 7.11. These are complicated semiparametric models and checking them requires experience. Moreover, interpreting and explaining these models to clinicians can be difficult. Nevertheless, the methodology is powerful and widely used. It is also a natural extension of the methods discussed thus far. If the Cox proportional hazards model is fitted with a term for the treatment effect and there are no adjusting variables, then the test that the coefficient of the treatment term is zero is the log-rank test introduced in the previous subsection.

In the same way that the Mantel–Haenszel procedure is an alternative to the logistic regression for adjusting binary outcomes — there are alternative ways to adjust survival analyses for baseline observations, although these are more relevant to categorical variables. The main such test is the stratified log-rank test. If the data are divided into $K$ strata, then the quantity $U$ and its variance $V$ defined in the previous subsection can be computed separately in each stratum, giving $K$ pairs of values $(U_1, V_1)$, ..., $(U_K, V_K)$, and then the test statistic is computed as

$$
L_{\text{strat}} = \frac{\left( \displaystyle\sum_{k=1}^{K} U_k \right)^2}{\displaystyle\sum_{k=1}^{K} V_k}
$$

This still has a $\chi^2$ distribution on one degree of freedom if the null hypothesis is true. In this case, the hypothesis allows the survival curves to differ between strata — it is simply that there must be no difference between treatments within each stratum.

There is a stratified counterpart to the simplified version of the log-rank statistic given in Equation 7.10. Suppose that expected and observed numbers of events on treatment 1 in stratum $k$ are written as $E_{1k}$ and $O_{1k}$, respectively, with $E_{2k}$ and $O_{2k}$ being the corresponding quantities for treatment 2. The simplified version is then

$$
\frac{\left( \displaystyle\sum_{k=1}^{K} O_{1k} - \sum_{k=1}^{K} E_{1k} \right)^2}{\displaystyle\sum_{k=1}^{K} E_{1k}} + \frac{\left( \displaystyle\sum_{k=1}^{K} O_{2k} - \sum_{k=1}^{K} E_{2k} \right)^2}{\displaystyle\sum_{k=1}^{K} E_{2k}}
$$

which also has a $\chi^2$ distribution on one degree of freedom if the null hypothesis is true.

## Example 7.1: (Part III) Survival Analysis in the PUVA vs. TL-01 Trial after Adjusting for Plaque Size

The following shows an analysis in R of the number of visits in the trial using a model that includes a term for the treatment effect and a term for the plaque size. The model used is the Cox proportional hazards model. The main item of interest is the hazard ratio adjusted for plaque size, the confidence interval, and the $P$-value. These are found on the second line marked treatment, showing that the hazard ratio adjusted for plaque size is 3.16, with confidence interval (1.95, 5.14). The $P$-value is given on the first line marked treatment as 0.0000034. The term for plaque size is also significant but is of no direct interest.

```
coxph(formula = Surv(visits, clear) ~ 1 + Treatment +
plaque, data = Survdat)
```

```
    n = 100
```

|            | coef  | exp(coef) | se(coef) | z     | p       |
|------------|-------|-----------|----------|-------|---------|
| Treatment  | 1.151 | 3.163     | 0.248    | 4.65  | 3.4e-06 |
| Plaque     | 0.975 | 0.377     | 0.253    | -3.86 | 1.1e04  |

|            | exp(coef) | exp(-coef) | lower.95 | upper.95 |
|------------|-----------|------------|----------|----------|
| Treatment  | 3.163     | 0.316      | 1.95     | 5.141    |
| Plaque     | 0.377     | 2.652      | 0.23     | 0.619    |

```
Rsquare = 0.285 (max possible = 0.996)
Likelihood ratio test   = 33.5 on 2 df,   p = 5.24e-08
Wald test               = 32.2 on 2 df,   p = 1.03e-07
Score (logrank) test    = 34.3 on 2 df,   p = 3.49e-08
```

The stratified log-rank test can be summarized by showing the observed and expected numbers of events within each stratum, and these are calculated using the method described in the previous subsection.

| Plaque Size | Treatment | Observed Events | Expected Events |
|-------------|-----------|-----------------|-----------------|
| Small       | TL-01     | 23              | 33.92           |
| Small       | PUVA      | 25              | 14.08           |
| Large       | TL-01     | 9               | 16.07           |
| Large       | PUVA      | 16              | 8.93            |

Applying the simplified version of the stratified log-rank statistic amounts to summing across the plaque size categories and then applying the simplified formula in Equation 7.10 to the aggregated table.

| Summed Over Plaque Size | Observed Events | Expected Events |
|-------------------------|-----------------|-----------------|
| TL-01                   | 32              | 49.99           |
| PUVA                    | 41              | 23.01           |

The simplified statistic is then

$$\frac{\left(32 - 49.99\right)^2}{49.99} + \frac{\left(41 - 23.01\right)^2}{23.01} = 20.54$$

The full version of the stratified log-rank statistic for these data is 22.84. It should be noted that the variances needed to compute this value cannot be calculated from the summary of the data given here.

Both statistics give $P < 0.0001$ and are in line with the findings of the preceding Cox regression. The square of the $z$ statistic for treatment given in the Cox regression, i.e., $4.65^2 \approx 21.62$ is close to the log-rank statistics presented earlier.

## 7.6   Analyses Using Randomization Models

Although ways of analyzing randomized clinical trials have been described in this and the previous chapter, the randomization has had no direct impact on the way the analyses have been performed. When two groups are to be compared with respect to a continuous outcome, then a $t$-test is often used, and this can be done whether or not the groups have been formed by randomization. Of course, the randomization entitles us to infer that any differences found can be ascribed to the effect of the treatment, and the randomization will generally result in balanced groups, but these are not requirements of the $t$-test. It is usually necessary to make some assumptions to ensure the validity of the tests used, and the analyst will have to check these in the course of the analysis. These assumptions are made about the population from which the data are supposed to have come and, in this sense, the application of these models to trial data does not differ from their application to suitable data obtained without the use of randomization. This approach to analyzing clinical trials could therefore be called a *population model* approach.

There is another approach that does not assume a model for the outcome variable and instead relies for its validity on the act of randomization used to produce the groups. It is widely applicable and powerful, though it is perhaps better suited to performing tests of hypotheses than producing point or interval estimates. The need to allow for the stratification of the treatment allocation in the analysis arises very naturally with this approach. Some of the key ideas and some simple applications will be discussed briefly in this section: further development can be found in the excellent text by Rosenberger and Lachin (2002). This approach could be referred to as the *randomization model* approach.

### 7.6.1   Randomization Models: Simple Randomization

The basis of this approach is to assume that the data observed in the trial are the data that would have been observed on these patients regardless of any treatment allocation. This is essentially the null hypothesis of no treat-

**TABLE 7.11**

Data from Hommel et al. Rewritten for a Randomization Analysis

| | | | Treatment Allocations | | |
|---|---|---|---|---|---|
| Patient | Baseline | Outcome | Actual Allocation | Alternative Allocation I | Alternative Allocation II |
| 1 | 147 | 137 | C | P | P |
| 2 | 129 | 120 | C | P | C |
| 3 | 158 | 141 | C | C | C |
| 4 | 164 | 137 | C | C | C |
| 5 | 134 | 140 | C | C | P |
| 6 | 155 | 144 | C | C | C |
| 7 | 151 | 134 | C | P | C |
| 8 | 141 | 123 | C | C | P |
| 9 | 153 | 142 | C | P | P |
| 10 | 133 | 139 | P | C | P |
| 11 | 129 | 134 | P | P | C |
| 12 | 152 | 136 | P | P | P |
| 13 | 161 | 151 | P | C | C |
| 14 | 154 | 147 | P | C | P |
| 15 | 141 | 137 | P | C | C |
| 16 | 156 | 149 | P | P | P |
| $|t \text{ statistic}|$ | | | 1.65 | 0.93 | 0.44 |

*Note:* The patients are numbered in a single sequence not within treatment groups as in Table 6.1.

*Source:* Hommel, E. et al. (1986), Effect of Captopril on kidney function in insulin-dependent diabetic patients with nephropathy, *British Medical Journal*, 293, 467–470.

ment difference, but it also embodies the notion that the data are fixed. This is in distinction to the population model approach, in which the data are realizations of random variables described in the specified model and refers to conditions on the parameters of the model. With the randomization model, the only random component is the treatment allocation, and it is this which is used to drive the inferences.

The data in Table 7.11 are the data presented in Chapter 6 on the Captopril trial run by Hommel et al. (1986) but written in a form more suitable for the current discussion. The difference between the treatment groups was assessed by computing a *t* statistic and this is shown again in Table 7.11 at the foot of the column headed "Actual Allocation." The analysis in Chapter 6 assumed a population model, namely, that the data are from a normal distribution with common variance for the two groups; on the basis of this a *P*-value of 0.12 was obtained.

In the randomization analysis, the outcomes are taken as fixed and it is the treatment allocation labels that provide the randomness. The difference between the groups is measured by some statistic $D = D(a_k)$, where $a_k$ is an allocation of treatments to patients. In the following we will take $D$ to be the usual *t*-statistic but, in principle, any suitable measure could be used. Suppose that the possible allocations that could be made are the set $S = \{a_1, a_2,$

..., $a_K$}, then the allocation procedure generates a probability distribution over this set, and if $A$ denotes a random variable with this distribution then we can write this as

$$\Pr(A = a_k) = p_k, \, k = 1, \, ..., \, K$$

The allocation actually made can be written as $a_{obs} \in S$, and $D_{obs} = D(a_{obs})$ is the observed value of the statistic measuring the difference between the samples. Under the null hypothesis that the allocation has no effect on the observed outcomes, the $P$-value ascribed to the test is the probability that $D$ is as or more extreme than $D_{obs}$. This can be written as

$$P = \sum_{k=1}^{K} I(D(a_k) \geq D_{obs}) \Pr(A = a_k) \tag{7.12}$$

where $I(E)$ is the indicator function of the event $E$. This is simply a way of writing the sum of the probabilities of allocations that lead to measures $D$ as least as extreme as the observed measure.

Evaluating $P$ requires several things to be specified. In principle, we need to know the probability distribution induced on $S$ by the allocation procedure, i.e., the $\Pr(A = a_k)$. We also need to choose the measure $D$, and the set $S$ also requires some thought.

If the trial was run using simple randomization, then all the allocations that could arise might be thought to be the relevant set $S$. For the Captopril vs. placebo trial, $S$ would comprise all possible sequences of length 16, {$T_1, \, ..., \, T_{16}$}, where each $T_i$ was equally likely to be C (Captopril) or P (placebo). There are $2^{16} = 65,536$ such sequences and each one is equally likely, so for this allocation, Equation 7.12 is simply the proportion of these allocations that give rise to differences between the treatment groups, which exceed the observed value.

Next to the actual allocation in Table 7.11 are two columns with alternative allocations and the corresponding value of the modulus of the $t$-statistic. To implement the preceding randomization test for this trial, we would have to generate in turn all $2^{16}$ possible allocations and compute $|t|$ for each. The $P$-value would then be the proportion of these allocations that gave values of $|t| \geq 1.65$.

There are two aspects of this approach that deserve comment, one practical and one statistical. The practical problem is that systematically generating all 65,536 possible allocations, though not onerous for modern computers, is not something that is easily done in most general statistical packages. Specialist routines are available (e.g., Chase, 1970) but are not widely used. One reason is that evaluating every term in Equation 7.12 requires 65,536 terms to be evaluated, and this is from a very small trial. A trial of 500 patients would give rise to $2^{500} \approx 3.3 \times 10^{150}$ possible allocations, and evaluating all these would be impossibly onerous, even for modern computers. Fortunately, it would also be unnecessarily onerous as alternative approximations to the sum in Equation 7.12 are possible. A further problem is that complete evaluation requires the analyst to handle the two extreme allocations in which all patients are allocated to the same treatment, in which case $D$ cannot be evaluated.

This leads on to the statistical issue. Under simple randomization over the set $S$ just described, the number of patients allocated to Captopril, $N_C$, say, is a random variable. As $N_C$ is a statistic that contains no information about the difference between the treatments, it is an ancillary statistic, and the principle of ancillarity alluded to in Subsection 6.4.5 suggests that inferences would be improved if the analysis conditioned on the observed value, $n_C$, of $N_C$. This amounts to redefining the set $S$ as the set of all possible ways in which 9 of the 16 patients can be given Captopril and 7 can be given placebo. The sum in Equation 7.12 is now over just these allocations and there are $K$

$$= \binom{16}{9} = 11{,}440 \text{ possibilities, each with equal probability. In Table 7.11 the}$$

column headed "Alternative Allocation I" gives an example of an allocation that would be in both versions of $S$. The allocation in the column headed "Alternative Allocation II" is an example that would be in the first definition of $S$ but not the second, because it allocates 8 patients to each of Captopril and placebo. This approach leads to an analysis with better theoretical credentials and also neatly avoids the problem of extreme allocations in which only one treatment is allocated.

Even with such a small trial and with the reduced set $S$, the sum in Equation 7.12 still has 11,440 terms. The corresponding sum for a trial of 200 patients, with 100 allocated to each treatment, would require over $9 \times 10^{58}$ terms. Fortunately, complete enumeration of this sum is not necessary because adequate approximations are available. Looking again at the sum in Equation 7.12, it can be seen that $P$ is simply the expected value of $I(D(A) \geq D_{obs})$ over the distribution of $A$ induced by the allocation procedure. It can, therefore, be approximated by randomly sampling from this distribution, evaluating $I(D(A) \geq D_{obs})$ for each allocation chosen, and then computing the mean of these values, that is

$$\hat{P}_J = \frac{\sum_{j=1}^{J} I(D(a_j) \geq D_{obs})}{J}$$

This is a randomization test of the null hypothesis. We simply generate $J$ random allocations from the set $S$ and estimate $P$ by the proportion of these random allocations that lead to a value of $D$ exceeding $D_{obs}$.

This has been done for this example taking $S$ to be the set with 9 allocations to Captopril and 7 to placebo; the histogram of the $J = 2000$ values is shown

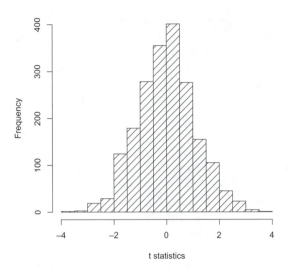

**FIGURE 7.6**
Histogram of 2000 t-statistics, each formed by comparing the treatment groups for a random allocation of 9 patients to Captopril and 7 patients to placebo.

in Figure 7.6. The modulus of the *t*-statistic obtained from the data actually observed is 1.65 and, of the 2000 randomly chosen allocations, 277 gave a *t*-statistic with modulus $\geq 1.65$. Therefore, a two-sided *P*-value can be calculated as $277/2000 = 0.1385$. This is similar to the value of $P = 0.12$ reported in Section 6.2, but this new value depends for its validity only on the act of randomization and not on any assumption of normality.

The value of $J$ was chosen rather arbitrarily. A heuristic basis for choosing $J$ is to approximate how accurately $\hat{P}_J$ estimates $P$ in Equation 7.12 by noting that the variance of $\hat{P}_J$ will be approximately $P(1-P)/J$, and this must be less than or equal to $1/(4J)$. Therefore, with $J = 2000$, the standard error of $\hat{P}_J$ will not exceed $1/\sqrt{(8000)} \approx 0.011$; so the estimate should be within about 0.02 of the value of $P$. The approximations are because this calculation is based on binomial sampling of an infinite population, but it should be reasonably good provided $J$ is not close to $K$, the size of the set $S$.

## 7.6.2  Randomization Models: Stratified Randomization

The principle of ancillarity was used to restrict the set $S$ to those allocations that have the same number of patients on each treatment as in the observed allocation. This is reasonable if simple randomization is used, but what if some form of restricted randomization was used? In this case, the set $S$ should be the set of allocations that could have arisen under the particular restricted scheme that was used in the trial.

Consider as an example the binary outcome that the patient cleared in the period of treatment in the PUVA vs. TL-01 trial. The preceding randomization analysis can also be applied here. The null hypothesis is that the outcomes,

**TABLE 7.12**

Structure of Data from the Tl-01 vs. PUVA Trial, Shown Separately for
Patients with Small and Large Plaques

| | Small Plaques | | | Large Plaques | | |
|---|---|---|---|---|---|---|
| | Cleared | Not Cleared | Total | Cleared | Not Cleared | Total |
| TL-01 | $48 - x$ | $x - 19$ | 29 | $25 - y$ | $y - 3$ | 22 |
| PUVA | $x$ | $28 - x$ | 28 | $y$ | $21 - y$ | 21 |
| Total | 48 | 9 | 57 | 25 | 18 | 43 |

*Note:* Observed values of $x$ and $y$ are 25 and 16, respectively.

cleared or not cleared, are taken as fixed and that they are unaffected by which
treatment label is allocated to the patient. In the trial, 51 patients are allocated
to TL-01 and 49 to PUVA. When the set $S$ is being constructed, it is necessary
to ensure that only allocations with 51 patients on TL-01 and 49 on PUVA are
used. However, it also has to be taken into account that the allocation was
stratified by the patient's plaque size, and the principle of ancillarity applies
within each stratum. Once this is taken into account, the only allocations that
can be permitted in $S$ are those that keep the numbers fixed on each treatment
within each stratum. Also, the total number of patients who clear within each
stratum will be fixed under the null hypothesis. This is because under the
null hypothesis, the outcomes are fixed, and it is only the allocation of treatments that is random. Consequently, the possible tables are shown in Table
7.12, where $x$ and $y$ are integers in the ranges $19 \leq x \leq 28$ and $3 \leq y \leq 21$, respectively. Therefore, $S$ can be generated as the set of allocations which 28 PUVA
and 29 TL-01 labels to the 57 patients with small plaques and 21 PUVA and
22 TL-01 labels to the 43 patients with large plaques.

One candidate for the role of $D(a_i)$ in Equation 7.12 is the Mantel–Haenszel
statistic, namely

$$MH = \frac{\left[ (r_{P1} + r_{P2}) - (e_{P1} + e_{P2}) \right]^2}{v_{P1} + v_{P2}}$$

This is calculated for each of the allocations in $S$ or for each of the randomly
sampled allocations if a randomization test is used. The $P$-value is the proportion of these statistics that exceed the value for the observed statistic. In
calculating this proportion, some simplifications are possible. Fixing the sizes
of the treatment groups and the number of patients clearing within each
stratum means that $v_{Pk}$ and $e_{Pk}$, $k = 1, 2$, are the same for each allocation in
$S$. In determining the relative sizes of the statistics, the denominator is
unimportant and the numerator simplifies to $T(x, y) = (x + y - 35.788)^2$.

An alternative and natural approach might be to consider the adjusted
OR, as estimated by the Mantel–Haenszel estimator, as a measure of the
difference between the groups. For this example, the Mantel–Haenszel odds
ratio can be written as

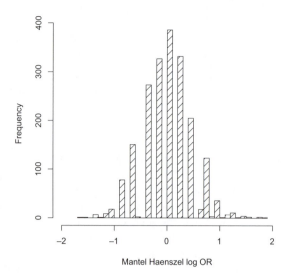

**FIGURE 7.7**
Values of log OR for 2000 random allocations, stratified by plaque size, for the PUVA vs. TL-01 trial. The observed value is 1.197.

$$OR(x,y) = \frac{43x(x-19) + 57y(y-3)}{43(48-x)(28-x) + 57(25-y)(21-y)}$$

For the measure based on the test statistic, an allocation with values $x$ and $y$ is counted as being at least as extreme as the observed value, $T(x_{obs}, y_{obs})$ = $T(25,16)$, if $T(x, y) \geq T(x_{obs}, y_{obs})$. However, if the odds ratio is used, care is needed to accommodate the aspects of this scale of measurement, which were mentioned in Subsection 7.3.2. An allocation is counted as being at least as extreme as the observed value if $OR(x,y) \geq OR(x_{obs}, y_{obs})$ (assuming that, as here, the observed odds ratio is calculated in the direction that gives a value greater than or equal to one), or if $OR(x,y)^{-1} \leq OR(x_{obs}, y_{obs})^{-1}$ or, equivalently, but more succinctly, if $|\log OR(x,y)| \geq |\log OR(x_{obs}, y_{obs})|$.

The results of 2000 random allocations, each stratified by plaque size, are shown in Figure 7.7. Thirty-six of these allocations gave an OR at least as extreme as the observed value, giving a $P$-value of 0.018. This is close to the values reported in Subsections 7.4.3 and 7.4.3 for the population model approach. If the measure used was the test statistic, then 39 of the allocations were at least as extreme as the observed value ($P = 0.0195$); this included the 36 cases that were more extreme under the other measure together with three other cases. These three cases all had $x + y = x_{obs} + y_{obs}$; two had $x = 24$ and one had $x = 23$. This close agreement arises because most of the variation in $OR(x, y)$ occurs only as $x + y$ changes, a feature that is illustrated by the contour plot in Figure 7.8.

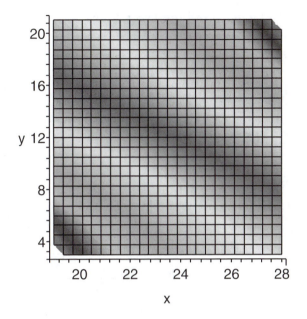

**FIGURE 7.8**
Contour plot of log $OR(x, y)$; colors change with modulus of the plotted value. Predomination of bands from NW to SE indicate that $OR(x, y)$ changes little as coordinates change subject to $x + y$ = constant.

Figure 7.7 is much more discrete than the histogram shown in Figure 7.6. This is because of the discrete nature of the sample space, namely, integer values subject to $19 \leq x \leq 28$ and $3 \leq y \leq 21$. This means that only $10 \times 19 = 190$ values of $OR(x, y)$ are possible and many of these may occur with such low probability that they may not arise in a sample of 2000 allocations. For $T(x, y)$ the situation is even more marked because this statistic depends only on $x + y$, and there are only 28 possible values for this sum.

In Equation 7.12 we were rather cavalier about whether to use the condition $I(D(a_k) \geq D_{\text{obs}})$ or $I(D(a_k) > D_{\text{obs}})$ and, for distributions that do not exhibit discreteness, the difference is minor. For cases such as those just encountered, some authors make a compromise by using the mid-P-value, in which cases with $D(a_k) = D_{\text{obs}}$ are only counted as $^1/_2$ toward the number exceedances, i.e.,

$$P_{\text{mid}} = \sum_{k=1}^{K} I(D(a_k) > D_{\text{obs}}) \Pr(A = a_k) + \frac{1}{2} \sum_{k=1}^{K} I(D(a_k) = D_{\text{obs}}) \Pr(A = a_k)$$

For the tests based on $OR(x, y)$, and $T(x, y)$ the mid-P-values are 0.01675 and 0.01475, respectively. Further details on mid-P-values can be found in Section 4.4 of Armitage, Berry, and Matthews (2002).

#### 7.6.2.1 Stratified Randomization: Exact Analysis

Consider for a moment only those patients with small plaques in the PUVA vs. TL-01 trial. If $X$ denotes the random variable underlying the observation $x$ in Table 7.12, then the distribution of $X$ induced by the random allocation can, in this case, be worked out explicitly. To do this, consider the $n_1$ patients with small plaques written out schematically as follows, each box representing a patient. The patients have been numbered so that those who clear occupy the first $r_1$ boxes.

| 1 | 2 | $r_1$ | $r_1+1$ | | | | $n_1$-1 | $n_1$ |
|---|---|---|---|---|---|---|---|---|

The random allocation places $n_{P1}$ Ps (for PUVA) and $n_{T1} = n_1 - n_{P1}$ Ts (for TL-01) in the boxes shown, for example, as

| P | T | T | T | P | T | P | P | T | P | T | P | T | T |
|---|---|---|---|---|---|---|---|---|---|---|---|---|---|
| 1 | 2 | | | | $r_1$ | $r_1+1$ | | | | | | $n_1$-1 | $n_1$ |

There are $n_1$ places where $n_{P1}$ P labels have to be placed, and this can be done in $\binom{n_1}{n_{P1}}$ ways. The $\Pr(X = x)$ can be found as the proportion of these allocations that have $x$ P labels in the first $r$ boxes (i.e., among the patients who cleared). The number of ways that $x$ of the P labels can be allocated among the $r_1$ boxes representing the cleared patients is $\binom{r_1}{x}$. For each of these allocations, there are $\binom{n_1 - r_1}{n_{P1} - x}$ ways of allocating the remaining $n_{P1} - x$ P labels among the $n_1 - r_1$ patients who did not clear. Therefore, the number of allocations that give $X = x$ is $\binom{n_1 - r_1}{n_{P1} - x}\binom{r_1}{x}$, giving

$$\Pr(X = x) = \frac{\binom{n_1 - r_1}{n_{P1} - x}\binom{r_1}{x}}{\binom{n_1}{n_{P1}}}$$

This shows that $X$ has a hypergeometric distribution, just as in the population models. The corresponding distribution for patients with large plaques is also hypergeometric and independent of the first distribution. Therefore, for this example, the randomization and the population models coincide, even though the derivations are quite different. Any differences in the

P-values obtained will simply reflect the adequacy of the normal approximation to the hypergeometric distribution invoked in Subsection 7.4.3 of this and the number of random allocations employed in the randomization tests.

### 7.6.2.2   Blocked Allocations

In specifying the set $S$ of allowed random allocations, the main principle was to include only those allocations that could have occurred under the random allocation scheme used. If a trial comparing two treatments recruits $4n$ patients and $2n$ are allocated to each treatment, then the foregoing discussion would suggest that $S$ would contain all $\binom{4n}{2n}$ possible ways of allocating $2n$ patients to each treatment. However, this will not be appropriate if the allocation has used a restricted scheme such as random permuted blocks (RPBs, cf. Section 4.2). This method of allocation would not, for example, allow the first $2n$ patients to be allocated to one treatment and the last $2n$ patients to the other, but this allocation would be counted in the total

of $\binom{4n}{2n}$ mentioned before. If RPBs with blocks of length 4 are used, then there are 6 possible blocks and, therefore, the number of possible allocations is $6^n$. This is much smaller than $\binom{4n}{2n}$. In many randomization analyses this feature is ignored, although this is probably done more for convenience than to deliberately ignore the principle involved.

---

## Exercises

1. Show that $X^2$ (Equation 7.4) and $G^2$ (Equation 7.5) are asymptotically equivalent under the null hypothesis that the clearance rates are the same in the two treatment groups. It may help to note that $G^2$ can be written as

$$2\sum e\log\left(\frac{o}{e}\right)+2\sum(o-e)\log\left(\frac{o}{e}\right)$$

2. Show that Newcombe's method (Subsection 7.3.2.2) for the confidence interval for the difference in two proportions never results in limits that are outside [-1,1].

3. In the example considered in the first four sections of this chapter
   the outcome was a binary variable, 1 meaning that the patient
   cleared and 0 meaning that they did not. From a mathematical point
   of view, the values 0 and 1 are essentially arbitrary and just serve
   as labels to the two possible outcomes. Suppose the outcome associated with 1 had not been cleared and 0 meant cleared, then the $\pi$
   parameters would measure the probability of not clearing and the
   principal estimates would have been:

   The proportion of patients not clearing on PUVA is estimated to be
   $p_P = 8/49 = 0.16$

   The proportion of patients not clearing on TL-01 is estimated to be
   $p_T = 19/51 = 0.37$

   Compute the table corresponding to Table 7.4 for this new definition
   of the parameters. Comment on what you find.

4. Show how Equation 7.8 can be used to derive the formula for the
   CI for the log OR given in Subsection 7.3.2 of this chapter.

5. Derive the formula for the variance of the hypergeometric distribution quoted in Subsection 7.4.4 of this chapter.

6. For exponential survival times, show that the parameter $\lambda$ is the
   hazard rate. It is usual to compare hazard rates in two groups
   through the hazard ratio. Use likelihood methods to derive a test
   that the hazard ratio is one, and show that this is equivalent to the
   test given in Subsection 7.5.2. Find a confidence interval for the
   hazard ratio. You may find it useful to write $\lambda_T = \psi\lambda_P$ and work with
   the parameterization $(\lambda_P, \psi)$. Interested readers may wish to investigate the concept of profile likelihood and apply it to this problem.

7. Show that the simpler version of the log-rank test statistic is smaller
   than that defined in Subsection 7.5.2 as $U^2/V$. You may wish to note
   that because $d_j$ is a positive integer

$$v_j = \frac{n_{1j}n_{2j}d_j(n_j - d_j)}{n_j^2(n_j - 1)} \leq \frac{n_{1j}n_{2j}d_j}{n_j^2} = v'_j$$

8. Look up Stirling's approximation to $n!$ and use it to find an approximation to the ratio of the sizes of two randomization sets for a trial
   comparing two groups, each with $2n$ patients. The first set considers
   all possible allocations of $2n$ patients to each treatment group and
   the second only allocations that could have arisen from the use of
   random permuted blocks with blocks of length 4.

# 8

## Monitoring Accumulating Data

### 8.1 Motivation and Problems with Repeated Analysis of Data

Clinical trials generally run for many months or even years. A consequence of this is that, for a trial with a fixed size (as outlined in Chapter 3), the results for the patients who enter at the start of the trial will become available before the patients entering the trial later are recruited. Trials are undertaken when the investigator does not have evidence whether one treatment is superior to another, but it is conceivable that this situation will change as the trial proceeds. Adequate evidence to settle which treatment is superior may have accumulated long before the trial runs to its planned conclusion. If this is so, and the investigator does not take notice of this evidence, then the patients entered into the trial after this point, and who receive the inferior treatment, will be receiving a treatment that could have been known to be inferior on the basis of the evidence from the first part of the trial. It is therefore important in maintaining an ethically defensible trial to take account of this issue. However, if a trial is stopped early on the basis of naïve methods, serious statistical problems arise that can undermine the results of the study. In extreme cases, the medical community may feel it has to discount the results from the trial and that a new trial is justified. If this happens, then the net effect may be that, in total, many more patients are exposed to the inferior treatment than might have been the case had the original trial run to its planned conclusion.

The only way to decide whether the information already collected is sufficient to determine if a treatment is superior is to analyze the data in hand. However, if this is done in an uncontrolled way, the suspicion will arise that the trial has been stopped because one treatment appears better than the other. This is indeed why the exercise would be undertaken, but it must be remembered that any difference found is a statistical difference, and these can arise by chance, even when no genuine difference exists. Indeed, the

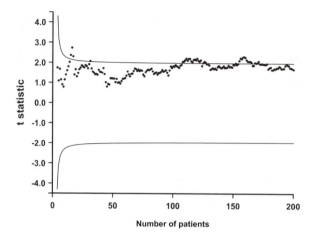

**FIGURE 8.1**

Accumulated *t*-statistics against combined sample size for simulated data in which null hypothesis is true.

main problem with repeatedly analyzing accumulating data is that the chance that a type I error will occur rises substantially.

Figure 8.1 illustrates this point. Outcomes from a trial of 200 patients were simulated from a single normal distribution. The patients were allocated to one of two treatments using random permuted blocks of length four. The two groups were compared with a *t*-test using just the first four patients. A second *t* statistic was found using the first five patients, a third using six patients, and so on until finally all 200 were compared. The resulting *t*-statistics are plotted against the number of patients used in the comparison, together with the 95% limits for the relevant *t*-distribution. The data are from a single distribution so the null hypothesis is known to be true, but out of 197 *t*-tests, 39 are significant at the 5% level. If this represented data from a real trial, then analyzing the data after the results from each patient became available would lead to the conclusion of a difference by the 15th patient. Even if stopping so early were proscribed, there would have been subsequent opportunities to conclude that there was good evidence of a treatment effect. If the trial had been allowed to run its course to 200 patients, the *P*-value would not have been below 0.05. It is clearly important that any credible scheme for repeatedly scrutinizing data during the course of a trial must take account of the potential this process has to inflate the type I error rate.

Although repeatedly inspecting the data can lead to false claims of a treatment difference where none exists, the ethical, practical, and financial advantages of stopping a trial early, if there is a genuine difference, means that it is worth pursuing methods that allow this possibility. Some of these will be discussed in the following sections.

## 8.2 Sequential and Group Sequential Methods

### 8.2.1 Using Repeated Significance Tests

Sequential methods intended for use in clinical trials were pioneered by Armitage (1975). They often use procedures that are collectively known as the *repeated significance test* method. In many of these, it is assumed that the trial compares two treatments, A and B, and patients are recruited in pairs with one member of each pair being randomly allocated to A and the other to B. The data are analyzed as the results from each pair become available.

The procedure is to stop the trial when a significance test yields a (two-sided) $P$-value less than $\alpha'$, or when $N$ pairs have been recruited, whichever happens sooner. The values of $\alpha'$ and $N$ are chosen so that the whole procedure has a type I error rate $\alpha$ and power $1 - \beta$ to detect a specified treatment difference. The value $\alpha'$ is often called a *nominal* significance level, because obtaining a $P$-value less than $\alpha$ does not entitle the analyst to assert "$P < \alpha$" in the usual way, instead the user can only claim "$P < \alpha'$". If the trial terminates when $N$ pairs have been recruited, the trial has not obtained evidence against the null hypothesis. Repeated tests at the $\alpha'$ level will give rise to a type I error rate that is in excess of $\alpha'$, and the procedure chooses $\alpha' < \alpha$ such that the inflated type I error rate comes out at $\alpha$. The value of $\alpha'$ that corresponds with a given $\alpha$ depends on how many times you might end up inspecting the data, i.e., $\alpha'$ depends on $N$ as well as $\alpha$. Moreover, the calculation that determines $\alpha'$ from $N$ and $\alpha$ is not straightforward, because the successive $P$-values computed in this procedure, being based on datasets that differ by only two observations, are highly correlated.

If the outcome is binary, in the sense that the result from treating each pair of patients is "A is superior to B" or "B is superior to A" (with ties discounted), then the null hypothesis corresponds to $\pi = 1/2$, where $\pi = \Pr(A$ is superior to B). A trial that has 95% power to detect a value of $\pi = \pi_1$ and with overall type I error of 0.05 would have the values of $N$ and $\alpha'$ given in Table 8.1.

**TABLE 8.1**

Values for Sequential Binary Trial

| $\pi_1$ | $\alpha'$ | $N$ |
|---------|-----------|-----|
| 0.95 | 0.0313 | 10 |
| 0.85 | 0.0193 | 25 |
| 0.75 | 0.0118 | 61 |
| 0.70 | 0.0081 | 100 |

*Source:* Data from Armitage, P., Berry, G., Matthews, J.N.S. (2002), *Statistical Methods in Medical Research*, 4th ed., Blackwell, Oxford, p. 618.

However, trials using this methodology are seldom used in practice. This is largely because of practical difficulties: patients rarely present in pairs; results for patients often take some time to become available; the organization required to analyze the data after every one or two patients should not be underestimated, especially in a large multicenter study. An alternative is to use a group sequential design (Pocock, 1977; O'Brien and Fleming, 1979). In this kind of design the data are inspected after every successive group of $2n$ patients have been recruited. The group size, $2n$, is often 20, 30, or even larger. Each group will contain patients receiving both treatments and, indeed, the use of a technique such as random permuted blocks could ensure that $n$ patients receive each treatment. Consequently, there is a natural comparison available from each group that replaces the need for patients to be recruited in pairs.

Group sequential trials proceed in a manner analogous to the fully sequential version. At the outset, the overall type I error rate, $\alpha$, and the power, $1 - \beta$, to detect a specified departure from the null hypothesis are set. After the results for each successive group of $2n$ patients has become available, the treatments are compared using an appropriate hypothesis test. If $P < \alpha'$, a nominal significance level, then the trial is stopped and a difference significant at $P < \alpha'$ is declared. There is a maximum number of groups $N$, and if $P < \alpha$ is not obtained by the time these results are analyzed, the trial is stopped with the conclusion that no evidence against the null hypothesis has been found at the $100\alpha\%$ level. The successive analyses are usually referred to as *interim analyses*.

The value of $\alpha'$ is essentially determined by the values of $\alpha$ and $N$, and as $N$ is now the number of groups, it will generally be much smaller than the values for $N$ under a fully sequential procedure. Values for $N$ between 2 to 10 are not uncommon.

Suppose that the outcome has a normal distribution with standard deviation $\sigma$ and that the difference in the treatment means is $\tau$. It will be seen in the next subsection that the power of the trial $1 - \beta$ will depend on $N$, $\alpha$, $\alpha'$, and $\mu = (\tau\sqrt{n}) / (\sigma\sqrt{2})$. The relationship among these five quantities cannot be expressed in closed form, and numerical integration is needed to determine the power given the rest. From tables of these integrations, it is possible to apply linear interpolation techniques to obtain tables of $\mu$ as a function of $1 - \beta$, $N$, $\alpha$, $\alpha$, and these are valuable in the design of group sequential trials. Table 8.2 gives the values of $\mu$ and $\alpha'$ for a few values of $N$ for a trial with $\alpha = 0.05$ and $1\beta = 0.90$ (Pocock, 1977).

In practice Table 8.2 would be used as follows. Suppose the intention is to run a trial having type I error of 5% and with a power of 90% to detect a treatment difference of 0.25 standard deviation. It follows that $\tau/\sigma = 0.25$, and hence $\mu = 0.25\sqrt{(1/2n)}$. The number of patients to be recruited for each treatment in each group is then given by solving:

1. $0.25\sqrt{(1/2n)} = 2.404$ (so $n = 185$) if a maximum of two interim analyses are planned $(N = 2)$

**TABLE 8.2**

Some Important Values for Group Sequential Designs with 5% Type I
Error and 90% Power (Pocock, 1977)

| N | 1 | 2 | 3 | 4 | 5 | 10 | 15 | 20 |
|---|---|---|---|---|---|----|----|----|
| m | 3.242 | 2.404 | 2.007 | 1.763 | 1.592 | 1.156 | 0.956 | 0.835 |
| $\alpha'$ | 0.05 | 0.0294 | 0.0221 | 0.0182 | 0.0158 | 0.0106 | 0.0086 | 0.0075 |

2. $0.25\sqrt{(1/2n)} = 1.592$ (so $n = 81$) if a maximum of five interim analyses
   are planned ($N = 5$)

3. $0.25\sqrt{(1/2n)} = 1.156$ (so $n = 43$) if a maximum of ten interim analyses
   are planned ($N = 10$)

In case 1, two analyses are performed and the trial stopped if the $P$-value
obtained is less than 0.0294. With more planned analyses, each test gets
stricter, so with $N = 10$, an interim analysis would have to yield $P < 0.0106$
for a difference to be declared at the 5% level.

Obviously, different numbers of planned interim analyses could be
explored. It should be noted that the case $N = 1$ (only one analysis is planned)
is the usual fixed sample size trial envisaged in Chapter 3. When planning
a group sequential trial, it is important to be aware of the total number of
patients your trial will require if it does not terminate early, which is $2nN$.
For the preceding three cases, this value is 740, 810, and 860, respectively.
These figures compare with that for the fixed size trial of 672 ($N = 1$). In
other words, in order to maintain a given power, there is a price to be paid
for repeated inspection in terms of the maximum possible sample size.
However, it should be remembered that in the case $N = 1$, the investigator
is guaranteed to require all 672 patients, whereas in the other designs there
is a chance that fewer will be needed.

## 8.2.2 Some Theory for Group Sequential Designs with Normal Outcomes

In the preceding subsection it has been asserted that there is a relationship
between the power of the trial $1 - \beta$, the type I error rate, $\alpha$, the nominal
type I error rate, $\alpha'$, the standardized treatment difference $\tau/\sigma$, the group size
$2n$, and the maximum number of interim analyses, $N$. The nature of the
relationship will now be examined. The theory that follows is much more
transparent if it is assumed that $\sigma$ is known. This apparently unrealistic
stance will be adopted, both because of the clarity it brings and because, in
practice, estimating $\sigma$ has a negligible effect on the quantities that will be
derived. The approach followed is that of Armitage, McPherson, and Rowe
(1969) and McPherson and Armitage (1971).

Suppose the mean responses to treatments A and B in the $i$th group
are $\bar{x}_{Ai}, \bar{x}_{Bi}$, respectively, each based on $n$ patients. The outcome variable is
assumed to have a normal distribution with standard deviation $\sigma$
and $\bar{d}_i = \bar{x}_{Ai} - \bar{x}_{Bi}$ then has a normal distribution with mean $\tau$ and variance

$2\sigma^2/n$. The hypothesis test based on the observed treatment means from the first $M$ groups is performed using

$$S_M = \sum_{j=1}^{M} \frac{\bar{d}_j}{\sqrt{2\sigma^2/n}} = \sum_{j=1}^{M} \bar{\delta}_j$$

which has mean $M\mu = (M\tau\sqrt{n})/(\sigma\sqrt{2})$ and variance $M$. Under the null hypothesis, $S_M$ has zero mean and the trial terminates at the first $M$ such that $|S_M| > a_M$ or when $M = N$. If each interim analysis tests at the $\alpha'$ level then $a_M = z_{1/2\alpha'}\sqrt{M}$, where $z_{\alpha/2}$ is the two-sided $100\alpha\%$ point of the standard normal distribution. However, for reasons that will become clear in the next subsection, it will be convenient to use the more general notation $a_M$ for the critical point of this interim analysis.

It is clear that $S_1$ has a normal distribution and also that for $M > 1$

$$S_M = S_{M-1} + \bar{\delta}_M \text{ , provided } |S_{M-1}| \leq a_{M-1} \tag{8.1}$$

It is this proviso that complicates the determination of the distribution of $S_M$, which would otherwise be normal, being the sum of independent normal random variables. The density function of $S_M$ can be found recursively from the formula for the density of the sum of two random variables.

If $X$ and $Y$ are two random variables with density functions $f_X$ and $f_Y$, respectively, then the density of $Z = X + Y$, $f_{X+Y}$, is given by

$$f_{X+Y}(z) = \int f_X(u)f_Y(z-u)du \tag{8.2}$$

where the integration ranges over the range of $X$ or an appropriate subset thereof.

If we use $\phi$ to denote the density of a standard normal variable,

$$\phi(x) = \frac{1}{\sqrt{2\pi}} \exp(-\tfrac{1}{2}x^2)$$

then $f_1 = \phi$. The density of $S_M$, $f_M(S_M)$ (or $f_M(S_M;\mu)$ if the dependence on the parameter $\mu$ needs to be emphasized), can be found by applying Equation 8.2 to Equation 8.1:

$$f_M(S_M;\mu) = \int_{-a_{M-1}}^{a_{M-1}} f_{M-1}(u;\mu)\phi(S_M - \mu - u)du; \ (M = 2, ..., N)$$

the integration ranges from $a_{M-1}$ to $a_{M-1}$ because $S_M$ is only defined if $S_{M1}$ lies in that range. There is no closed form solution to this set of equations and numerical integration is needed to evaluate a general $f_M(.)$.

The probability that the trial terminates without giving a significant result at the $100\alpha\%$ level is simply $\Pr(|S_N| \le a_N)$; so the chance of a type I error is the complement of this probability when $\mu = 0$, i.e.,

$$\alpha = \Pr(\text{Type I error}) = 1 - \int_{-a_N}^{a_N} f_N(u; 0) du \qquad (8.3)$$

This is implicitly an equation in $N$ variables, namely, $a_1, a_2, \ldots, a_N$. In order to solve the equation, extra information is required. One way to supply this is to assume that each interim analysis is performed at the same significance level, $100\alpha\%$ so $a_M = z_{\alpha/2}\sqrt{M}$, for $M = 1, \ldots, N$, and now Equation 8.3 is an equation for a single variable $\alpha$. It is the numerical solution to an equation of this type that provides the entries in the last row of Table 8.2.

Using the values of $a_1, a_2, \ldots, a_N$ obtained from the solution of Equation 8.3, the power of the trial can be found by computing the probability of obtaining a significant result when the mean treatment difference, and hence $\mu$, is not zero. This gives

$$1 - \beta = 1 - \int_{-a_N}^{a_N} f_N(u; \mu) du \qquad (8.4)$$

Numerical methods are again needed to solve this equation, either for $1 - \beta$, given $\mu$, or for $\mu$, given $1 - \beta$. This explains the remark in Subsection 8.2.1 of this chapter that the power of the trial depends on the treatment difference $\tau$ through $\mu = (\tau\sqrt{n}) / (\sigma\sqrt{2})$. It is through the solution of equations of a type similar to Equation 8.4 that the second line of Table 8.2 is obtained.

It should be noted here that if a trial terminates early, then there are problems with obtaining an unbiased estimate of the effect of treatment. The difference in means is simply $KS_M / M$ with $K = \sigma\sqrt{2} / n$, and though this is an unbiased estimator of $\tau$ for a fixed-size trial, it is not so in a sequential trial. This is because the relevant expectation is actually $(K / M)E(S_M \mid |S_M| > a_M, |S_k| \le a_k, k = 1, \ldots, M-1)$ which will not, in general, be $\tau$. Methods for attempting to correct the bias are available but are beyond the scope of this book.

### 8.2.3   Other Forms of Stopping Rule

The collection of critical points $a_1, a_2, \ldots, a_N$ defined earlier constitute a stopping rule, in the sense that a trial is stopped early if an interim analysis provides a test statistic that exceeds the relevant $a_M$. The rule in which each test uses the same nominal significance level, i.e., $a_M = z_{1\alpha'}\sqrt{M}$, is often associated with the name of Pocock, who was the first to propose its use (Pocock, 1977).

The Pocock boundaries have two related properties that may, in some circumstances, be disadvantageous. The first is that it is not difficult for a trial to be halted early using this scheme. As part of the rationale for adopting a sequential approach was that it should be possible to stop a trial early if it turns out that one treatment was noticeably more beneficial, it may be surprising to see this property listed as a potential problem. However, some authors have argued that it would be unwise to allow a trial to stop very early unless there was an overwhelming (and unsuspected) benefit attached to one treatment. If a trial stops very early on the basis of a difference that is any less than this, then it may be viewed as uncompelling by other workers in the field. If a trial is stopped early, but near to its planned maximum size, then there is at least a substantial body of data available for analysis. If a trial is stopped after, say, one or two of a maximum of ten planned analyses, little data will have been collected. The effort involved in the mounting the trial could be wasted if other workers in the field do not accept that it was justified to stop the trial so early.

A second difficulty with the Pocock boundaries is more to do with communication with colleagues who are not in the field of statistics. The final interim analysis is made at the same level of significance as all the others so, for example, with 10 planned analyses, a test is only significant for an overall type I error of 5% if $P \leq 0.0106$. Suppose the trial terminates after ten analyses with $P > 0.0106$ in each interim analysis but with the $P$-value for the final analysis (i.e., based on the whole trial) equal to 0.03. Had you not performed any interim analyses, then you could have legitimately claimed the results were significant at the 5% level, but you cannot do so now, simply because you have analyzed these data throughout their collection. Many clinicians find this point, which emerges from the frequentist approach to significance testing, difficult to accept.

A way to avoid both these problems is to make the early tests of significance at a much more stringent level than the later tests, with the overall type I error rate, determined through Equation 8.3, held at the same value as before, usually 5%. A significant result arises at an early test only if there is a very large difference observed between the treatments. A consequence of maintaining the overall type I error rate at its usual level is that the later tests become less stringent and therefore closer to the value for a fixed-size trial. It is consequently less likely that a trial will terminate after $N$ groups in such a way that the final analysis is embarrassingly different from the fixed-size result.

The Pocock boundaries were derived from Equation 8.3 by imposing the constraint $a_M = z_{1_\alpha} \cdot \sqrt{M}$ on the $a_1, a_2, \ldots, a_N$. Alternative boundaries are found by imposing different constraints. As $S_M$ is a sum, the Pocock boundaries maintain a constant significance level by allowing the $a_M$ to increase as $\sqrt{M}$. The so-called O'Brien–Fleming boundaries (O'Brien and Fleming, 1979) allow decreasing levels of significance to terminate the trial at increasing $M$ by specifying $a_1 = a_2 = \ldots = a_N$. Using this stopping rule the nominal significance level used as the critical point for the $M$th interim analysis changes with $M$. An example for $N = 5$ is given in Table 8.3. Notice that the final nominal significance level for the O'Brien–Fleming rule is much closer to 0.05 than it is for the Pocock rule.

**TABLE 8.3**

Nominal Significance Levels for $M$th Interim Analysis for Various Stopping Rules with $\alpha = 0.05$

| $M$ | 1 | 2 | 3 | 4 | 5 |
|---|---|---|---|---|---|
| Pocock | 0.0158 | 0.0158 | 0.0158 | 0.0158 | 0.0158 |
| O'Brien–Fleming | $5 \times 10^6$ | 0.0013 | 0.0085 | 0.0228 | 0.0417 |
| Haybittle–Peto | 0.001 | 0.001 | 0.001 | 0.001 | 0.05 |
| Fleming, Harrington, and O'Brien | 0.0038 | 0.0048 | 0.0053 | 0.0064 | 0.0432 |

Other rules are also possible. An informal one associated with the names of Haybittle (1971) and Peto et al. (1976) is to use a very stringent level of significance for the first $N - 1$ tests, such as $P = 0.001$ if $N > 3$ (perhaps $P = 0.01$ if $N = 2$ or 3), with the final test being conducted at the level of the overall type I error, $\alpha$. This rule was proposed on heuristic grounds before the preceding, more formal approach had been derived. The idea is that the effects of repeated testing at the 0.001 level are negligible and need not be reflected in the level of the final test. The overall type I error will now exceed 0.05. This could, in principle, be corrected by determining a value for $a_N$ from Equation 8.3 when for $M < N$, $a_M = z_{0.0005}\sqrt{M}$ but the difference from $z_{0.025}\sqrt{N}$ would be practically unimportant. Some statisticians do, however, perform the final analysis at the 4.9% level.

A further boundary due to Fleming, Harrington, and O'Brien (1984) is to ensure that the probability of a type I error at the $M$th analysis (i.e., the trial stops erroneously at the $M$th interim analysis when $\tau = 0$) is constant for $M = 1, \ldots, N - 1$, with the final significance level being chosen to ensure that the overall type I error is $\alpha$. To be specific, for $M < N$,

$$\pi_M = \Pr(\,|S_M| > a_M;\,|S_K| \le a_K, K = 1, \ldots, M - 1\,|\,H_0)$$

$$= \int_{-\infty}^{-a_M} f_M(u;0)du + \int_{a_M}^{\infty} f_M(u;0)du$$

is the probability of a type I error occurring at the $M$th analysis. This boundary demands $\pi_M = \pi_1$, $M < N$ and $\pi_N = \alpha - (N - 1)\pi_1$. As it stands, these constraints do not determine the boundaries. The analyst has the freedom to set $\pi_N$ so that it is close to $\alpha$ and this has been done in Table 8.3. The boundary was introduced to be intermediate between the Pocock and O'Brien–Fleming boundaries because the latter were felt to be too strict in the early stages.

A more flexible approach is to perform interim analyses in such a way that they "spend" the type I error rate, $\alpha$, a little at a time as the review process continues. This method does not require the maximum number of interim analyses to be specified in advance. A description of the method is beyond the scope of this book but interested readers can find an account in Lan and DeMets (1983).

## 8.3  Other Approaches to Accumulating Data

### 8.3.1  SPRT and Triangular Test

The classical approach to the sequential testing of data is Wald's sequential probability ratio test (SPRT). In its simplest form, this test attempts to distinguish between two specific hypotheses, $H_0$ and $H_1$, under which the accumulating data, $x_1, x_2, \ldots, x_n, \ldots$, have densities $f_0(x_1, x_2, \ldots, x_n, \ldots)$ or $f_1(x_1, x_2, \ldots, x_n, \ldots)$, respectively. The SPRT works by computing successively

$$L_n = \exp(l_n) = \frac{f_1(x_1, x_2, \ldots, x_n)}{f_0(x_1, x_2, \ldots, x_n)} \tag{8.5}$$

If $A < L_n < B$, then the test requires that another observation be obtained and the test repeated. If $L_n \leq A$, then the procedure is terminated and $H_0$ is accepted; if $L_n \geq B$ then $H_1$ is accepted. The user is required to specify beforehand the error probabilities that will be acceptable. These are the probabilities of declaring for $H_0$ when it is false and for $H_1$ when that is false. From these probabilities, values of $A$ and $B$ can be found from simple formulae.

If the data are normally distributed with variance $\sigma^2$ and mean $\mu_i$ under $H_i$ then Equation 8.5 becomes

$$l_n = \{(\mu_1 - \mu_0)t_n - \tfrac{1}{2}n(\mu_1^2 - \mu_0^2)\} / \sigma^2$$

where $t_n = x_1 + x_2 + \ldots + x_n$.

The procedure can be implemented by plotting $t_n$ against $n$ and following the sample path until it crosses one of the boundaries, which can be plotted on the chart as the lines

$$t_n = \sigma^2 \log A / (\mu_1 - \mu_0) + \tfrac{1}{2}n(\mu_1 + \mu_0)$$

and

$$t_n = \sigma^2 \log B / (\mu_1 - \mu_0) + \tfrac{1}{2}n(\mu_1 + \mu_0)$$

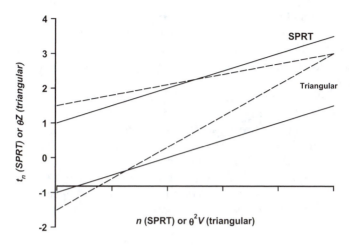

**FIGURE 8.2**
Continuation regions for SPRT and triangular test.

These are parallel lines and an example of such boundaries is shown in Figure 8.2. It follows that there is no finite upper bound on the sampling region, and the procedure cannot be guaranteed to terminate by any pre-specified time (it can, however, be shown that the procedure does terminate at some stage with probability 1).

The inability to specify a time by which a trial must terminate is a serious practical shortcoming of the simple SPRT. Various alternative methods have been proposed, one of the most popular being the triangular test, which is advocated by Whitehead (1992). The method works with quantities based on the likelihood, namely the score statistic, $Z$, and the observed information, $V$. This has the advantage that the method can be applied readily to different types of outcome measure, not just those with a normal distribution (although it should be noted that the methods in Subsection 8.2.1 can also be adapted to nonnormal responses). If the parameter under investigation is $\theta$, then to a good approximation, $Z \sim N(\theta V, V)$, and it is assumed that the null hypothesis is $\theta = 0$. The trial is run assuming an error probability $\alpha$, where this is both the probability of obtaining a significant result when $\theta = 0$ (i.e., the type I error) and of not obtaining a significant result when $\theta = \theta_M$, the analogue of the minimal clinically important difference $\tau_M$ from Chapter 3 (i.e., $1 - \alpha$ is the power). The successive points are plotted on a graph of $\theta_M Z$ vs. $\theta_M^2 V$ and the trial terminates when one of the following boundaries is crossed:

$$\theta_M Z = 2\log(2\alpha) + \tfrac{3}{4}\theta_M^2 V \quad \text{(lower boundary)};$$

$$\theta_M Z = -2\log(2\alpha) + \tfrac{1}{4}\theta_M^2 V \quad \text{(upper boundary)}.$$

These are straight lines, but unlike for the SPRT, they are not parallel, so they meet when $V = V^*$, say, and the trial cannot continue beyond this point. In most trials, $V$ is proportional to $n$, the number of patients recruited, so this effectively imposes an upper limit on the number of patients that could be recruited.

An example is given in Figure 8.2. If the upper boundary is crossed then the null hypothesis is rejected, whereas if the lower boundary is crossed it is not. As shown in Figure 8.2 the triangular test is a one-sided test, that is, the test is of $H_0 : \theta = 0$ vs. $H_1 : \theta > 0$ (cf. Subsection 3.2.3). Modifications that implement two-sided test are available.

The triangular tests have many advantages and are very flexible. They are, however, technically rather more complicated than the repeated significance test methods outlined earlier in this chapter.

### 8.3.2 Bayesian and Likelihood Approaches

In the Bayesian approach to the analysis of data, inferences about the parameter of interest, $\theta$, say, are based on the posterior density of $\theta$, given the data observed. The process starts with the analyst quantitatively specifying his or her beliefs about $\theta$ in a prior distribution, which has density $\pi(\theta)$. If the data available at time $t$ are $x(t)$, with likelihood $L(x(t)|\theta)$, then the posterior density, $\pi(\theta|x(t))$, is

$$\pi(\theta|x(t)) \propto L(x(t)|\theta)\pi(\theta) \tag{8.6}$$

with the constant of proportionality set so that $\pi(\theta|x(t))$ integrates to one over the parameter space. This gives a natural way for updating information about $\theta$ in the light of new data. Suppose $\theta$ is a parameter measuring the effect of a treatment, then it may be that the evidence about $\theta$ contained in $\pi(\theta|x(t))$ is insufficient to terminate the study, and data are collected until time $t' > t$. If $x(t') - \{x(t)\}$ is used to denote the new data collected between $t$ and $t'$, then the new posterior is obtained by updating the old posterior using Equation 8.6, i.e.,

$$\pi(\theta|x(t')) \propto L(x(t') - \{x(t)\}|\theta)\pi(\theta|x(t))$$

Sequential analysis, therefore, fits naturally with a Bayesian approach to the analysis of clinical trials. Unlike the frequentist approach, sequential Bayesian analysis differs little from nonsequential Bayesian analysis. This is, in part, due to the lesser importance attached to hypothesis testing in the Bayesian framework.

Bayesian methods for RCTs are still not widely used in practice, but they are undoubtedly becoming more prominent and in years to come, things may be very different (see Spiegelhalter, Abrams, and Myles [2003] for a fuller discussion of this approach to RCTs). The reliance of Bayesian methods on prior distributions perhaps hinders its adoption in RCTs more than in other fields. Although there are undoubtedly prior beliefs held about treatments, there are at least three broad reasons why a Bayesian approach may not be readily accepted. First, the prior beliefs, though undoubtedly present, might be difficult to quantify. Second, different experts will have different prior beliefs. Much work is in progress on these matters. A third and perhaps more fundamental issue is the nature of the distinction between belief and evidence. In a sense, there are only beliefs in a Bayesian analysis, albeit ones expressed precisely using the language of probability theory. The Bayesian viewpoint sees Equation 8.6 as the means of modifying one's beliefs in the light of the data. Many clinicians see the collection of data in an RCT as a means of collecting definitive evidence about the relative efficacies of treatments, untainted by anyone's beliefs. In practice, there may be little substance to this objection, as most RCTs are likely to be so large that the posterior in Equation 8.6 will be dominated by the contribution from the likelihood for all but the most absurdly concentrated priors, but it may be more difficult to persuade clinical colleagues to accept the underlying principles.

The advantages that the Bayesian approach holds for sequential analysis largely stem from the likelihood principle that is implicit in this approach, namely, that all information relevant to inference is encapsulated in the likelihood function. Some statisticians hold to this principle without subscribing to a Bayesian viewpoint. They too have an easier time with sequential analysis than does the frequentist.

### 8.3.3 Adaptive Allocation

Adaptive allocation is when the chance a patient receives a treatment depends on the outcomes of previous patients. Although this topic is not strictly about sequential analysis, it shares many of its features. In particular there is an underlying intention to limit the number of patients allocated to the inferior treatment. Various methods have been proposed, such as the simple "play-the-winner" rule. This method assumes that allocation is made by selecting balls from an urn. If there are two treatments, say black and white, then there are balls of these two colors in the urn. Initially, there is one ball of each color. If the treatment allocated, say white, is successful, then another white ball is added to the urn; otherwise a black ball is added to the urn. Therefore, in the long run, patients will be more likely to receive the more effective treatment. This method assumes that the result of the previous patient is available when the next patient needs to be allocated (and that it is reasonable to summarize how they fared using a binary outcome). To judge by their prevalence in actual use, such methods have greater theoretical than practical appeal. They can lead to groups that are of very different sizes, and the final inferences about treatment effects can be difficult to make.

A recent and widely discussed example of this kind of trial was used to compare a new form of treatment for severe lung disease in newborn infants. Conventional respiratory support was compared with a way of oxygenating blood outside the body, known as *extracorporeal membrane oxygenation* (ECMO). The trial was designed as follows. Patients were allocated to treatment using randomly permuted blocks of size 4 until 4 deaths occurred on one of the treatments. At that point, all subsequent patients were allocated to the other treatment, until 4 patients die on the new treatment or until the testing procedure in the trial established the superiority of that treatment. In this case, the statistical methodology required that at least 28 patients receiving ECMO survive before the fourth death on ECMO during the nonrandomized phase of the study. The figure of 28 was computed on the basis of the results in the randomized phase, in which 4 out of 10 patients died on conventional therapy and 0 out of 9 died on ECMO. In the second (ECMO-only) phase, only 20 patients were actually recruited and only one of them died.

The results from this trial gave rise to wide-ranging discussion of the attendant statistical methodology with a bewildering range of conclusions. The lack of a statistical consensus on how to handle these designs cannot encourage their acceptance in the medical community, and for the present they are likely to remain little used. Interesting discussions of the issues can be found in articles by Ware (1989) and Begg (1990).

## 8.4   Data Monitoring Committees

Section 8.2 and Section 8.3 of this chapter only scratch the surface of a wealth of statistical techniques that have been devised for the problem of repeatedly analyzing data accumulating in an RCT. Despite this apparent embarrassment of methodological riches, none of the methods is wholly satisfactory. The problem is essentially that the methods are too formalized to reflect the huge complexity of the process that surrounds the decision whether or not to terminate a trial, particularly a major trial, early. The methods usually examine a single variable for evidence that one treatment is superior to the others. Most of the frequentist methods are concerned with controlling the type I error rate. In the background to many of these methods, there is a suggestion that once the trial has been terminated with evidence in favor of a treatment, then that treatment will generally be adopted in medical practice henceforth. Such a conception is certainly too simplistic.

In practice, matters are much less one-dimensional than this. The decision to terminate a trial must take into account many features. The trial may well have to stop early, not because one treatment is plainly more efficacious with respect to, say, levels of blood pressure, but because one treatment is associated with a worryingly high incidence of cases of irregular heartbeat. A trial may present evidence that the new treatment is noticeably less efficacious than the existing treatment. A treatment may have an impact on an outcome variable other than the one it was thought likely to affect. Should investigators be as ready to abandon a study in the light of unexpected evidence (which they might argue is more likely to represent chance variation) than if things turn out to be as extreme but in the anticipated direction?

A more contentious issue concerns the degree of evidence that investigators want to present. Some triallists have argued that in order for the results of a study to change medical practice, the levels of evidence required are more extreme than is often realized, but if such evidence is not adduced, then the trial has been pointless. This has led some trials to continue until differences with $P < 0.0000001$ have been achieved. It could be argued that the superior treatment could have been identified much earlier in the study, so some patients have been exposed unnecessarily to inferior treatment. The argument turns on what is seen as the end of the trial and what is necessary to achieve it. The conflict between the individual and collective ethics that it presents is not an easy one to resolve.

These issues imply that the decision to terminate a study early depends on many factors, and it is risible to suppose that they can be summarized in a sequence of hypothesis tests. In major trials, it is now good practice to have a data and safety monitoring committee. The responsibility of this committee is to periodically review the evidence currently available from the trial and to recommend to those running the trial whether the trial should continue, perhaps in a modified form, or terminate. The multidisciplinary nature of the decision to terminate a major trial should be reflected in the membership of the committee, which should include both doctors and statisticians, and possibly others with relevant expertise. Such membership emphasizes that statistical thinking is an essential component of the process, but should not dominate it. The decision of this committee will carry less conviction if those making it were too closely involved with the trial, thus the members of the committee should not be trial investigators. The deliberations of the committee must be attended by the trial statistician in order to have the relevant interim analyses available, but other trial investigators should not be involved.

One of the possible decisions that a data and safety monitoring committee may make is to agree to have an additional interim analysis. This can be very awkward for designs with stopping rules such as Pocock or O'Brien–Fleming, where $N$ is specified in advance. It may, therefore, be helpful to have the additional flexibility of the Haybittle–Peto boundary or the alpha spending function approach when designing a trial.

A valuable discussion of these complex issues can be found in Pocock (1993) and a fuller discussion in the book devoted to this topic by Ellenberg, Fleming, and DeMets (2002).

## Exercises

1. A group sequential design for a normally distributed outcome uses Pocock boundaries with overall type I error rate of 5% and is planned to have a maximum of 5 analyses and a power of 90%. If 20 patients are recruited to each arm of the study in each group, what size of treatment difference can be found (give your answer in units of the standard deviation of the outcome)? If this size of effect is to be found from a similar trial with $N = 10$, how many patients are needed on each treatment in each group? Compare the maximum possible number of patients.

2. If a group sequential design comparing treatments A and B is to recruit twice as many patients to treatment B than A in each group, how should the theory in Subsection 8.2.2 be amended?

3. Although the functions $f_M(.)$ were derived from formula for a density, they are not conventional densities and some care is needed in their interpretation. For example

$$\int_{-\infty}^{-a_N} f_N(u)du + \int_{-a_N}^{\infty} f_N(u)du \neq 1 - \int_{a_N}^{a_N} f_N(u)du$$

Describe precisely what the event is whose probability is determined by $f_M(.)$. (You may find it helpful to work through the case $N = 2$ in detail.)

4. What event has probability defined by $\int_{-\infty}^{-a_N} f_N(u)du + \int_{a_N}^{\infty} f_N(u)du?$

5. Write down an expression for the mean number of patients required in a group sequential trial.

6. In a group sequential trial using Pocock boundaries, with overall type I error 0.05 and $N = 2$, what is the expected number of patients required?

7. Show explicitly that

$$\int_{-\infty}^{\infty} f_N(u;0)du = \Pr(|S_M| \leq a_M, M = 1,...,N-1)$$

for $N = 2$.

# 9

## Subgroups and Multiple Outcomes

### 9.1 The Role of Subgroups in Randomized Clinical Trials

The discussion of RCTs so far has focused on comparisons of two (or more) groups of patients. The results of the trial will, usually, be generalized to a wider population as defined by the eligibility criteria used when the patients were recruited. As such, the results will be taken to apply equally to all the patients in the trial.

However, the patients will not all be the same: they may be male or female, they may be adults or children, they may be breast-fed or bottle-fed, they may have tumors that have spread beyond the primary site or not. Moreover, it may occur to the investigators that the treatment might have different effects on the different types of patients. Indeed, it is natural for doctors to ask this type of question as they do not treat "average" patients — they treat the patient before them, and if the patient is female and they think that the drug may not work so well in females, then it is certainly relevant to ask if this really is the case. These more homogeneous groupings of patients are referred to as *subgroups*.

Although quite reasonable, this way of thinking needs to be approached carefully. The doctor not only knows that the patient is female but that she is a child, was bottle-fed as a baby, her parents do not have the disease, etc. If you try to find how the treatments compare using only the data on little girls who were bottle-fed and had no family history of the disease, you will probably find very few, if any, patients of this kind in your trial and little can learned about the treatment effect on them. You need to adopt a sensible compromise between, on the one hand asking questions about subgroups that are so refined they are too small to provide worthwhile evidence and, on the other hand, failing to find differences between important subgroups.

The analysis of subgroups of patients is essentially a secondary exercise. The number of patients needed for a trial will almost always be determined on the basis of the number of patients as a whole and not on the numbers in certain subgroups. It follows that analyses of subgroups will necessarily have less power to detect the difference originally postulated as important when the trial was planned.

There are two distinct problems when considering subgroup analysis, which are as follows:

1. Given the different subgroups, how do you assess if the treatment effect differs between them?
2. How do you choose the subgroups in the first place?

These questions will be addressed in turn.

## 9.2   Methods for Comparing Subgroups

In the following subsections a method for comparing simple subgroup effects is described. Throughout these sections, it is worth bearing in mind that we are not concerned directly with the size (or indeed the existence) of a treatment effect *per se*, but with the homogeneity of any effect there might be across the subgroups.

In the examples in this chapter, we will be concerned exclusively with subgroups that have two levels: male or female, breast-fed or bottle-fed, etc. However, subgroups can be determined with many levels: ABO blood group, eye color or, indeed, with a continuum of levels, as with age. We are interested in assessing whether the effect of one factor, the treatment group, is different at different levels of the factor or covariate determining the subgroup. In terms of statistical models, we are considering treatment by covariate interactions. For subgroups defined by a continuous variable or having more than two levels, the usual methods for testing interactions in statistical models can be applied. Although these can also be used for subgroups with just two levels, we develop some simple alternatives as described in the following text.

### 9.2.1   Approximate Theory

For a variable defining two subgroups of patients (you can think of them as males, M, and females, F), a simple piece of theory that gives an approximate test of the null hypothesis of equal treatment effect in the two subgroups and is applicable to several different kinds of outcome can be derived. The theory assumes the parameter estimates have normal distributions and that variation in estimates of standard errors can be ignored. This is usually sensible when the trial has reasonable size. It is foolish to attempt serious subgroup analyses in small trials as the subgroups will then be even smaller, and the whole exercise is likely to be fruitless.

Suppose the expectation of the outcome in subgroup $F$ is

$$\theta_A^F \text{ when given treatment A}$$

$$\theta_B^F \text{ when given treatment B}$$

Similar definitions for subgroup $M$ apply to $\theta_A^M, \theta_B^M$. The estimates of these quantities are, respectively, $\hat{\theta}_A^F, \hat{\theta}_B^F, \hat{\theta}_A^M, \hat{\theta}_B^M$, and the corresponding variances are $v_A^F, v_B^F, v_A^M, v_B^M$. The treatment effect in subgroup $F$ is $\tau_F = \theta_A^F - \theta_B^F$ and in $M$ is $\tau_M = \theta_A^M - \theta_B^M$.

The null hypothesis of interest is $\tau_F = \tau_M$ and a natural test statistic for this is

$$Z = \frac{(\hat{\theta}_A^F - \hat{\theta}_B^F) - (\hat{\theta}_A^M - \hat{\theta}_B^M)}{s.e.(numerator)}$$

and, under the null hypothesis, this will have a standard normal distribution. This is usually referred to as a *test of interaction*. Because $\hat{\theta}_A^F, \hat{\theta}_B^F, \hat{\theta}_A^M, \hat{\theta}_B^M$ are independent, the denominator of the preceding is found to be

$$\sqrt{(v_A^F + v_B^F) + (v_A^M + v_B^M)}$$

so a test of the null hypothesis is obtained by referring:

$$Z = \frac{(\hat{\theta}_A^F - \hat{\theta}_B^F) - (\hat{\theta}_A^M - \hat{\theta}_B^M)}{\sqrt{(v_A^F + v_B^F) + (v_A^M + v_B^M)}} \tag{9.1}$$

to a standard normal distribution. A 95% confidence interval for the difference between the treatment effects is

$$(\hat{\theta}_A^F - \hat{\theta}_B^F) - (\hat{\theta}_A^M - \hat{\theta}_B^M) \pm 1.96\sqrt{(v_A^F + v_B^F) + (v_A^M + v_B^M)}$$

Note that this is a difference in treatment effects: it is not a difference between those treated with A and those with B but of how the difference between the treatments does itself differ between the subgroups $F$ and $M$.

This theory will now be illustrated using two examples.

## 9.2.2 Practice: Continuous Outcomes

A controlled trial of vitamin D supplementation for the prevention of neonatal hypocalcemia (low levels of calcium, which can lead to rickets and

**TABLE 9.1**

Data from Neonatal Hypocalcemia Trial

|  | Breast-Fed | | Bottle-Fed | |
|---|---|---|---|---|
|  | Supplement | Placebo | Supplement | Placebo |
| Treatment mean | 2.445 | 2.408 | 2.300 | 2.195 |
| Number of babies n | 64 | 102 | 169 | 285 |
| SE | 0.0365 | 0.0311 | 0.0211 | 0.0189 |
| Treatment effect | 0.037 | | 0.105 | |
| SE | 0.0480 | | 0.0283 | |
| P-value | 0.44 | | 0.0002 | |

*Note:* All calcium levels in mmol/l.

other skeletal problems) was reported (Cockburn et al. 1980). Expectant mothers received either supplements of vitamin D or placebo. Several end-points were measured, but we will consider only the serum calcium of the baby at 1 week of age. It was thought that the effect of vitamin D supplementation might be different in babies who were breast-fed from those who were bottle-fed. Table 9.1 is based on data from the study.

The $\hat{\theta}_A^F, \hat{\theta}_B^F, \hat{\theta}_A^M, \hat{\theta}_B^M$ are the simple treatment means, given in the row "treatment mean" in Table 9.1. The sample variances of the treatment means, the $v_A^F, v_B^F, v_A^M, v_B^M$s of the previous subsection, are simply the usual variance for a mean, $s^2 / n$ and the SEs for the preceding treatment means are just the square roots of these.

The "treatment effect" row shows $\hat{\theta}_A^F - \hat{\theta}_B^F$ and $\hat{\theta}_A^M - \hat{\theta}_B^M$, and the corresponding standard errors are $\sqrt{v_A^F + v_B^F}$ and $\sqrt{v_A^M + v_B^M}$. To test the null hypothesis that the effect of vitamin D is the same for breast-fed and bottle-fed babies, we compute the quantity in Equation 9.1, namely

$$Z = \frac{0.037 - 0.105}{\sqrt{0.0365^2 + 0.0311^2 + 0.0211^2 + 0.0189^2}} = -\frac{0.068}{0.0557} = -1.22$$

which gives $P = \Phi(-1.22) + [1 - \Phi(1.22)] = 0.22$.

Thus, there is no evidence that vitamin D supplementation affects bottle-fed and breast-fed babies differently.

### 9.2.2.1   An Erroneous Analysis

At this point, it is worth taking a moment to discuss a flawed method for assessing subgroup effects. The P-values in Table 9.1 are those relevant to testing the null hypotheses:

$\theta_A^F = \theta_B^F$, i.e., no treatment effect in the breast-fed group

$\theta_A^M = \theta_B^M$, i.e., no treatment effect in the bottle-fed group

**TABLE 9.2**

Percentages and Proportions of Babies with RDS in Trial of Antenatal Steroid Therapy

| Pre-eclampsia Groups | Steroid Group | Placebo Group | P-Value |
|---|---|---|---|
| With pre-eclampsia | 21.2% 7/33 | 27.3% 9/33 | .57 |
| Without pre-eclampsia | 7.9% 21/267 | 14.1% 37/262 | .021 |

and are found by referring $(\hat{\theta}_A^F - \hat{\theta}_B^F) / \sqrt{v_A^F + v_B^F}$ and $(\hat{\theta}_A^M - \hat{\theta}_B^M) / \sqrt{v_A^M + v_B^M}$ to a standard normal distribution.

The *P*-values obtained for the breast-fed and bottle-fed groups are, respectively, 0.44 and 0.0002. The temptation is to say that there is a clear effect of vitamin D supplementation in bottle-fed babies but not in breast-fed babies, so the treatment works for the former but not the latter. This contradicts the analysis we have just presented, so which is correct? The answer is that the comparison of the two *P*-values does not demonstrate a subgroup effect. The value of 0.44 in the breast-fed group does not establish that there is no effect in this group, but merely that we have no evidence — perhaps the breast-fed group was too small to provide such evidence.

### 9.2.3 Practice: Binary Outcomes

When applying the methods from Subsection 9.2.1. To binary outcomes, the role of $\theta_A^F$, etc., is taken by the proportion of successes $\pi_A^F$ and

$$v_A^F = \frac{\pi_A^F(1 - \pi_A^F)}{n_A^F}$$

where $n_A^F$, etc., are the numbers of patients in the different groups.

The example of a subgroup effect when there is a binary outcome comes from a controlled trial of maternal steroids for the prevention of neonatal respiratory distress syndrome (RDS) in the baby. It is a trial of giving a drug (a steroid, dexamethasone) or a placebo to expectant mothers to see if using steroids in this way led to fewer of their babies having severe breathing difficulties. Unlike the previous example, the outcome is binary, i.e., whether or not the baby had RDS (Collaborative Group on Antenatal Steroid Therapy, 1981).

The subgroups to be studied here are whether or not the mother developed preeclampsia during her pregnancy (dangerously high blood pressure), see Table 9.2.

If we use $F$ to denote the mothers with pre-eclampsia and $M$ for the remainder, and A for steroid and B for placebo then:

$$\pi_A^F = 7/33 = 0.212 \quad v_A^F = 0.212 \times 0.788/33 \qquad \pi_B^F = 9/33 = 0.273 \quad v_B^F = 0.273 \times 0.727/33$$
$$= 0.00506 \qquad\qquad\qquad\qquad = 0.00601$$

$$\pi_A^M = 21/267 = 0.079 \quad v_A^M = 0.079 \times 0.921/267 \qquad \pi_B^M = 37/262 = 0.141 \quad v_B^M = 0.141 \times 0.859/262$$
$$= 0.000273 \qquad\qquad\qquad\qquad = 0.000462$$

The quantity from Equation 9.1 can now be written as

$$Z = \frac{(0.212 - 0.273) - (0.079 - 0.141)}{\sqrt{0.00506 + 0.00601 + 0.000273 + 0.000462}} = \frac{0.001}{0.109} = 0.0092$$

and $P = \Phi(-0.0092) + 1 - \Phi(0.0092) = 0.99$. This large $P$-value means there is no evidence that antenatal steroid therapy affects babies born to mothers suffering from preeclampsia differently from the way it affects babies born to mothers who do not suffer from this condition. Again comparison of $P$-values would have led us astray (see final column of Table 9.2). The treatment effects are similar in the two subgroups (as measured by the ARD, see subsection 7.3.1) and the difference in $P$-values arises from the different SEs, which in turn arises from the difference in the sizes of the two subgroups.

## 9.3    Methods of Selecting Subgroups

A subtle but important problem in the analysis of subgroups in RCTs is the question of how the subgroups arose in the first place. The patients in virtually any trial will exhibit many features that could be used to define subgroups. If the results of comparing treatment effects using many subgroups are reported, those reading the report will need to know why the comparisons were made. If subgroups defined by 20 variables are compared, then even if the null hypothesis is true, so that there is no treatment effect, you would expect one of the analyses to yield a result significant at the 5% level. This is intuitively obvious and can be seen more formally as follows. Suppose the $P$-value for the analysis testing the null hypothesis that treatment effect is the same for all subgroups determined by the $i$th variable is $P_i$. Define

$$I_i = 1 \text{ if } P_i < 0.05, \quad 0 \text{ otherwise}$$

As there is no treatment effect, for all $i$ $\Pr(I_i = 1) = 0.05$. The expected number of significant tests is

$$\mathrm{E}\left(\sum_{i=1}^{20} I_i\right) = \sum_{i=1}^{20} \mathrm{E}(I_i) = \sum_{i=1}^{20} \Pr(I_i = 1) = \sum_{i=1}^{20} 0.05 = 1$$

(Note that we do not assume that the $I$s are independent.) Thus, if there is indiscriminate identification of many subgroups, there is the chance that someone will appear to suggest a difference where none really exists. The critic will be suspicious that the investigator trawled through the data looking for something positive to report: these suspicions will be heightened if the overall result of the trial failed to reach a conventional level of statistical significance.

However, there may well be occasions when there is good reason to believe that the treatment effect is not the same for patients in different subgroups. In other trials marked differences in treatment effect may be observed and, if genuine, could be a finding of considerable importance. We must distinguish two sorts of subgroups.

1. Subgroups that were identified as being of potential interest before the data were collected. These should be limited in number, and there should be an apparent clinical or biological reason for the interest. For example, in the comparison of different types of compounds used to treat breathing difficulties in very premature babies, the timing of the administration of treatment is critical and closely controlled for babies born in the center running the trial. However, the close control of timing may not have been possible for babies born elsewhere and subsequently transferred to the center. The "outborn" and "in-born" babies form subgroups that are identified at the outset of the trial, and there is good prior reason to suspect that the effect of treatment may differ between these subgroups.

2. Subgroups whose apparent importance is *post hoc*, and arises only through the result of performing analyses on the data.

If the treatment effect appears to differ across subgroups identified as in 1, then the phenomenon should be taken much more seriously than if the subgroups came to light through the process in 2.

## Example 9.1: Subgroups Reported in the Antenatal Steroid Trial (Collaborative Group on Antenatal Steroid Therapy (1981))

Subgroups based on the following variables were reported.

1. Sex of baby: male, female
2. Mother developed preeclampsia or did not develop preeclampsia

3. Mode of delivery: vaginal, cesarean (in labor), cesarean (not in labor)
4. L/S ratio (a measure of maturity of baby): immature, not assessed
5. Race: White (not Hispanic), Black (not Hispanic), other
6. Duration in study: <24 h, 24 h to 1 week, >1 week
7. Gestational age at delivery: < 30 weeks, 30 to 34 weeks, > 34 weeks
8. Premature rupture of membranes: yes, no

Example 9.1 demonstrates the range of subgroup analyses that are sometimes reported for a trial. There is no indication in the paper how these subgroups were selected. A difference in the treatment effect between boys and girls was reported. However, no similar difference has been found in any subsequent trials of ante-natal steroid therapy (Crowley et al., 1990). This illustrates the hazardous nature of making inferences about subgroups.

## 9.4 Qualitative Interactions

A useful distinction between qualitative and quantitative interactions or subgroup differences has been made. In the latter, the size of the treatment effect varies between the subgroups, but it is always in the same direction, whereas in the former, one treatment is better for some patients and the other treatment is better for the remaining patients. It has been argued that quantitative interactions are not surprising and, indeed, can be functions of the scale on which the response is expressed, e.g., if a main effects model is appropriate once the response has been log-transformed, then it is inappropriate on the original scale. On the other hand, a qualitative interaction (sometimes called a *crossover* interaction) cannot be an artifact of the scale of measurement and, moreover, if it is genuine, it is clearly of great clinical importance. This is illustrated in Figure 9.1.

The figure represents a trial comparing two treatments split into two subgroups: the origin is no treatment effect in either group, and the diagonal shows equal treatment effects in the two subgroups. Quantitative, or non-crossover, interactions are represented by the unhatched parts not on the diagonal, whereas points in the shaded area showed interactions in which different treatments were superior in the two subgroups, that is, qualitative or crossover interactions.

An example in which the possibility of a qualitative interaction arose was the National Surgical Adjuvant Breast and Bowel Project trial that compared treatments for breast cancer with acronyms PFT and PF (PF is a chemotherapeutic agent and PFT is PF plus tamoxifen) in 1891 patients (Fisher et al., 1983). The following table (Table 9.3) is taken from Gail and Simon (1985) and shows the variation of treatment effect with age (above or below 50 years) and progesterone receptor status (PR: above or below 10 fmol).

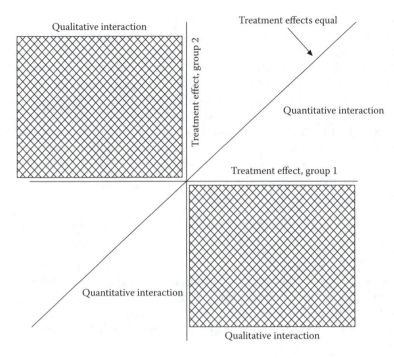

**FIGURE 9.1**

The regions in which interactions are quantitative or qualitative.

**TABLE 9.3**

Results from the National Surgical Adjuvant Breast and Bowel Project Trial

|  | Age < 50 PR < 10 | | Age ≥ 50 PR < 10 | | Age < 50 PR ≥ 10 | | Age ≥ 50 PR ≥ 10 | |
| --- | --- | --- | --- | --- | --- | --- | --- | --- |
|  | PF | PFT | PF | PFT | PF | PFT | PF | PFT |
| Proportion disease free at 3 years | 0.599 | 0.436 | 0.526 | 0.639 | 0.651 | 0.698 | 0.639 | 0.790 |
| SE | 0.0542 | 0.0572 | 0.0510 | 0.0463 | 0.0431 | 0.0438 | 0.0386 | 0.0387 |
| D | 0.163 | | −0.114 | | −0.047 | | −0.151 | |
| s | 0.0788 | | 0.0689 | | 0.0614 | | 0.0547 | |
| $D^2/s^2$ | 4.28 | | 2.72 | | 0.59 | | 7.58 | |

In this table, $D$ is the difference in proportions disease free between the treatment groups and $s$ is its SE.

At first sight, there appears to be an advantage to PF for women under 50 with PR < 10 but with PFT preferable for the other three groups. A standard test for interaction is highly significant ($P = 0.0097$). Clearly, such a conclusion would have a major impact on how the results of the trial were used. In such circumstances, it is important to use the most appropriate statistical procedure.

A problem with the standard test for interaction can be described as follows. Suppose there are $k$ subgroups and the treatment effects are $\theta_1,\dots,\theta_k$:

the standard test for interaction tests the null hypothesis $H_0 : \theta_1 = \theta_2 = \ldots = \theta_k$ against a general alternative, that is, one that includes both qualitative and quantitative interactions. A more specific test that is easily applied and based on a likelihood ratio test is available. This replaces the preceding null hypothesis with the hypothesis of no qualitative interaction, that is the vector of $\theta$s must lie in either the set of all positive effects or all negative effects, that is, $O^+ \cup O^-$ with $O^+ = \{\theta : \theta_i \geq 0 \text{ all } i\}$ and $O^- = \{\theta : \theta_i \leq 0 \text{ all } i\}$.

To apply the procedure, obtain estimates of the $\theta_i$ and their standard errors, say $D_i$ and $s_i$, and compute ($I(E)$ is the indicator function of event $E$)

$$Q^+ = \sum (D_i^2 / s_i^2) I(D_i > 0)$$

$$Q^- = \sum (D_i^2 / s_i^2) I(D_i < 0)$$

If $\min\{Q^+, Q^-\}$ exceeds $c(\alpha, k)$, then we can reject the hypothesis of no qualitative interaction; value of $c$ can be found in Gail and Simon (1985).

When applied to the preceding table, values obtained for $Q^+, Q^-$ are, respectively, 10.89 and 4.28, and as $c(0.05,4) = 5.43$ and $c(0.1,4) = 4.01$, we find $0.05 < P < 0.1$, so the evidence of a qualitative interaction is weaker than it was for a general interaction.

Qualitative interactions need careful analysis and the method of Gail and Simon is worth considering in these circumstances.

---

## 9.5   Multiple Outcomes

Thus far we have considered RCTs as experiments in which we assess the effect of a treatment on an outcome variable. The variable is carefully chosen to measure some important aspect of the disease being studied. However, in more general and colloquial terms, we are interested in which of the treatments makes the patient better or makes them get better more quickly. Being made better, although unquestionably relevant, is usually too subjective and difficult to define for scientific purposes. We reduce the problem to the measurement of an outcome variable in an attempt to make the task of measuring improvement in health more easily defined and reproducible. However, this reduction is achieved at the cost of trying to measure a very complex process, the well-being of a patient, in a single variable.

In fact, most clinical trials do not try to measure the well-being of a patient in a single variable but actually measure numerous variables relevant to the condition being studied. However, this raises statistical problems similar to those encountered when several subgroups are compared.

## Example 9.2: Outcome Measures for a Trial of Open vs. Laparoscopic (Key-Hole) Appendicectomy (Tate et al., 1993)

| | |
|---|---|
| 1. Doses of pethidine in first 24 h | 2. Total doses of pethidine (a pain killing drug) |
| 3. Hospital stay in days | 4. Wound infection |
| 5. Wound erythema (redness) | 6. Prolonged pyrexia (temperature) |
| 7. Time to reintroduction of liquid diet | 8. Urinary retention |
| 9. Requirement of analgesia | 10. VAS* score for pain in first 24 h |
| 11. VAS score for nausea in first 24 h | 12. Reintroduction of solid diet |
| 13. Respiratory complications | 14. Ileus (temporary paralysis of the bowel) |

* VAS = Visual analogue scale, marking a 10-cm line to represent severity of symptom.

The measurement of several outcomes is universal. In cardiovascular trials, it is common to record variables such as mortality (all causes), mortality (from ischemic heart disease [IHD]), incidence of myocardial infarction (heart attack), presence of IHD, cardiac output, ejection fraction, and walking distance. In cancer trials, as well as all causes mortality and disease specific-mortality, survival at several conventional times (usually 1, 2, and 5 years), tumor response, various cytometric measures of cell proliferation and, increasingly, measures of quality of life are recorded. In asthma trials measures of quality of life and frequency of attacks may often accompany the vast range of lung function and other tests, such as FEV1, PEFR, FVC, PD20 (all measurements of lung function).

One of the concerns that investigators have is that if there are several outcome variables, then the chance that at least one of them will provide a significant *P*-value will be larger than the nominal Type I error rate. Corrections for this have been devised and a rather crude one is described in the following section. However, two general comments should be made at this stage.

1. The severity of the problem should not be overstated. Although aimed at the overall goal of improving the health of the patient, it may be entirely legitimate to enquire what effect the treatment has on variables that often measure quite different aspects of the disease process. Put more crudely, if you ask 4 questions, you should expect 4 answers. Problems are most acute when the 4 questions are based on variables that measure very similar aspects of the disease.

2. You would tend to expect treatment effects to be consistent across the variables. For example, an exercise and diet program designed to improve cardiovascular fitness would be expected to: reduce blood pressure, lower blood cholesterol, and increase various measures of lung function. Techniques beyond the scope of this course are available that take account of such expectations.

## 9.6   Correction of $P$-Values

### 9.6.1   Boole's Inequality

It is useful to remind oneself of the following. Suppose $A_1, A_2, \ldots, A_k$ are events, then Boole's inequality is

$$\Pr\left(\bigcup_{i=1}^{k} A_i\right) \le \sum_{i=1}^{k} \Pr(A_i)$$

This is proved as follows. It is well-known and easy to show that for any events $A$ and $B$

$$\Pr(A \cup B) = \Pr(A) + \Pr(B) - \Pr(A \cap B) \le \Pr(A) + \Pr(B)$$

The proof of Boole's inequality follows by induction. It is clearly true for $k = 1$. If it is true for $k - 1$, then the preceding result for $A$ and $B$ applied with

$$B = \bigcup_{i=1}^{k-1} A_i$$

$A = A_k$ shows it is true for $k$, hence the result.

### 9.6.2   Application to RCTs

If there are $k$ outcomes and the corresponding treatment comparisons yield $P$-values $P_1, P_2, \ldots, P_k$ then even if the treatment has no effect on any of the outcomes, simply by chance, one of the $P$-values may be small. If we aim for an overall type I error rate of $100\alpha\%$, then it is not sufficient to consider a trial as confirming the superiority of one treatment simply if a single $P$ falls below $\alpha$. The Bonferroni inequality states that if the treatment has no effect then:

$$\Pr\left(\text{smallest } P \text{ value } \le \frac{\alpha}{k}\right) \le \alpha$$

The inequality follows by noting that under the null hypothesis, a $P$-value has a uniform distribution on $[0,1]$, so $\Pr(P_i \le \alpha / k) = \alpha / k$ for each $i$. The inequality follows by setting $A_i = \{P_i \le \alpha / k\}$, noting that the event that the smallest $P$-value is less than $\alpha / k$ is

$$\bigcup A_i$$

and applying Boole's inequality. Note that we do not assume the $P$s are independent, and indeed they are unlikely to be so as they arise from data collected on the same patients.

This inequality is used is to deem that a test is not significant at the $100\alpha\%$ level unless the corresponding $P$-value is less than $\alpha / k$.

The approach is not satisfactory for a variety of reasons. Perhaps the most important is that by concentrating on the minimum $P$-value, the method is very conservative. For example, if a trial had four outcomes and the resulting $P$-values were 0.01, 0.7, 0.8, 0.9 then the preceding procedure would consider the trial significant at the 5% level, whereas one with $P$-values 0.03, 0.04, 0.05, 0.05 would not be significant, despite a pattern that may seem to provide more consistent evidence against the null hypothesis.

Several alternative approaches exist and some of these are outlined briefly in Section 9.7 of this chapter. However, they are often not necessary because a commonsense approach can cause an important reduction in the scale of the problem. An extreme form is to designate one variable as the variable that will be subject to a hypothesis test. This is often too extreme and variables could be grouped such that each group measures a common aspect of the disease.

An example is provided by the appendicectomy trial in Example 9.2. The 14 variables come in different groups, each group measuring a specific aspect. The table in Example 9.2 can be rearranged to show the variables grouped according to whether variables measure aspects of "pain," "diet," "stay in hospital" and "complications in hospital," and "late complications" (see Table 9.4). As all the variables within a group will attempt to measure aspects that are related, they will often exhibit high correlations. This could lead to interpretational problems of several similar $P$-values. It may be possible to restrict hypothesis testing to one, preselected, variable within each group. Although there will still be several hypothesis tests, the problem is much more manageable with five as opposed to 14 tests.

## 9.7   Some Alternative Methods for Multiple Outcomes

This section outlines some of the more sophisticated methods that are available for dealing with multiple outcome measures in RCTs. They make use of statistical methods that are not needed elsewhere in this book and are not fully explained in this text. Some readers may wish to omit this section.

**TABLE 9.4**

Outcomes in Appendicectomy Trial Arranged by Outcome Type

---

**Outcome Measures in Open vs. Laparoscopic Appendicectomy Trial**

---

*Pain*

  1. Doses of pethidine in first 24 h      2. Total doses of pethidine
  3. Requirement of analgesia            4. VAS score in first 24 h

*Diet*

  5. Reintroduction of liquid diet      6. Reintroduction of solid diet
  7. VAS score for nausea

*Stay*

  8. Hospital stay

*Complications in hospital*

  9. Ileus                           10. Retention of urine
11. Respiratory complications      12. Prolonged pyrexia
13. Wound erythema

*Late complications*

14. Wound infection

---

### 9.7.1　Extension to Bonferroni Inequality

It was mentioned that the Bonferroni inequality outlined in Subsection 9.6.2 was conservative because it considered only the smallest $P$-value. A modified Bonferroni procedure, proposed by Simes (1986), is based on all the ordered $P$-values, $P_{(1)} \leq P_{(2)} \leq \ldots \leq P_{(k)}$ rather than just $P_{(1)}$: the trial is considered positive if $P_{(j)} \leq j\alpha/k$ for any $j = 1, \ldots, k$. If the $P$-values are independent, then the procedure has overall type I error of $\alpha$. In the general case, unlike with the classical Bonferroni inequality, the procedure is not conservative. However, the procedure has type I error rate much closer to $\alpha$ than the classical version for a wide variety of correlation patterns. Under this procedure the second set of $P$-values in Subsection 9.6.2 would be considered significant.

### 9.7.2　Multivariate Methods

A more general approach to the problem of multiple outcomes is to consider that the outcome from each patient is a $k$-dimensional vector, that is, all the outcomes are considered simultaneously. The null hypothesis when comparing treatments A and B would then be $\tau = \mu_A - \mu_B = 0$, with each element in this equation now a $k$-dimensional vector. The multivariate analogue of the $t$-test is Hotelling $T^2$ test, which refers:

$$\frac{n_A n_B (n-k-1)}{nk(n-2)} (\bar{x}_A - \bar{x}_B) S^{-1} (\bar{x}_A - \bar{x}_B)$$

to an $F$ distribution with $k$ and $n - k - 1$ degrees of freedom. Here $\bar{x}_A, \bar{x}_B$ are the sample means on treatments A and B, based on $n_A, n_B$ patients, respectively, and $S$ is the pooled sample dispersion matrix and $n = n_A + n_B$.

It is very unlikely that all outcomes from an RCT will be continuous, so the assumption this method makes that all the outcomes have a normal distribution is unrealistic. Even if this were the case, the test will lack power. This is because the test is of $\tau = 0$ vs. $\tau \neq 0$. The alternative to the test, therefore, accepts deviations from the null hypothesis in any direction for each outcome. In practice, if a treatment is superior, it will tend to change related outcomes in consistent ways. For example, in Example 9.2, an earlier reintroduction of a solid diet would be expected to be associated with a lower VAS for nausea.

O'Brien (1984) has proposed several tests that attempt to focus attention on alternative hypotheses which indicate consistent departures from the null hypothesis. The method described here attempts to combine information across variables that will be defined on different scales, so the variables must first be transformed to a common scale. This is done by taking the difference from the variable's mean, computed ignoring the treatment groups, and divided by the pooled within-treatment standard deviation. In the following, it is assumed that this has already been done.

The procedure can be motivated by the model

$$\mu_A = \mu + \beta 1 \text{ and } \mu_B = \mu - \beta 1$$

where 1 is the $k$-dimensional vector of ones. This model effectively states that we expect similar deviations on all (standardized) variables. If this is the case, then it is intuitive that we can get a more sensitive test of a treatment effect by looking at the mean of the standardized variables on each patient. This amounts to testing the null hypothesis $\beta = 0$ by referring

$$\frac{n_A n_B \{1^T (\bar{y}_A - \bar{y}_B)\}^2}{n 1^T S 1}$$

to $F$ on 1 and $n - 2$ degrees of freedom. In this formula, $\bar{y}_i$ is the sample mean vector of the standardized variables in the group receiving treatment $i$. If the $j$th standardized variable on patient $\ell$ is $y_{\ell j}$, then the preceding amounts to a simple univariate two sample $t$-test of the two sets of within-patient means, $\bar{y}_\ell = k^{-1}(y_{\ell 1} + y_{\ell 2} + ... + y_{\ell k})$. Modifications of the tests to allow variation from the null hypothesis in different, but still prespecified directions, have been discussed and amount to replacing the vector 1 in the preceding with a different, but known vector.

### 9.7.3 O'Brien's Rank-Based Method

It is commonplace to find that several important outcomes are not normally distributed; for example, outcomes will often be categorical. The following rank-based approach is a useful and efficient method that should work with a range of variables from normal through non-normal continuous to categorical, provided that the grouping of the last is not too coarse. Suppose that the data are arranged as follows:

| Treatment Group | Patient | Variable 1 | Variable 2 | ... | ... | Variable k |
|---|---|---|---|---|---|---|
| A | 1 | $Y_{A11}$ | $Y_{A12}$ | | | $Y_{A1k}$ |
| A | 2 | $Y_{A21}$ | $Y_{A22}$ | | | $Y_{A2k}$ |
| B | 1 | $Y_{B11}$ | $Y_{B12}$ | | | $Y_{B1k}$ |
| | | | | $Y_{ijk}$ | | |
| B | $n_B$ | $Y_{Bn_B1}$ | $Y_{Bn_B2}$ | | | $Y_{Bn_Bk}$ |

The procedure starts by replacing each observation with its within-column rank, that is, by its within-variable rank (that is the only rank one could sensibly take, you cannot rank a blood pressure and a heart rate!). The result is shown in the following table, where the $S_{ij}$ are the within-patient sums of ranks, namely:

$$S_{Xi} = \sum_{\ell=1}^{k} R_{Xi\ell}$$

where X = A or B. If a treatment tends to produce a favorable effect across the variables, then the ranks across the variables will be lower in this treatment group, and so the rank sums will also be lower in that treatment group. The test is accomplished by performing a *t*-test to compare the $S_{ij}$ between $i$ = A and $i$ = B.

The method can be used for more than two groups, in which the $S_{ij}$ are compared using a one-way analysis of variance.

| Treatment Group | Patient | Ranks of Variables 1 | Ranks of Variables 2 | ... | ... | Ranks of Variables k | Rank sum |
|---|---|---|---|---|---|---|---|
| A | 1 | $R_{A11}$ | $R_{A12}$ | | | $R_{A1k}$ | $S_{A1}$ |
| A | 2 | $R_{A21}$ | $R_{A22}$ | | | $R_{A2k}$ | $S_{A2}$ |
| B | 1 | $R_{B11}$ | $R_{B12}$ | | | $R_{B1k}$ | $S_{B1}$ |
| | | | | | | | $S_b n_b$ |
| B | $n_B$ | $R_{Bn_g1}$ | $R_{Bn_g2}$ | | | $R_{Bn_gk}$ | |

## Exercises

1. In a trial to compare the effects of a diuretic (D) and beta-blocker (B) on blood pressure, the null hypothesis of no treatment effect was tested separately in males and females, giving $P$-values of 0.03 and 0.4, respectively. Does this provide evidence that the treatment affects males and females differently? Justify your answer.

2. A clinical trial is performed to compare two treatments, A and B, that are intended to treat psoriasis (a scaly, itchy skin condition). The outcome shown in the following table is whether the patient's skin cleared within 16 weeks of the start of treatment, i.e., a binary variable. The data are shown separately for those with fair and dark skins.

|  | Fair Skin | | Dark Skin | |
| --- | --- | --- | --- | --- |
|  | Treatment A | Treatment B | Treatment A | Treatment B |
| Cleared | 9 | 5 | 10 | 3 |
| Did not clear | 17 | 21 | 15 | 20 |

*Source*: Data available by kind permission of Professor P.M. Farr, Department of Dermatology, Royal Victoria Infirmary, Newcastle upon Tyne, U.K.

a. Test, separately for patients with fair and dark skin, the null hypothesis that the proportion of patients whose skins cleared is the same for the two treatments. Present your analyses. Does this provide evidence that the treatment affects patients with fair and dark skins differently?

b. Test the null hypothesis that the treatment effect is the same for patients with fair and dark skins. Give a $P$-value and a 95% confidence interval for a suitably defined quantity.

# 10

## *Protocols and Protocol Deviations*

### 10.1 Protocols: Their Nature and Role

There are virtually no RCTs run today that do not have a trial protocol. The trial protocol is a document that serves several purposes. Broadly, these fall into three groups.

1. The reasons why a trial needs to be run in the first place are documented in the protocol: this will include descriptions of the inadequacies of existing therapies and of the ways the new treatment or treatments might improve matters.

2. The protocol is an operations manual for the trial. For example, how the patients are assessed for eligibility and by whom, where blood samples are to be sent, how treatment allocations are to be made, what treatments are to be used and their doses, who is allowed to know who gets what treatment, when outcomes are to be assessed — all these should and more be specified in the protocol.

3. The protocol is the scientific design document for the trial. The methods for allocation, the ways of assessing outcomes, the size of the trial are all justified in the protocol. In addition, the conduct of a clinical trial is improved if certain decisions are taken, and are seen to be taken, before data are collected. Such decisions are documented in the protocol.

The protocol can be a complicated document that evolves through several stages before the first patient is recruited. Different agencies will have interests that require them to accord different emphases to the different aspects of the protocol. Ethics committees and funding bodies will often concentrate on 1, whereas editors of medical journals and regulatory authorities (which assess certain types of trial to see if drugs can be put on the market) will scrutinize 3. Those involved in the trial on a day-to-day basis will concentrate on 2.

The way a trial is reported is of the utmost importance if those in the wider community are to learn about the results and to be convinced by them. A group of those interested in good trial methodology, together with editors of leading medical journals have cooperated to produce the CONSORT statement, which amounts to guidelines regarding how a trial should be reported. A convincing (and honest) report of a study can only arise from a convincing study, so the guidelines are well worth consulting when designing a trial and writing the accompanying protocol. The output of the CONSORT group can be found at http://www.consort-statement.org.

It is not the intention of this book to prepare readers immediately to take on the role of a trial statistician, so we will say much less about protocols than could be said, and roles 1 and 2 will be ignored. Discussion of role 3 will be brief, but there are statistical issues that should be mentioned.

Numerous problems that might be termed *problems of multiplicity* occur in the conduct of an RCT. Examples of these which have been mentioned already in this book are the following:

1. Which subgroups should be examined to see if differences in treatment effect exist?
2. Which of the outcome variables is of primary importance and which are secondary?
3. Should outcomes be compared using baseline information, and if so, how? Should the outcome variable be transformed?

If answering these questions is left until after the data are collected, then the results of the trial may be given less credence than might otherwise be the case. This is because the results will be open to the suspicion that the choices made in 1 to 3 may have been made to enhance the apparent effect of one treatment at the expense of the others. The choices do not need to have been made in this way for the trial to be less compelling — the inability of the investigators to exclude the possibility of this form of bias is sufficient to damage the trial. If the choices were all made and documented in the protocol, then they could not have been influenced by the results, and the trial would command greater respect. Indeed, some journals now make a preliminary decision to publish a trial on the basis of the protocol, not soley on the basis of the results, as a means of avoiding publication bias (cf. Subsection 2.2.4).

---

## 10.2  Protocol Deviation

The protocol describes which patients should be recruited to the trial, how they are treated and monitored during the trial, and how they are assessed at its conclusion. However, even in the best-run trials, things will happen that ensure that not all patients adhere to the protocol. Patients may not take the tablets in the quantities and at the times specified in the protocol, they may not turn up at the clinic for outcome measurements to be assessed or they may assert their right to withdraw from the study. If such problems affect a high proportion of the patients in the trial, then the whole study could be undermined. Such protocol deviations have serious and sometimes surprisingly subtle consequences. We will illustrate these by considering two specific forms of protocol deviation, namely treating patients that are not eligible for the trial and those given a treatment other than that which was allocated by the randomization.

### 10.2.1 Ineligible Patients

In 1966, the British Medical Research Council (MRC) conducted an RCT to compare surgery and radiotherapy for the treatment of operable lung cancer. Only patients who were thought to be suitable for surgery were entered into the trial, but in 1966 the imaging technology available to help to assess suitability for surgery was much less advanced than it is now.

The situation illustrated in Figure 10.1 arose. Some patients with inoperable tumors were entered into the study because the preoperative assess-

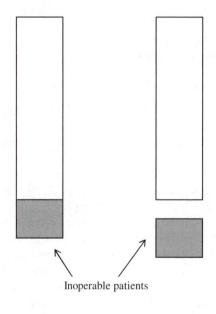

Inoperable patients

Radiotherapy
group

Surgery group

**FIGURE 10.1**
An example of ineligible patients in a trial.

ment of the status of the tumor was mistaken. Often this would be because of the precise location of the tumor within the lung or thorax. If allocated to surgery, the surgeon would, at operation, be able to identify the patient as one on whom the operation could not proceed as planned, and the mistaken assessment of an operable tumor would be revealed. However, if the patient had been allocated to the radiotherapy group, the mistake would not have come to light.

This poses a major problem for the trial. The patients in the unshaded surgery group in Figure 10.1 (those on whom the surgeon could operate) cannot be compared with those in the unshaded radiotherapy group because we cannot identify these patients. Randomization ensures that similar proportions of patients with inoperable tumors appear in both treatment groups. However, patients with inoperable tumors are likely to have more advanced cancer and have a shorter life expectancy. Consequently, comparing the unshaded surgery group with the entire radiotherapy group will bias the comparison in favor of surgery because the radiotherapy group contains a subgroup of patients with poorer prognoses that has been excluded from the surgery group.

An approach to dealing with this problem is outlined in Section 10.3 of this chapter.

### 10.2.2    Administration of Treatment Other than That Allocated

Patients sometimes receive treatments other than the one allocated at randomization. This can occur for several reasons, including:

1. Refusal by the patient to take the allocated treatment.
2. Failure to comply with the treatment regimen specified in the protocol.
3. The doctor imposes a change in the interests of the well-being of the patient.

An example of problems arising from 3 is shown in Table 10.1, which relates to a trial in which medical and surgical treatments for angina were compared (European Coronary Surgery Study Group, 1979). Patients were randomly allocated to surgical or medical groups but surgery was performed on some of the patients allocated to medical treatment and some patients allocated to surgery did not have an operation and received medical treatment. Numbers of patients in these groups, together with the numbers who did receive the treatment to which they were allocated, are given in Table 10.1.

An important outcome variable was whether or not the patient was alive 2 years after they entered the study. The percentage of patients in each category who died within 2 years of entry to the study is also shown in the table.

**TABLE 10.1**

Outcomes in Angina Trial

| | Allocated to Surgical Treatment | | Allocated to Medical Treatment | |
|---|---|---|---|---|
| | Actually Received Surgical Treatment | Actually Received Medical Treatment | Actually Received Surgical Treatment | Actually Received Medical Treatment |
| Number of patients | 369 | 26 | 48 | 323 |
| Two-year mortality rate (number and percentage) | 15  4.1% | 6  23.1% | 2  4.0% | 27  8.4% |

*Source:* European Coronary Surgery Study Group (1979), Coronary-artery bypass surgery in stable angina pectoris: survival at two years, *Lancet*, i, 889–893.

If we compare the groups who actually received the treatment they were intended to have, we find that the 2-year mortality on surgery (4.1%, 15 deaths out of 369 patients) compares favorably with that on medical treatment (8.4%, 27 deaths out of 323 patients). Applying a $\chi^2$ test gives $P = 0.018$, suggesting that the difference has not arisen by chance.

On the other hand if we compare the groups as they were formed by randomization, then surgical treatment does not appear to do so well.

$$\text{Mortality for those allocated to surgical treatment is } \frac{6 + 15}{26 + 369} = 5.3\%$$

$$\text{Mortality for those allocated to medical treatment is } \frac{2 + 27}{48 + 323} = 7.8\%$$

Applying a $\chi^2$ test gives $P = 0.16$, so chance now becomes a plausible explanation of the observed difference between the treatments.

A clue about what might be going on comes from the high mortality (23.1%) attached to patients randomized to surgery but who received medical treatment. It is a strong possibility that these patients were sufficiently ill that the surgeon did not believe that an operation was in their best interests — their chances of surviving it were too low to proceed — so they were given the medical option. Similar patients allocated to medical treatment would simply proceed with their allotted treatment. Hence, in the comparison between those who received the treatments to which they were allocated, a group of high-risk patients has been removed from the surgery group. It follows that this comparison is biased and potentially misleading.

A safer option is to compare the groups as formed by randomization, notwithstanding the fact that some of those allocated to surgery got medicine and vice versa. A rationale for this, both mathematical and clinical, is given in the next section.

## 10.3   Analysis by Intention-to-Treat

### 10.3.1   Informal Description

When faced with all manner of deviations from the protocol, not just the preceding descriptions, there is no entirely satisfactory solution. However, there is a guiding rule that should only be broken in the full knowledge of the potential consequences. The principle is that you should compare the groups as they were formed by randomization, regardless of what has subsequently happened to the patients. You are not necessarily analyzing the patients according to how they were treated, but according to how you intended to treat them. Because of this, the principle is often referred to as the dictum of *analysis by intention-to-treat*.

The justification of the approach is that any other way of grouping the patients cannot be guaranteed to have been comparable at the start of the study. Admittedly, you will often compare groups that are "contaminated" in some way — in the example in Subsection 10.2.2, each allocated treatment group contains a few patients who are given the other treatment.

Although there are no fully satisfactory solutions, comparing apparently strange groups can often be viewed in ways that make the comparison seem less strange. In the example in Subsection 10.2.1, if surgery turned out to be the treatment of choice in the future, then patients found to have inoperable tumors only at surgery would continue to arise. We would need to decide how to treat such patients; in the MRC trial they were offered radiotherapy. In other words, there will never be a time in clinical practice when surgery is appropriate for all patients, and the provision of alternatives for those whose tumors cannot be excised is implicit in the allocation of surgery. Consequently, a more realistic approach is to view the trial as comparing "the policy of offering surgery but accepting that some will need to resort to radiotherapy with the policy of offering radiotherapy."

The comparison of the groups as randomized is then an appropriate way to compare these policies.

## 10.3.2 Theoretical Description

A more mathematical description can be given. It is rather simplistic but illustrates the issues quite clearly. For definiteness, we will use the example of the surgery vs. radiotherapy trial, although the principle applies more widely.

The outcome, survival time, $X$, is supposed to have different means for different types of patients and these are listed below.

1. Operable tumors allocated to radiotherapy have mean, say, $\mu_O + \tau_R = E(X \mid O, R)$
2. Operable tumors allocated to surgery have mean $\mu_O + \tau_S = E(X \mid O, S)$
3. Inoperable tumors allocated to radiotherapy have mean $\mu_I + \tau_R = E(X \mid I, R)$
4. Inoperable tumors allocated to surgery have mean $\mu_I + \tau_R = E(X \mid I, S)$

The terms $\mu_O, \mu_I$ represent the mean survival time for the patients with, respectively, operable and inoperable tumors (and it is likely that $\mu_O > \mu_I$). The change in mean survival time that surgery and radiotherapy confer are, respectively, $\tau_S, \tau_R$, and the aim of the trial is to estimate $\tau_R - \tau_S$. Note that the mean in group 4 contains the term $\tau_R$ rather than $\tau_S$ because patients in the surgery group with inoperable tumors receive radiotherapy.

Suppose that the proportion of patients who have inoperable tumors is $\lambda$, which, because of randomization, we expect to be the same in the two groups. We write $\Pr(I) = \lambda$ for the probability that a patient has an inoperable tumor, and $\Pr(O)$ for the complementary probability.

The mean survival time in the radiotherapy group is

$$E(X \mid R) = \Pr(I)E(X \mid I, R) + \Pr(O)E(X \mid O, R)$$
$$= \lambda(\mu_I + \tau_R) + (1 - \lambda)(\mu_O + \tau_R)$$
$$= \lambda\mu_I + (1 - \lambda)\mu_O + \tau_R$$

If the radiotherapy group were compared with the group of patients who actually received surgery, then we would be comparing this mean with a group that has mean $\mu_O + \tau_S$. Consequently, the difference in treatment means would have expectation:

$$E(X \mid R) - E(X \mid O, S) = \lambda\mu_I + (1 - \lambda)\mu_O + \tau_R - (\mu_O + \tau_S)$$
$$= \lambda(\mu_I - \mu_O) + \tau_R - \tau_S$$

As we do not expect $\mu_O$ to equal $\mu_I$, the comparison of these groups provides a biased estimator. Moreover, the presence of the $\mu$ parameters means that we have little idea how this quantity relates to the quantity of interest $\tau_R - \tau_S$.

The mean survival time for the group allocated to surgery, regardless of which treatment they actually received, is

$$E(X \mid S) = \Pr(I)E(X \mid I, S) + \Pr(O)E(X \mid O, S)$$
$$= \lambda(\mu_I + \tau_R) + (1 - \lambda)(\mu_O + \tau_S)$$
$$= \lambda\mu_I + (1 - \lambda)\mu_O + \lambda(\tau_R - \tau_S) + \tau_S$$

and the difference between the means of the groups as randomized is, therefore:

$$E(X \mid R) - E(X \mid S) = [\lambda\mu_I + (1 - \lambda)\mu_O + \tau_R] - [\lambda\mu_I + (1 - \lambda)\mu_O + \lambda(\tau_R - \tau_S) + \tau_S]$$
$$= (1 - \lambda)(\tau_R - \tau_S)$$

Again we get a biased result, but this time, the bias only depends on the quantity of interest, $\tau_R - \tau_S$ and $\lambda$. We know that $(1 - \lambda)(\tau_R - \tau_S)$ is an attenuated version of $\tau_R - \tau_S$, as $0 < \lambda < 1$. Also, we see that the comparison is unbiased when $\lambda = 0$, i.e., when there are no patients with inoperable tumors (so there would not have been a problem in the first place). The groups are identical if $\lambda = 1$, i.e., if all patients have inoperable tumors so no one ends up with surgery and the comparison is then vacuous.

The preceding derivation makes many dubious assumptions, so it would be unwise to suppose that in these (and related) circumstances, the comparison of randomized groups necessarily leads to an attenuated estimate of the treatment effect. Nevertheless, the results are not without an aspect of realism and do serve to illustrate the nature of the difficult problem that the intention-to-treat dictum attempts to address.

Because comparisons of the groups as randomized is the only comparison that is based on comparable groups, it should always be presented in the report of the trial. Other analyses, such as the comparison of the groups of patients who were actually treated as specified in the protocol (usually called the *per protocol* analysis) can be presented but should be interpreted cautiously.

---

## Exercises

1. Pain from muscle strains generally lasts about two weeks. A trial was performed to compare a fortnight of treatment with one of two types of painkiller for the relief of pain from this condition. One treatment was paracetamol (acetaminophen) with codeine (C) and the other was indomethacin (I). About 20% of the patients randomized to I complained of stomach pains within 2 d of starting treatment and had to stop taking the treatment. Your clinical colleague suggests comparing those allocated to C with those who completed two weeks taking I. What is wrong with this strategy? What comparison should be made? This would be an instance of what dictum?

# 11

## Some Special Designs: Crossovers, Equivalence, and Clusters

The trials considered so far have all been of a simple kind, often referred to as *parallel group designs*, in which individual patients are allocated to one of the treatments under investigation, and the intention is to assess if the treatments used differ. However, there are many other kinds of trials, and three more specialized designs will be described in this chapter. In crossover trials, patients may receive, in turn, several of the treatments under investigation. In cluster randomized trials, it is not individual patients but groups of patients or other subjects who are randomized to different treatments. Equivalence trials seek to establish equivalence, rather than difference, between treatments.

## 11.1 Crossover Trials

In all the trials considered so far in this book, each patient has received just one of the treatments being compared. This is natural for a majority of diseases and conditions. Investigation of a new material for use in the construction of plasters for fractures, new approaches to removing the appendix and antithrombolytic treatment (preventing blood clots) following heart attacks are examples of trials in which each patient will have the opportunity of only one treatment. However, what about conditions such as asthma and diabetes, which cannot be cured? What about comparing different dialyzer membranes for patients having kidney dialysis thrice a week? Such patients could be given several treatments.

Trials in which the aim is not to cure a condition present the possibility of giving more than one treatment to each patient. Such trials are known as *crossover trials*.

The main advantage of using a crossover trial is that the outcome of a patient when given treatment A is not compared to the outcome from some different patients given treatment B but to the outcome from the same patient when given B. Crossover trials therefore seem to offer the possibility of obtaining more precise treatment comparisons.

## 11.2 The AB/BA Design

For two treatments, the simplest form of crossover design would be to give each patient treatment A and then follow it with B. However, the results would be ambiguous for a reason that has two forms.

1. If A appeared worse than B, it may be that the treatment given second does better, whatever it is, and had we given the treatments in the opposite order, it would have been B that fared worse. This is not entirely fanciful; if blood pressures are measured serially, they are commonly found to be higher the first few times they are measured.
2. If all the patients start the trial at the same time, there may be a trend that affects the outcomes. One instance might be if all the readings from the laboratory were higher on Monday than Tuesday.

To overcome this, the simplest form of crossover trial that is used randomly allocates patients to two groups. Patients in group 1 receive the treatments in the order AB, whereas those in group 2 receive them in the opposite order. The times when treatments are given are referred to as *treatment periods* or simply, *periods*. The design is represented schematically in the following table.

Treatment Allocations in the AB/BA Design

|         | Period 1 | Period 2 |
| ------- | -------- | -------- |
| Group 1 | A        | B        |
| Group 2 | B        | A        |

This design overcomes the problems described in 1 and 2. If A appears to do worse than B in group 1, this can only be ascribed to an order or period effect if B appears to do worse than A in group 2.

## 11.3 Analysis of AB/BA Design for Continuous Outcomes

### 11.3.1 The Theory

An analysis needs to take account of several features.

1. It should ensure that pairs of measurements from a single patient be kept together, in some sense.
2. There may be systematic differences between the treatment periods as well as treatment effects.

In the following it is assumed that the numbers of patients allocated to groups 1 and 2 are $n_1$ and $n_2$, respectively. It will also be assumed that the outcome has a normal distribution.

The analysis starts from a model for the outcome. In group 1, the outcome on patient $i$ ($i = 1, \ldots, n_1$) in period $j$ ($j = 1,2$) is assumed to be $x_{ij}$. For $i = 1, \ldots, n_1$,

$$x_{i1} = \mu + \pi_1 + \tau_A + \xi_i + \varepsilon_{i1} \text{ (period 1) and } x_{i2} = \mu + \pi_2 + \tau_B + \xi_i + \varepsilon_{i2} \text{ (period 2)}$$

Here, $\pi_j$ ($j = 1,2$) is the systematic effect of period $j$, $\tau_A, \tau_B$ are the systematic effects of treatment, and $\mu$ is a general mean. The term $\xi_i$ represents the effect of the $i$th patient. Patients may have a tendency to always give a high or low response, and we model this by taking $\xi_i$ to be a normal random variable with mean 0 and variance $\sigma_B^2$. Note that the same realization of $\xi_i$ appears in the outcome for both periods. The $\varepsilon$ terms are independent error terms with zero mean and variance $\tilde{\sigma}^2$.

For group 2, an identical argument gives, for $i = n_1 + 1, \ldots, n_1 + n_2$,

$$x_{i1} = \mu + \pi_1 + \tau_B + \xi_i + \varepsilon_{i1} \text{ (period 1) and } x_{i2} = \mu + \pi_2 + \tau_A + \xi_i + \varepsilon_{i2} \text{ (period 2)}$$

The term $\xi_i$ represents the variability that exists between patients. However, this should not affect our analysis as the adoption of a crossover design has effectively eliminated this source of variation. This gives the clue on how to proceed most simply. We can remove $\xi_i$ from the analysis by taking differences within each patient. The differences in group 1 are:

$$d_i = x_{i1} - x_{i2} = \pi + \tau + \eta_i \quad i = 1, \ldots, n_1$$

where $\pi = \pi_1 - \pi_2$, $\tau = \tau_A - \tau_B$, and $\eta_i = \varepsilon_{i1} - \varepsilon_{i2}$. The first of these parameters measures the difference between the treatment periods, the second is what we are interested in, namely, the difference between the treatments, and the third is another error term, with zero mean and variance $\sigma^2 = 2\tilde{\sigma}^2$. In group 2, the differences are:

$$d_i = x_{i1} - x_{i2} = \pi - \tau + \eta_i \quad i = n_1 + 1, \ldots, n_1 + n_2$$

Therefore, the expected value of the differences in group 1 is $\pi + \tau$ and in group 2 is $\pi - \tau$. If there is no treatment difference, then $\tau = 0$, and the two sets of differences have the same expectation. In other words, the hypothesis of no treatment difference in the AB/BA design is tested simply by using a two-sample $t$-test to compare the two sets of within-patient differences.

If the mean sample difference in group $k$ is $\bar{d}_k$, $k = 1,2$ then $E(\bar{d}_1 - \bar{d}_2) = 2\tau$. So, an estimate of the treatment difference $\tau$ is $\frac{1}{2}(\bar{d}_1 - \bar{d}_2)$. A confidence interval for $\tau$ can be found by dividing the ends of the usual confidence interval for the difference between the means of the two sets of differences by 2. This procedure is illustrated in the following text.

Note that the term $\xi_i$ was eliminated from the analysis by taking differences. Hence, the precision of the results depends only on the variance of the $\varepsilon$s, $\tilde{\sigma}^2$ and not on the variance of $\xi_i$, $\sigma_B^2$. For outcomes that differ much more between individuals than within individuals, the elimination of a relatively large variance component $\sigma_B^2$ from analysis is valuable. This is a mathematical expression of the intuitive observations that it is better to use a patient as his or her own control.

### 11.3.2    An Application

Children suffering from enuresis (bed wetting) are given a drug to alleviate their problem. The drug is given for a fortnight, and the outcome is the number of dry nights (out of 14) observed. The control drug is a placebo. Patients are allocated to group 1, in which the drug is given for a fortnight. At the end of this period, a placebo is administered for a fortnight and the same outcome variable is recorded. In group 2, the placebo is given first followed by the drug. The data for 29 patients are shown in Table 11.1.

The mean differences in the two groups are

$$\text{Group 1: } \bar{d}_1 = 2.824 \quad \text{Group 2: } \bar{d}_2 = -1.25$$

The mean in group 1 is positive, and as this is the mean of differences (drug-placebo), it suggests that the number of dry nights is larger on the drug than the placebo. The mean in group 2 is negative, and as this is the mean of differences (placebo-drug), it again suggests that the number of dry nights is larger on the drug than the placebo.

Does this stand up to more careful scrutiny? To do this we compare the two sets of differences using a two-sample $t$-test. Doing this in Minitab, with group 1 differences in a column named *Group 1*, etc., we obtain the following output:

```
Two-Sample T for Group 1 vs. Group 2
N          Mean     StDev      SE     Mean
Group 1    17       2.82      3.47    0.84
Group 2    12      -1.25      2.99    0.86
```

**TABLE 11.1**

Data from Enuresis Trial: Number of Dry Nights out of 14

| | Group 1 Drug > Placebo | | | | Group 2 Placebo > Drug | | |
|---|---|---|---|---|---|---|---|
| Patient | Period 1 | Period 2 | Difference | Patient | Period 1 | Period 2 | Difference |
| 1 | 8 | 5 | 3 | 18 | 12 | 11 | 1 |
| 2 | 14 | 10 | 4 | 19 | 6 | 8 | -2 |
| 3 | 8 | 0 | 8 | 20 | 13 | 9 | 4 |
| 4 | 9 | 7 | 2 | 21 | 8 | 8 | 0 |
| 5 | 11 | 6 | 5 | 22 | 8 | 9 | -1 |
| 6 | 3 | 5 | -2 | 23 | 4 | 8 | -4 |
| 7 | 13 | 12 | 1 | 24 | 8 | 14 | -6 |
| 8 | 10 | 2 | 8 | 25 | 2 | 4 | -2 |
| 9 | 6 | 0 | 6 | 26 | 8 | 13 | -5 |
| 10 | 0 | 0 | 0 | 27 | 9 | 7 | 2 |
| 11 | 7 | 5 | 2 | 28 | 7 | 10 | -3 |
| 12 | 13 | 13 | 0 | 29 | 7 | 6 | -1 |
| 13 | 8 | 10 | -2 | | | | |
| 14 | 7 | 7 | 0 | | | | |
| 15 | 9 | 0 | 9 | | | | |
| 16 | 10 | 6 | 4 | | | | |
| 17 | 2 | 2 | 0 | | | | |

*Source:* Data from Armitage P., Hills, M. (1982), The two-period crossover trial, *The Statistician*, 31, 119–131.

```
95% CI for mu Group 1 - mu Group 2: (1.54, 6.61)

T-Test mu Group 1 = mu Group 2 (vs. not =): T = 3.29
P = 0.0028 DF = 27

Both use Pooled StDev = 3.28
```

We see that the test of the null hypothesis that the means in the two groups are the same, i.e., $\tau = 0$, yields $P = 0.0028$, indicating that the drug does appear to alleviate the problem.

The difference in means, $\bar{d}_1 - \bar{d}_2 = 4.074$, and the preceding output shows that an associated 95% confidence interval is (1.54, 6.61).

At the end of Subsection 11.3.1, The Theory, it was shown that $E(\bar{d}_1 - \bar{d}_2) = 2\tau$, i.e., $\bar{d}_1 - \bar{d}_2$ is an unbiased estimator not of the quantity of interest but of twice that quantity. Consequently, the estimator of $\tau$ is $\frac{1}{2}(\bar{d}_1 - \bar{d}_2) = 2.037$ nights. A 95% confidence interval for $\tau$ is ($1/2 \times 1.54$, $1/2 \times$ 6.61) = (0.77, 3.31) nights.

## 11.4 The Issue of Carryover

An obvious potential problem with a crossover trial is that the effects of the treatment given in period 1 may still persist during period 2. Such a persistence of a treatment effect is known as a *carryover effect*. What might be the effect if such a phenomenon were present?

A way to investigate this is to adapt the model presented in Subsection 11.3.1. This can be done as follows, using the notation of that subsection.

In group 1, so for $i = 1, ..., n_1$, we leave the model for period 1 unchanged (carryover cannot affect the first period), but add a term $\gamma_A$ to the model for period 2.

$$x_{i1} = \mu + \pi_1 + \tau_A + \xi_i + \varepsilon_{i1} \qquad \text{(period 1) and}$$

$$x_{i2} = \mu + \pi_2 + \tau_B + \gamma_A + \xi_i + \varepsilon_{i2} \quad \text{(period 2)}$$

The response in period 2 might be affected by the persistent effect of treatment A given in period 1, and $\gamma_A$ is a parameter that represents this effect. Similarly for $\gamma_B$, so the model for responses in group 2, i.e., for $i = n_1 + 1, ..., n_1 + n_2$, becomes

$$x_{i1} = \mu + \pi_1 + \tau_B + \xi_i + \varepsilon_{i1} \qquad \text{(period 1) and}$$

$$x_{i2} = \mu + \pi_2 + \tau_A + \gamma_B + \xi_i + \varepsilon_{i2} \quad \text{(period 2)}$$

If we did not take any notice of this amended form of the model and decided to estimate treatment effect as before, i.e., using $\frac{1}{2}(\bar{d}_1 - \bar{d}_2)$, what would we actually be estimating?

From the amended model, it follows that $E(\bar{d}_1) = \pi + \tau - \gamma_A$ and $E(\bar{d}_2) = \pi - \tau - \gamma_B$, and hence, $E[\frac{1}{2}(\bar{d}_1 - \bar{d}_2)] = \tau - \frac{1}{2}\gamma$, where $\gamma = \gamma_A - \gamma_B$. Therefore, if there is a carryover effect, i.e., $\gamma \neq 0$, and it is ignored in the analysis, the estimator of $\tau$ is biased.

What can be done about this? One proposal that was widely followed for many years was to perform a preliminary analysis to test the null hypothesis that $\gamma = 0$. Such a hypothesis test is simple to implement: it is a two-sample $t$-test comparing the sums $s_i = x_{i1} + x_{i2}$ between groups 1 and 2. The procedure continued as follows:

1. If the test rejected the null hypothesis $\gamma = 0$ then the data from period 1 only were compared using the usual $t$-test for a parallel group trial (to which this study has now been reduced).

2. If the test could not discredit $\gamma = 0$ then the procedure described in Section 11.3 of this chapter is followed.

This approach is not recommended now because there are several problems. The most transparent one is that $\xi_i$ has not been eliminated from the test of $\gamma = 0$. So this test is affected by between-patient variation. This is likely to be large, and as the size of the trial would be determined by a sample size calculation based on the smaller variance $\tilde{\sigma}$, it is likely that the test of $\gamma = 0$ has poor power. Consequently, the decision to follow the procedure in Section 11.3 of this chapter may well be taken even in the presence of a substantial nonzero value of $\gamma$.

The recommended approach is not to use this particular crossover design when there is a possibility of a carryover effect. You should try to use nonstatistical arguments, perhaps based on the half-lives of drugs, etc., to decide how long treatment effects are likely to persist. The AB/BA design can then be used if the treatment periods are separated by "washout periods" whose duration is sufficient to ensure that carryover cannot occur.

## 11.5 Equivalence Trials

### 11.5.1 General Remarks

There are circumstances when the aim of a trial is not to detect differences between the treatments under study but to establish that, for all practical purposes, the efficacy of two treatments is equivalent. It may be that one treatment might be thought to be safer than another, one might be cheaper, or there may be advantages in terms of convenience.

A fundamental feature of an equivalence trial is that the usual hypothesis test is of little value. Failing to establish that one treatment is superior to the other is not the same as establishing their equivalence; see Subsection 3.2.1. On the other hand, a difference that is detected may have little importance and could well correspond to clinical equivalence.

The usual method when determining the equivalence of two treatments, A and B, is to compute a 95% confidence interval or, in general, a $100(1 - \alpha)\%$ interval for the difference in the treatment means, $\mu_A$ and $\mu_B$. For the purposes of illustration, it will be assumed that the standard deviation of the outcomes, $\sigma$, is known. If $n_A$ and $n_B$ patients are recruited to each group, then the confidence interval is

$$(\bar{d} - z_{\frac{1}{2}\alpha}\sigma\lambda, \bar{d} + z_{\frac{1}{2}\alpha}\sigma\lambda) \tag{11.1}$$

where $\bar{d}$ is the difference in the sample means, $z_\xi$ is such that $\Pr(Z > z_\xi) = \xi$, where $Z$ is a standard normal variable and, as in Chapter 3, $\lambda = \sqrt{n_A^{-1} + n_B^{-1}}$.

A commonly used method is to consider the treatments to be equivalent if both ends of the interval in Equation 11.1 lie within the prespecified interval of equivalence $(-\delta, \delta)$. If this does not occur, then equivalence has not been established. There is a more general formulation using an interval $(\delta_L, \delta_U)$, which can be helpful when comparing a new treatment with a standard, and there is less concern if the new treatment is better than the standard. This refinement of the methodology will not be pursued here. The specification of $\delta$ must be made in close collaboration with clinical experts and is, in some ways, analogous to specifying $\tau_M$ in a conventional parallel groups trial (cf. Chapter 3).

The methods explained in Chapter 3 for determining the size of a conventional RCT do not apply directly to equivalence studies, because they are focused on a test of the hypothesis $\tau = \mu_A - \mu_B = 0$, which is inappropriate in this setting. The calculations and associated error probabilities required for equivalence trials are set out in the following subsection.

### 11.5.2 Sample Sizes for Equivalence Trials with Normally Distributed Outcomes

It should be recalled that the null hypothesis can only be discredited, it cannot be shown to be true. In the context of an equivalence trial, it is therefore useful to think in terms of the null hypothesis representing difference and the alternative being equivalence. These hypotheses might be written as

$$H_0 : |\tau| > \delta \text{ vs. } H_1 : |\tau| \leq \delta$$

It should be noted that there is no point in trying to establish exact equivalence, $\delta = 0$, as there will always be some uncertainty in our estimates, and such a null hypothesis would never be discredited. As with conventional trials, two kinds of mistakes can be made when conducting an equivalence trial: it can be concluded that the treatments are equivalent when they are not, or it can be concluded that genuinely equivalent treatments are not equivalent. In terms of the preceding hypotheses, these are the type I and type II errors, respectively. As with conventional trials, the sample size is set to place acceptable values on these error probabilities.

Two treatments will be deemed equivalent if the interval in Equation 11.1 lies within $(-\delta, \delta)$. This amounts to requiring that $\bar{d} \in (-\varsigma, \varsigma)$ where $\varsigma = \delta - z_{1\alpha}\sigma\lambda$. Note that it would be impossible to assert equivalence if $\delta < z_{1\alpha}\sigma\lambda$. The distribution of $\bar{d}$ is normal with mean $\tau$ and standard deviation $\sigma\lambda$, so

$$\Pr(\bar{d} \in (-\varsigma, \varsigma)) = \Phi(\frac{\varsigma - \tau}{\lambda\sigma}) - \Phi(\frac{-\varsigma - \tau}{\lambda\sigma}) = \Phi(\frac{\delta - \tau}{\lambda\sigma} - z_{\frac{1}{2}\alpha}) - \Phi(\frac{-\delta - \tau}{\lambda\sigma} + z_{\frac{1}{2}\alpha}) \quad (11.2)$$

The chance of asserting equivalence when the treatments are not equivalent (which in terms of parameters we take to mean $|\tau| \geq \delta$), i.e., the type I error rate varies with $\tau$, reaching a maximum over the region of difference,

$|\tau| \geq \delta$, when $|\tau| = \delta$. The type I error rate is taken to be the value of Equation 11.2 when $\tau = \delta$, which is

$$\Phi(-z_{\frac{1}{2}\alpha}) - \Phi\left(z_{\frac{1}{2}\alpha} - \frac{2\delta}{\lambda\sigma}\right) = \frac{1}{2}\alpha - \Phi\left(z_{\frac{1}{2}\alpha} - \frac{2\delta}{\lambda\sigma}\right) \tag{11.3}$$

The power of the trial, $1 - \beta$, is the probability of declaring the treatments are equivalent when they really are equivalent. For this purpose, the power is defined as the value of Equation 11.2 when there is exact equivalence, i.e., $\tau = 0$. Hence

$$1 - \beta = 2\Phi\left(\frac{\delta}{\lambda\sigma} - z_{\frac{1}{2}\alpha}\right) - 1$$

and, therefore,

$$1 - \frac{1}{2}\beta = \Phi(z_{\frac{1}{2}\beta}) = \Phi\left(\frac{\delta}{\lambda\sigma} - z_{\frac{1}{2}\alpha}\right)$$

It follows that

$$\delta/(\lambda\sigma) = (z_{\frac{1}{2}\alpha} + z_{\frac{1}{2}\beta}) \tag{11.4}$$

so if the two treatment groups have the same size, $n$, we have

$$n = 2\frac{\sigma^2}{\delta^2}(z_{\frac{1}{2}\alpha} + z_{\frac{1}{2}\beta})^2 \tag{11.5}$$

Substituting $\delta/(\lambda\sigma) = (z_{\frac{1}{2}\alpha} + z_{\frac{1}{2}\beta})$ into Equation 11.3 gives the type I error rate as

$$= \frac{1}{2}\alpha - \Phi(-z_{\frac{1}{2}\alpha} - 2z_{\frac{1}{2}\beta}) \approx \frac{1}{2}\alpha$$

assuming a reasonable power, say, >70%. Therefore, if equivalence is based on a $100(1 - \alpha)\%$ confidence interval, then the type I error rate is $100(^1/_2\alpha)\%$, so a 95% confidence interval has type I error 2.5%.

### 11.5.3   Comparison of Conventional and Equivalence Trials

The roles of $\tau_M$, the minimal clinically important difference, and $\delta$ are similar, especially in the way they appear in the formulae in Subsection 11.5.2 of this chapter. However, it will often be prudent to use a value of $\delta$ substantially smaller than a value of $\tau_M$ used in a related but conventional trial. In a trial looking for a difference, a clinician may only be interested in changing treatments if the new therapy offers a substantial advantage. In an equivalence trial, evidence is sought to support the interchangeability of the two treatments, and it may then be appropriate to demand a closer agreement in their mean response. A further reason why equivalence trials are often larger than conventional trials can be found from comparing formulae in Equation 3.3 of Chapter 3 and Equation 11.4. The term $z_\beta$ in Equation 3.3 of Chapter 3 becomes $z_{\frac{1}{2}\beta}$ in Equation 11.4 and as $z_{\frac{1}{2}\beta} > z_\beta$, this will increase the required sample size.

There are many less technical issues surrounding equivalence trials but these will not be discussed in depth. A general comment that is often made concerns the standard of execution of these studies. In a conventional trial, sloppy conduct is not at all in the interests of the investigator: e.g., poor data recording and checking will increase $\sigma$ and make it more difficult to find genuine differences. In an equivalence study, sloppiness tends to increase the chances that the investigator will be unable to discover a difference, which is now the aim of the study. This is certainly true if part of the sloppiness includes an inappropriate analysis. However, if the analysis is based on comparing the confidence interval in Equation 11.1 with a prespecified interval of equivalence, then poor technique will tend to widen Equation 11.1, thereby reducing the chance it will be contained within a properly chosen interval of equivalence. It is, nevertheless, worth reinforcing that poor technique, such as inadequate attention to blindness, can cause problems for an equivalence study that are every bit as severe as those caused to conventional trials.

## 11.6   Cluster Randomized Trials

### 11.6.1   Introduction and Rationale

The trials described up to this time have allocated each patient to a treatment, or in the case of crossover trials, a sequence of treatments. As RCTs have become more widely accepted as the method of choice for the assessment of treatment efficacy, there has been an increase in the areas in which investigators have wanted to use this methodology. However, application in areas different from the traditional use in clinical medicine, which essentially deals with the health of individual patients, often gives rise to a particular difficulty. This is that it is no longer appropriate to randomize individual patients but whole clusters, or groups of patients must be allocated en bloc to a given treatment. These are known as *cluster randomized* or *group randomized trials.*

One example is provided by a trial designed to assess the impact of improved methods for the treatment of sexually transmitted diseases (STDs) on the incidence of HIV infection in a rural region of Tanzania, near Mwanza (Grosskurth et al., 1995). The treatment comprised a program that among other things, involved the training of health center staff to manage STDs better, the provision of better laboratory facilities in Mwanza, and the provision of a reliable supply of effective drugs for the treatment of STDs. Twelve large communities, each being the catchment area of a health center, were involved in the study. The RCT had to apply the improved methods and compare these with the current methods. Individuals cannot be randomized as the methods are not applied to the patients but to the staff of the health centers, each serving many hundreds of patients. Therefore, the community and its health center were randomly allocated to receive the improved treatment scheme or the current scheme. With only twelve communities in the trial, if the communities exhibit substantial initial differences in their HIV incidences, it is clear that the randomization could lead to substantial differences between the two treatment groups. This was indeed the case: communities near to major roads or the shore of Lake Victoria did exhibit higher incidence of HIV infection than did more remote communities. To overcome this, the investigators formed six pairs from the communities, matched with respect to their location and a number of other factors. One member of each pair was randomly allocated to the new treatment scheme and the other received the standard treatment.

This illustrates a general feature of cluster randomized trials: the number of clusters is generally much lower than the number of patients in the usual individual-patient parallel group study. Often, small numbers of clusters arise when each cluster comprises many patients and, in these cases, the clusters may not be particularly heterogeneous, so important imbalances might not arise. However, as the preceding example shows, this is by no means always the case and, in these instances, paired designs such as that just described are used.

Another example is provided by a study that is similar insofar as it is aimed at assessing the effect of an intervention in primary care. The study is designed to assess whether additional training of nurses and GPs in a general practice would improve the care of patients with newly diagnosed type II diabetes mellitus (Kinmonth et al., 1998). Forty-one practices in the south of England were randomized to the status quo or to receive additional training for their staff. The outcomes were measures of quality of life and of diabetic control. In this trial there was no pairing of practices.

The main statistical problem that arises with this sort of study is that you cannot analyze the data as if the patients themselves had been individually randomized to treatment. It cannot be assumed, *ab initio*, that responses on patients that are from the same cluster are independent. Such a correlation could arise because of similarities in the way certain measurements are taken by the practice nurse, or that methods for sending samples to the laboratory might differ more between practices than they do within a practice. For variables such as measures of quality of life, less tangible aspects, such as the atmosphere within a practice, could have a bearing. If these responses have a positive correlation, then they will be more similar than would be expected if they were independent. If the method used for the analysis assumes that the individual responses are independent then the estimated variance will be too small. This can be seen more formally as follows.

Suppose the outcome of the $j$th individual in the $i$th cluster is represented by a continuous random variable $X_{ij}$ with mean $\mu_A, \mu_B$ in treatment groups A and B, respectively, and variance $\sigma^2$. Suppose also that responses within a cluster have correlation $\rho$ and that responses in different clusters are independent. The estimate of variance, computed from one of the treatment groups (so the mean of each response is the same), but without regard to the presence of clusters is

$$\hat{\sigma}^2 = \frac{\displaystyle\sum_{i=1}^{K}\sum_{j=1}^{n_i}(X_{ij} - \bar{X})^2}{N-1} \tag{11.6}$$

the $i$th cluster has size $n_i$ and $N = \displaystyle\sum_{i=1}^{K} n_i$, where there are $K$ clusters. The mean is computed without taking account of the clustering, so $\bar{X} = \displaystyle\sum_{i=1}^{K}\sum_{j=1}^{n_i} X_{ij} / N$.

Expanding the numerator of Equation 11.6 and taking expectations we obtain:

$$E(\{N-1\}\hat{\sigma}^2) = N\sigma^2 - N^{-1}E\left(\left[\sum_{i=1}^{k}\sum_{j=1}^{n_i}[X_{ij} - E(X_{ij})]\right]^2\right)$$

$$= N\sigma^2 - N^{-1}\,\mathrm{var}\left(\sum_{i=1}^{K} T_i\right)$$

$$= N\sigma^2 - \frac{1}{N}\sum_{i=1}^{K}\mathrm{var}(T_i)$$

as clusters are independent and $T_i$ is the sum of responses in cluster $i$. This variance can be computed as

$$\text{var}(T_i) = \sum_{j=1}^{n_i} \text{var}(X_{ij}) + \sum_{j \neq \ell} \text{cov}(X_{ij}, X_{i\ell})$$

$$= n_i \sigma^2 + n_i(n_i - 1)\rho\sigma^2$$

so the expectation of Equation 11.6 is $\sigma^2(1 - C\rho)$ where

$$C = \frac{\sum n_i(n_i - 1)}{N(N-1)}$$

Thus if the analyst supposed that Equation 11.6 was a valid estimate of error, then the analysis would be biased with too small a value used for the estimate of standard deviation, with a consequent exaggeration of the significance of treatment effects.

## 11.6.2 Methods of Analysis for Cluster-Randomized Trials

A valid method of analysis is to use the simple treatment means, $\bar{X}_A, \bar{X}_B$, found ignoring clustering and to adapt the preceding calculations so that a legitimate standard error for $\bar{X}_A - \bar{X}_B$ is used. The variance of a treatment mean is, in the notation of the previous subsection,

$$N^{-2} \text{var}\left(\sum_{i=1}^{K} T_i\right) = N^{-2} \sum_{i=1}^{K} \text{var}(T_i) = N^{-2} \sum_{i=1}^{K}(n_i\sigma^2 + n_i(n_i - 1)\rho\sigma^2)$$

$$= \frac{\sigma^2}{N}\left[1 + \rho\left(\frac{\sum n_i^2}{N} - 1\right)\right]$$

Thus the effect of clustering is to increase the variance of the sample mean by a factor $[1 + \rho(\Sigma n_i^2 / N - 1)]$. If the clusters all have the same size, $n$, then this factor becomes $[1 + \rho(n - 1)]$. Thus, the variance, $V$, of $\bar{X}_A - \bar{X}_B$ can be found as the sum of this expression for the two treatment groups and a test of the null hypothesis of no treatment difference can be made by referring $(\bar{X}_A - \bar{X}_B)/\sqrt{V}$ to a standard normal distribution.

There remains the problem of how to estimate the variance of an individual response, $\sigma^2$, and the within-cluster correlation $\rho$. Naïve methods for $\sigma^2$ have been shown to be misleading.

Maximum likelihood methods could be employed but a simpler approach can be used. In this a model is postulated for the outcomes from a cluster-randomized trial. The model has some similarities to the model proposed in Subsection 11.3.1 for a crossover trial. The idea is that the response on the $j$th individual in the $i$th cluster is modeled by

$$X_{ij} = \mu_T + G_i + \varepsilon_{ij} \tag{11.7}$$

where $T$ is either $A$ or $B$, depending on which treatment was applied in the $i$th cluster. The terms $\varepsilon_{ij}$ are independent random variables with zero mean and common variance $\sigma_W^2$. The term $G_i$ is a random variable, also with zero mean, independent of $\varepsilon_{ij}$, which measures the effect of the $i$th cluster. As with the random variable measuring the patient effect in a crossover trial, $\xi_i$, the same realization of $G_i$ is applied to each member of the cluster. The variance of $G_i$ is $\sigma_G^2$. Consequently, responses in a cluster that has a larger value of $G_i$ will all tend to be higher, and it is this feature of the model that induces the within-cluster correlation needed to make the model reasonable. More specifically, the variance of any member of a cluster is $\sigma^2 = \sigma_G^2 + \sigma_W^2$, and the covariance of any two members of the same cluster is, from Equation 11.7, for $j \neq \ell$:

$$E\left[(X_{ij} - \mu_T)(X_{i\ell} - \mu_T)\right] = E\left[(G_i + \varepsilon_{ij})(G_i + \varepsilon_{i\ell})\right] = \sigma_G^2$$

It follows that the within-cluster correlation $\rho = \sigma_G^2 / \sigma^2$.

Estimates of $\sigma_G^2$ and $\sigma_W^2$ can be found as the standard between- and within-group variance components applied in each treatment group, and the results averaged appropriately across the treatments. Alternatively, the mixed model in Equation 11.7 can be fitted directly to all the data. Estimates of $\sigma^2$ and $\rho$ can be found from their relationships with $\sigma_G^2$ and $\sigma_W^2$.

An alternative and simpler analysis is to compute the mean response within each cluster, $\bar{X}_i$, and use these means as if they were raw data in a $t$-test. The clusters are independent, so the analysis is free from the difficulties due to within-cluster dependency. A potential criticism is that a $t$-test assumes each number used in the test has the same variance. As the variance of the mean of the $i$th cluster is $\sigma_G^2 + \sigma_W^2 / n_i$, this is not true unless the clusters all have the same size. However, the analysis will lose only a little efficiency if either the clusters have similar sizes or if $\sigma_G^2$ is substantially larger than $\sigma_W^2$, in which case the term varying with cluster size is relatively unimportant.

## 11.6.3   Sample Size Estimation for Continuous Outcomes from Cluster-Randomized Trials

If the method of analysis is affected by the presence of clustering, so too is the manner in which sample sizes are estimated. In the absence of clustering, the formula for the size of each group is given by Equation 3.4 of Chapter 3

$$N = \frac{2\sigma^2(z_\beta + z_{\frac{1}{2}\alpha})^2}{\tau_M^2}$$

where $\alpha$ is the type I error rate, $1 - \beta$ is the power to detect a difference of $\tau_M$, and $\sigma^2$ is the variance of the response of an individual patient. The formula provides a link with $N$ because the variance of each treatment mean is $\sigma^2/N$.

For a cluster randomized trial, the variance of the treatment mean is not $\sigma^2/N$ but $(\sigma^2/N)[1+\rho(\Sigma n_i^2/N-1)]$. A difficulty with cluster-randomized trials is that the sizes of the clusters may well not be known when the trial is planned. In this case, it is essential to have some idea about this quantity, perhaps through an estimate of the likely average cluster size, $n_a$. If this is available, the variance of the mean is taken to be $(\sigma^2/N)[1+\rho(n_a-1)]$, and it is $\sigma^2[1+\rho(n_a-1)]$ that is used in place of $\sigma^2$ in the sample size formula; that is, the total number of patients in the clusters receiving each treatment should be

$$N = \frac{2\sigma^2(1+\rho(n_a-1))(z_\beta + z_{\frac{1}{2}\alpha})^2}{\tau_M^2} \tag{11.8}$$

As can be seen, the presence of clustering means that the planning of a cluster-randomized trial requires knowledge not only of all the quantities needed for Equation 3.4 of Chapter 3 but additional information about the size and effect of clustering, through $n_a$ and $\rho$.

An alternative approach is to base the calculation of sample size on the cluster means, giving a formula for the number of clusters that should receive each treatment. If the outcome follows the model in Equation 11.7, then the variance of the sample mean should be used in Equation 3.4 of Chapter 3 giving the number of clusters receiving each treatment as

$$\frac{2(\sigma_G^2 + \sigma_W^2/n_a)(z_\beta + z_{\frac{1}{2}\alpha})^2}{\tau_M^2} \tag{11.9}$$

### 11.6.4 General Remarks about Cluster-Randomized Trials

Cluster-randomized trials raise many complicated practical issues. The sample size estimates in the previous subsection are just one example. They require the specification of not only the usual quantities but of the cluster size and the intraclass correlation, which is likely to need extensive experience of the area of application before the trial can be planned adequately. Sensible assessment of the sensitivity of the required number of patients will generally require the statistician to investigate the effect of a range of values for $\rho$ in Equation 11.8.

Other issues, such as the way withdrawals and dropouts are handled, and the meaning of informed consent, present problems that are absent from conventional trials. On a more technical level, the foregoing discussion has concentrated on continuous outcomes for good reason. The technicalities presented by binary outcomes are rather more formidable. Recent developments in hierarchical data-analysis do, however, mean that the efficient analysis of cluster-randomized trials is becoming easier.

## Exercises

1. The following data are from an AB/BA crossover trial in which patients are treated with two bronchodilators (a widely used form of inhaled drug designed to help patients with asthma), namely salbutamol (S) and formoterol (F). The outcome presented in the following table is the peak expiratory flow (PEF) in liters per minute (l/min). Patients were randomized to receive the drug in the order F then S or S then F (Data from Senn and Auclair, *Statistics in Medicine*, 1990, 9, 1287–1302).

| Patient | PEF in Period 1 (l/min) | PEF in Period 2 (l/min) | Order (1 = FS, 2 = SF) |
|---------|-------------------------|-------------------------|-------------------------|
| 1 | 310 | 270 | 1 |
| 2 | 370 | 385 | 2 |
| 3 | 310 | 400 | 2 |
| 4 | 310 | 260 | 1 |
| 5 | 380 | 410 | 2 |
| 6 | 370 | 300 | 1 |
| 7 | 410 | 390 | 1 |
| 8 | 290 | 320 | 2 |
| 9 | 250 | 210 | 1 |
| 10 | 380 | 350 | 1 |
| 11 | 260 | 340 | 2 |
| 12 | 90 | 220 | 2 |
| 13 | 330 | 365 | 1 |

   Analyze the preceding data, assuming that there is no carryover effect of treatment; be careful to define the statistical model that you use. Make sure that your analysis includes a test of the null hypothesis that there is no difference in the mean treatment effect when treated with formoterol or salbutamol. You should also provide point and interval (95%) estimates of the treatment effect, making sure that you define clearly what you mean by this term. Compute similar quantities using the parallel group trial formed from the data in the first period and comment.

2. Suppose that the assumption of no carryover cannot be sustained on nonstatistical grounds and it is decided to try to use the data to assess if carryover is present. Suppose that the model for the responses is now:

$$x_{i1} = \mu + \pi_1 + \tau_F + \xi_i + \varepsilon_{i1} \qquad \text{(period 1) and}$$

$$x_{i2} = \mu + \pi_2 + \tau_S + \gamma_F + \xi_i + \varepsilon_{i2} \quad \text{(period 2)}$$

in the F then S group and in which the terms are as defined in Section 11.4 of this chapter but with A and B replaced by F and S to conform with the present application.

(a) What is the expectation of $S_i = x_{i1} + x_{i2}$? What is the corresponding expectation in the S and F group?

(b) What null hypothesis does a two-sample $t$-test between the two samples of $S_i$s test? Perform this test using the data from question 1. What conclusion can you draw?

(c) If you proceed with the analysis used in question 1 but the true model is that shown in this question, what is the expectation of the treatment estimator? What is a 95% confidence interval for the bias term?

3. The model for the outcomes on the $i$th patient from an AB/BA crossover trial is as follows:

| Sequence | Period 1 | Period 2 |
|---|---|---|
| AB ($i = 1, ..., n$) | $x_{i1} = \mu + \pi_1 + \tau_A + \xi_i + \varepsilon_{i1}$ | $x_{i2} = \mu + \pi_2 + \tau_B + \xi_i + \varepsilon_{i2}$ |
| BA ($i = n + 1, ..., 2n$) | $x_{i1} = \mu + \pi_1 + \tau_B + \xi_i + \varepsilon_{i1}$ | $x_{i2} = \mu + \pi_2 + \tau_A + \xi_i + \varepsilon_{i2}$ |

where $\mu$ is the general mean, $\pi_j$ is the effect of period $j$ (=1,2), the treatment effect of interest is $\tau = \tau_A - \tau_B$, and $\xi_i, \varepsilon_{ij}$ are independent residuals with zero mean and variances $\sigma_B^2, \sigma^2$, respectively.

(a) Define $d_i = x_{i1} - x_{i2}$ and let the mean of these in sequence AB be $\bar{d}_{AB}$ and similarly for $\bar{d}_{BA}$. Also let $\bar{x}_{1AB}, \bar{x}_{1BA}$ be the mean responses in period 1 for patients allocated to sequences AB and BA, respectively. Show that $\frac{1}{2}(\bar{d}_{AB} - \bar{d}_{BA})$ has the same expectation as $\bar{x}_{1AB} - \bar{x}_{1BA}$ and identify this quantity.

(b) Find the variance of $\frac{1}{2}(\bar{d}_{AB} - \bar{d}_{BA})$ and of $\bar{x}_{1AB} - \bar{x}_{1BA}$ and the ratio R of these quantities.

(c) If $\sigma_B^2 = 6\sigma^2$ evaluate R and comment on the implication of this value when deciding whether to use a crossover design or a parallel group design.

4. The type I error rate in an equivalence trial is given by Equation 11.2, with $|\tau| > \delta$. The actual value varies as $\tau$ changes within this region, reaching a maximum when $|\tau| = \delta$. Prove that this is true.

5. Suppose that the outcome in a cluster randomized trial follows Equation 11.7. Show if the required number of patients is estimated by Equation 11.8, then this is consistent with the number of clusters needed as computed by Equation 11.9.

6. A parameter $\theta$ is to be estimated and $M$ independent observations are available. Each observation has mean $\theta$ and the $i$th, $\hat{\theta}_i$, has variance $v_i$. It is proposed to estimate $\theta$ using a statistic of the form

$$\sum w_i \hat{\theta}_i$$

where the $w_i$ are positive weights that sum to one. Show that the estimator with minimum variance is

$$\left(\sum v_i^{-1}\right)^{-1} \left(\sum v_i^{-1} \hat{\theta}_i\right)$$

7. Apply the result of question 6 to the cluster-mean analysis of a cluster-randomized trial. Comment on the properties of the estimator derived.

# 12

## Meta-Analyses of Clinical Trials

### 12.1 What Are Meta-Analyses, and Why Are They Needed?

The early chapters of this book may have given the impression that an RCT is undertaken to establish whether one treatment is superior to another and, provided the trial is properly conducted and of adequate size, that at the conclusion of the trial there will be a clear-cut answer about which is the better treatment. Moreover, once such a study has been published, it is unlikely that it would be ethically defensible to run another similar trial. Thus, the reader might have been led to believe that clinical research largely comprises a collection of well-conducted studies which each settle once and for all, which of the particular treatments is superior for the condition under study. In reality things are quite different.

Even if the badly run studies are discounted, there are many reasons why several RCTs may be run that test virtually the same treatments for virtually the same type of patients. Studies do vary in the details of the treatments, perhaps using different doses or treating for different durations, or recruiting patients using different eligibility criteria. Even the best planned and executed studies can fail to recruit adequate numbers of patients; perhaps a trial has to be terminated early because of slow recruitment or the departure of key trial personnel. Studies can plan to recruit too few patients because the investigators overestimated the minimal clinically important difference; thus, although their study may have been nonsignificant, colleagues did not accept that it ruled out the possibility of a clinically important difference. Large studies are often run for a number of years, and even if one such should prove sufficiently decisive to make new trials unnecessary, many may still be in progress when these results are published. The decision about the continuation of an existing trial in the light of strong, new, but perhaps not fully digested results can be one of the most difficult decisions for the triallist.

The result of this environment is that the literature will contain many reports of trials that all aim to compare the same, or very similar treatments for more or less the same condition. There is the further complication that the results of some trials will not make it into the literature at all. This may be because no journal would accept the report, perhaps because the trial was too small, or because the investigators did not submit their work, possibly because they felt it was defective in some way or because it did not report a definitive result. This can give rise to the issue of publication bias mentioned in Subsection 2.2.4 of Chapter 2. A related, but slightly different problem is finding all published material: there are currently about 20,000 biomedical journals publishing around 2,000,000 articles each year, so locating all relevant articles is not a trivial task.

The clinician who wants to know what treatment to use for a given condition is then faced with an array of individual studies, each relevant, to a greater or lesser extent, but all slightly different. A natural response to this position is for experts in the field to write review articles that collate, compare, discuss, and summarize the current results in that field. Reviews, sometimes called *narrative reviews*, in which the author discusses the results selected have been around for decades. Meta-analyses or overviews of clinical trials have a much shorter history, stretching back only 15 to 20 years. These are quantitative reviews of all the available evidence. In some cases, meta-analyses try to obtain the original data from RCTs but, more commonly, they attempt to combine the published summaries of the results of a trial.

Meta-analyses attempt to combine results from trials and in this sense, serve a similar purpose to a narrative review: they attempt to present a digestible summary of numerous disparate pieces of research. However, by combining large and small studies, they are based on a larger number of patients than is found in any one trial, so there should, in principle, be benefits in terms of power to detect treatment differences and increased precision for estimates of treatment effect. In this way, the results from small, inconclusive studies can contribute to an overall picture that is very compelling. By combining results from several studies, each using its own treatment regimen and eligible patients, the clinician is able to put the results of the studies in a broader context. Even if the results of the trials are not identical, consistency of results across a broad range of patients and regimens can be very reassuring.

Many trials, even if they have adequate power overall, are not big enough to provide strong evidence about the effect of treatment in important subgroups of patients. A further advantage of meta-analyses is that they may allow such investigations in which previously it may have been thought necessary to run a new study. In general, it is becoming an important part of a trial protocol (see Section 10.1) to present a meta-analysis of studies in the area of the proposed trial, to demonstrate that a new trial is justified and the question being asked cannot be answered using data that have already been collected.

## 12.2 Some Methodology for Meta-Analysis

### 12.2.1 Data Collection

The way data are collected for inclusion in a meta-analysis is an issue of central importance to the subject. Indeed, the term *systematic review* seems to be gaining acceptance as the term for the means of attempting to collect all data from the research literature that are relevant to a particular question. Only once a systematic review has been completed can a meta-analysis proceed. Despite its pivotal position, the problems faced by those undertaking systematic reviews are more concerned with issues of information retrieval than statistics, so it is not central to the theme of this book and will not be given the attention that it actually warrants.

Most systematic reviews of medical topics these days start with a search of a computerized database of the medical literature. A widely used and important database is *Medline*. This can be searched for keywords in the title or keyword list of the paper. Although one of the best and most widely used databases, Medline is far from exhaustive and the process cannot stop once all the reports in Medline have been identified. Searching through the reports cited in the papers that have been identified typically results in several new studies coming to light. Knowledge of who are the active researchers in the field is also helpful, as these people can often supply further information: they are a particularly valuable source of information concerning unpublished studies.

Once all the studies have been identified, they can be subjected to a meta-analysis. There is some dispute about the extent to which the analyst can interfere with the selection of studies at this stage. Some authors argue that all identified trials must be included whereas others argue that it is wrong to include studies whose methodological quality is clearly inadequate. Some authors suggest scoring studies for quality and use this score either to decide on the inclusion of the study or to weight the study when it is included. One of the difficulties is that all studies will have some flaws, and omitting any studies will necessarily require the exercise of judgment. Although this will introduce some subjectivity, it is difficult to see how worthwhile aggregations of data can emerge without the exercise of some well-informed judgment.

### 12.2.2 Estimating the Overall Effect Using a Fixed-Effects Model

One of the aims of a meta-analysis is to adduce an estimate of the effect of the treatment being assessed based on all the trials that have been identified. The outcomes of trials differ widely and can be continuous or binary or some other measure. To make the following as general as possible, it will be assumed that the true overall effect is $\theta$ and the estimate from the $i$th study is $\hat{\theta}_i$, $i = 1, \ldots, k$. The $\theta$s could be differences of means, of proportions or, as is quite common, log odds ratios (the logarithm is used because log odds ratios have a distribution much closer to normal than does the odds ratio itself). It is also assumed that the only source of variability affecting $\hat{\theta}_i$ is sampling variability, which is measured by the usual sampling variance $v_i$.

This model is known as the *fixed-effects model* because the result from each study is considered to estimate the same quantity $\theta$, with deviations from this essentially reflecting differences in the size of the trial (and some other factors affecting the sampling variation). In some ways, this is reasonable; the $\hat{\theta}_i$ are all summaries from RCTs and, if the underlying methodology is sound, should all be unbiased estimates of the treatment effect.

The minimum-variance estimator of $\theta$ based on the $\hat{\theta}_i$ is

$$\hat{\theta}_F = \frac{\sum w_i \hat{\theta}_i}{\sum w_i}$$

where $w_i = v_i^{-1}$, and the subscript $F$ emphasizes that a fixed-effects model is in use. This estimator has variance $1/(\Sigma w_i)$, and, assuming $\hat{\theta}_i$ is reasonably close to normally distributed, a 95% confidence interval for $\theta$ is

$$\hat{\theta}_F \pm 1.96 / \sqrt{\sum w_i}$$

The example used in Subsection 9.2.3 was from a trial of the effect of giving steroids or placebo to expectant mothers to see if it had an effect on the incidence of respiratory complications in their babies. An overview in this area was reported by Crowley et al. (1990) and Table 12.1 gives the results from 12 of the trials reported in the overview. The aim of this particular analysis is to see if the use of steroids given before preterm birth had an effect on the number of deaths among very young babies.

The preceding method can be applied to these data. The first step is to compute the odds ratio, i.e., the odds of death if steroids are administered relative to the odds if a placebo is used. If the entries in columns 2 to 5 of one row of Table 12.1 are $a$, $b$, $c$, $d$, respectively, then the odds ratio is found as $[(a + \frac{1}{2})(d + \frac{1}{2})] / [(b + \frac{1}{2})(c + \frac{1}{2})]$, where halves have been added to obtain less biased estimates and to avoid difficulty in the case of trial 6.

The sampling variance for the natural log of this odds ratio is estimated by $(a + \frac{1}{2})^{-1} + (b + \frac{1}{2})^{-1} + (c + \frac{1}{2})^{-1} + (d + \frac{1}{2})^{-1}$. Computing the odds ratio for these trials gives the sixth column of Table 12.1. The weights for the fixed effect model can be found as described earlier, with $\hat{\theta}_i$ taken as the log odds ratio for the $i$th trial; they are presented in column 7 of the table. It can be seen that most weight is attached to the largest trials, as would be expected when weighting only takes account of sampling variation.

**TABLE 12.1**

Results from 12 Trials of the Effect of Maternal Steroid Therapy on Early Neonatal Death and Weights Applied by Fixed- and Random-Effects Meta-Analysis

| Trial | Steroid Group | | Control Group | | Odds Ratio | Weights | |
|---|---|---|---|---|---|---|---|
| | Dead | Alive | Dead | Alive | | Fixed | Random |
| 1 | 36 | 496 | 60 | 478 | 0.58 | 0.33 | 0.24 |
| 2 | 1 | 68 | 5 | 56 | 0.22 | 0.02 | 0.03 |
| 3 | 3 | 61 | 12 | 46 | 0.21 | 0.04 | 0.06 |
| 4 | 5 | 51 | 7 | 64 | 0.92 | 0.05 | 0.06 |
| 5 | 2 | 79 | 10 | 53 | 0.16 | 0.03 | 0.04 |
| 6 | 0 | 38 | 0 | 42 | 1.10 | 0.00 | 0.01 |
| 7 | 14 | 117 | 20 | 117 | 0.71 | 0.12 | 0.13 |
| 8 | 36 | 335 | 37 | 335 | 0.97 | 0.26 | 0.22 |
| 9 | 7 | 114 | 13 | 111 | 0.54 | 0.07 | 0.09 |
| 10 | 1 | 70 | 5 | 70 | 0.27 | 0.02 | 0.03 |
| 11 | 2 | 65 | 7 | 52 | 0.27 | 0.03 | 0.04 |
| 12 | 5 | 29 | 5 | 26 | 0.90 | 0.04 | 0.05 |

*Source:* Data from Crowley, P., Chalmers, I., Keirse, M.J.N.C. (1990), The effects of corticosteroid administration before preterm delivery: an overview of the evidence from controlled trials, *British Journal of Obstetrics and Gynaecology*, 97, 11–25.

The fixed-effect estimate of the overall log odds ratio is found to be –0.480, which corresponds to an odds ratio of 0.62. The 95% confidence interval expressed on the odds ratio scale is (0.48, 0.79).

## 12.2.3 Estimating the Overall Effect Using a Random-Effects Model

The idea that each $\hat{\theta}_i$ estimates the same quantity because each RCT provides an unbiased estimate of the treatment effect is not necessarily plausible. This argument overlooks the clinical heterogeneity of the trials — slightly different types of patient, slightly different treatment regimens, etc. — so it is probably unwise to assume that the only source of difference between the $\hat{\theta}_i$ is sampling variation. The hypothesis that the only difference between the $\hat{\theta}_i$ is sampling variation can be tested by computing:

$$Q = \sum_{i=1}^{k} w_i(\hat{\theta}_i - \hat{\theta}_F)^2$$

If the hypothesis is true, then $Q$ has a $\chi^2$ distribution with $k - 1$ degrees of freedom. However, this test has low power, and a nonsignificant result should certainly not be taken as evidence of homogeneity of the treatment effects in the $k$ trials. This hypothesis test is not all that valuable, and the real value of computing $Q$ will become clear in a moment.

If $\hat{\theta}_i$ does not estimate $\theta$, what does it estimate? It is, in fact, assumed to estimate $\theta_i$. However, if each trial has its own separate effect, what is the point of combining the studies at all? This would be the case if the $\theta_i$ were simply $k$ separate effects, but this formulation would not reflect the underlying situation. Although the trials may not all estimate the same thing, the studies are similar, and this must be reintroduced to the formulation in some way.

The usual approach, which is not without its oddities, is to assume that the underlying trial effects are actually a random selection from a population with mean $\theta$ and variance $\sigma^2$. This is known as the *random-effect model*. To be able to construct confidence intervals, it will also be assumed that the $\theta_i$ are normally distributed.

To be more precise, the random-effect model assumes that, given the $\theta_i$, the observed effects are $\hat{\theta}_i \sim N(\theta_i, v_i)$ and $\theta_i \sim N(\theta, \sigma^2)$. It follows that the $\hat{\theta}_i$ can be written $\hat{\theta}_i = \theta + \eta_i + \varepsilon_i$, where $\eta_i, \varepsilon_i$ are independent random variables with zero mean and variances $\sigma^2, v_i$, respectively. Hence $\text{var}(\hat{\theta}_i) = \sigma^2 + v_i = \tilde{w}_i^{-1}$, say. It follows that the random-effects estimator is $\hat{\theta}_R = \Sigma \tilde{w}_i \hat{\theta}_i / \Sigma \tilde{w}_i$, with variance $1/(\Sigma \tilde{w}_i)$. As with the fixed-effects model, the 95% confidence interval is

$$\hat{\theta}_R \pm 1.96 / \sqrt{\sum \tilde{w}_i}$$

Because $\tilde{w}_i \leq w_i$ for each $i$, it follows that the random-effects confidence interval is wider than the fixed-effects interval. This is to be expected, as the random-effects model has incorporated an extra source of variability into the analysis.

However, $\tilde{w}_i$ depends on $\sigma^2$, so an estimate of this quantity is needed before a random-effects analysis can proceed. This is provided by

$$\hat{\sigma}^2 = \max \left\{ 0, \frac{Q - (k-1)}{\sum w_i - \left( \sum w_i^2 \right) / \sum w_i} \right\} \qquad (12.1)$$

note that the formula uses weights $w_i$, not $\tilde{w}_i$. If the number of trials ($k$) is small, then this estimate will be imprecise.

The value of $Q$ computed for the data from Table 12.1 is 14.05, which gives $P = 0.23$. However, though there is little evidence of heterogeneity between the studies, the low power of this test means that it is sensible to estimate $\sigma^2$ and proceed to a random-effects analysis. The preceding formula gives $\hat{\sigma}^2 = 0.061$ and the random-effects weights are given in the final column of Table 12.1. Note that the larger trials still receive the most weight, but the weighting is less heavily in favor of the large studies. The random-effects estimate of the log odds ratio is –0.549, with corresponding odds ratio 0.58, and 95% confidence interval (0.42, 0.79). The confidence interval is wider than that for the fixed-effects analysis, but the difference is slight because the estimate of $\sigma^2$ is small.

## 12.3 Some Graphical Methods for Meta-Analysis

### 12.3.1 Meta-Analysis Diagrams

This is not an accepted term, but the diagrams that are to be described are ubiquitous in reports of meta-analyses, so the term seems appropriate. They are sometimes known as forest plots. Figure 12.1 shows summaries of the results from the trials in Table 12.1 in this widely seen format.

The vertical axis is arbitrary, being merely a way of displaying the data from the separate trials. For each trial, the odds ratio is shown by the plotted point, and the associated 95% confidence interval is shown by the length of the horizontal line. Care should obviously be taken to ensure that the plotted difference, whether an odds ratio as in this case, or a difference in means, is calculated in a consistent direction across all the trials. In Figure 12.1, all odds ratios have been arranged so that values less than 1 correspond to steroids being better than placebo. In this case, it is also sensible to display the odds ratios on a log scale. Note that the trial with a very wide confidence interval is the trial with zero deaths in either treatment group (trial 6 in Table 12.1).

The overall estimate of the odds ratio, and its associated confidence intervals, calculated using both fixed-effects and random-effects models are shown at the bottom of Figure 12.1.

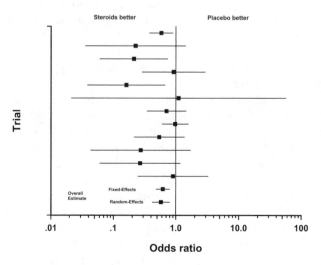

**FIGURE 12.1**
Plot of trials from Table 12.1.

One of the disadvantages of this way of displaying the data from the meta-analysis is that the most dominant features of the plot, such as the wide interval for trial 6, are actually the least important features of the data. The large trials that report estimates with highest precision (and hence are most important in determining the overall estimate) are the ones with the smallest confidence intervals and therefore are among the least conspicuous features of the plot. A simple device that goes some way to counteract this feature is to order the vertical axis such that the trials are listed in increasing order of the width of their associated confidence interval. This way the important trials appear first.

### 12.3.2   Sensitivity Plots for Random-Effects Analysis

Again, there is no widely accepted name for these plots. They are seen much less often than those described in Subsection 12.3.1 of this chapter and, indeed, much less often than they deserve to be seen. They are due to Thompson (1993).

The idea is that the definition of the overall estimate for the random-effects model, $\hat{\theta}_R = \Sigma \tilde{w}_i \hat{\theta}_i / \Sigma \tilde{w}_i$, depends on the unknown between-trial variance $\sigma^2$. Usually an estimate of this is provided by Equation 12.1 but, being a measure of the variation between just a few trials, this estimate is often imprecise. However, it is the estimate $\hat{\theta}_R$ that is of direct interest, not $\sigma^2$, so it is useful to investigate how $\hat{\theta}_R$ varies with different values of $\sigma^2$. It may be that quite a substantial variation in $\sigma^2$ about $\hat{\sigma}^2$ makes little difference to the value of $\hat{\theta}_R$, in which case imprecision in the estimate of $\sigma^2$ is unimportant.

The sensitivity plot computes $\hat{\theta}_R = \hat{\theta}_R(\sigma^2)$ for a range of values of $\sigma^2$, and the result is inspected. This is shown in Figure 12.2 (a) for $\sigma^2$ between 0 and 5 (recall $\hat{\sigma}^2 = 0.061$, so this range represents a substantial variation about the observed value).

It can be seen from Figure 12.2 (a) that the estimate of $\hat{\theta}_R$ obtained from the various values of $\sigma^2$ do not vary substantially, changing from 0.62 to 0.54 as $\sigma^2$ changes from 0 to 5.

A difficulty in producing one of these plots is to decide on the range of $\sigma^2$ that should be used. Obviously, the range will include $\hat{\sigma}^2$ and, usually, it will be appropriate to include $\sigma^2 = 0$ as this corresponds to the fixed-effects model (i.e., $\hat{\theta}_F = \hat{\theta}_R(0)$). It is often more difficult to decide on the limit at the upper end of the range. The case $\sigma^2 = \infty$ is interpretable because it corresponds to giving equal weight to each study, but is obviously impossible to include on a plot such as Figure 12.2(a). For this reason, it is sometimes convenient to plot $\hat{\theta}_R(\sigma^2)$ not against $\sigma^2$ but against $S^2 = \sigma^2 / (\sigma^2 + \hat{\sigma}^2)$, so the cases $S^2 = 0$, $\frac{1}{2}$, and 1 correspond to cases of fixed effects, random effects, and equal weighting, respectively. Such a plot appears in Figure 12.2(b). Inspection of the vertical scale of these plots shows that the overall estimate of the odds ratio changes little over most of the range of $\sigma^2$. For

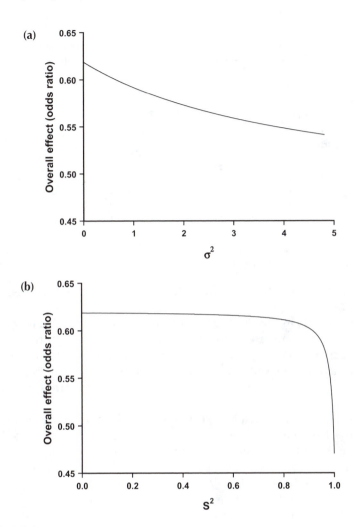

**FIGURE 12.2**
(a) Plot of sensitivity of $\hat{\theta}_R$ to changes in value of $\sigma^2$. (b) Plot of sensitivity of $\hat{\theta}_R$ to changes in value of $\sigma^2$ (transformed scale).

very large values of $\sigma^2$, Figure 12.2(b) shows that the estimate of effect changes much more rapidly than at smaller values of $\sigma^2$, but even here the change in the estimate is not that marked.

### 12.3.3 Funnel or Radial Plots

In these plots, that are sometimes also called *Galbraith plots* after their originator, the values of $\hat{\theta}_i / se(\hat{\theta}_i)$, sometimes called the *effect size*, are plotted on the vertical axis and the precision of each trial, $1 / se(\hat{\theta}_i)$, is plotted on

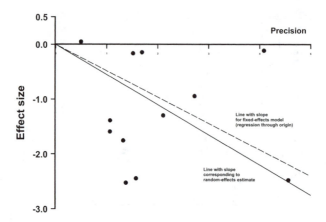

**FIGURE 12.3**
Plot of effect size against precision for trials in Table 12.1.

the horizontal axis. The trials from Table 12.1 are plotted in this way in Figure 12.3.

The estimate $\hat{\theta}_i$, in this application, the log odds ratio, can be found as the slope of the line joining the origin and the point for the $i$th trial. In some cases, a circular scale is appended so that by extrapolating the line from the origin to the $i$th point out to this scale, the odds ratio can be read directly. The use of such a radial scale is the basis of one of the names for this type of plot.

The regression line through the origin has slope equal to the overall effect size from a fixed-effects model. Figure 12.3 includes this and also the line with slope equal to estimate from the random-effects model. The link with regression shows means that the plot provides a clear method of identifying the trials that are important in determining the overall estimate, at least for the fixed-effects model.

It might be expected that the trials in this kind of plot would cluster symmetrically about the line representing some measure of the overall effect. The variability of each point in the vertical direction is the same by the construction of the effect size. However, one use of these plots is to attempt to detect publication bias. A plausible way publication bias might arise is if small studies that show positive effects are more likely to be published than small studies that do not show any positive effects. Large studies are less likely to have their publishability judged on their findings, as negative findings from a sufficiently large study may well be thought to be clinically important. In this case, the studies would not appear to cluster symmetrically about a regression through the origin. A method of detecting such asymmetry that has been proposed is to fit a regression that is not constrained to pass through the origin: the fitted intercept then becomes a measure of the asymmetry.

## 12.4 Some General Issues in Meta-Analysis

### 12.4.1 Random-Effects and Intertrial Variation

The fixed-effects model has been described earlier as implausible because it is thought unreasonable that different trials, with their differing designs, will necessarily estimate the same quantity, with the only variability being sampling error. The alternative is to use a random-effects model in which the size of effect that each trial is actually trying to determine is considered to be a sample from a population with given mean and variance. This is a slightly odd formulation — trials will have been designed quite deliberately to have the different characteristics that they actually possess, not because they have arisen by chance.

Of course, this does not preclude modeling the variation between trials by a random variable. In statistics generally the term *random variation* can apply to widely varying types of difference. At one extreme some random variation will be as genuinely unpredictable as it is possible to imagine, such as times of emissions of particles in radioactive decay. On the other hand some differences are consigned to random variation because we did not or could not delve deeper into what makes the items differ. If you can look deeper, then a more informative analysis may well emerge.

This is certainly the case with a meta-analysis. A random-effects model is really a first step — a comprehensive analysis would entail investigating why results from different trials might have differed. Studies with older patients may have systematically different effects from those treating younger patients; studies using surgical rather than medical treatments for heart disease may have different outcomes. The detection of such clinical heterogeneity is clearly important. Once statistical heterogeneity has been found, it is important to go back to the trials and try to identify sources of clinical heterogeneity that could account for these differences. However, the number of studies is often too small for a formal statistical modeling approach to be worthwhile, and simpler graphical methods can often be very valuable. Although of great importance, this topic will not be pursued here.

### 12.4.2 Position of Meta-Analysis

In medical circles, and particularly for RCTs, meta-analysis has rapidly gained a position of prominence. Many ethics committees and other relevant bodies now demand evidence in the form of a formal review of existing evidence before a trial can be permitted to proceed. Institutions have been established whose sole purpose is the collation and dissemination of research results. Despite this, it would be wrong to give the impression that the present role of meta-analysis is uncontroversial and universally accepted.

Critics cite many defects with meta-analyses (see, for example, Eysenck 1995). They dislike the aggregation of many studies whose qualities are widely different and are scornful of methods for weighting such studies according to some quality score. They also question the population to which the results of a meta-analysis can be applied.

Many studies actually measure related outcomes in ways that make them awkward to combine. For example, lung function might be measured as forced expiratory volume in 1 sec (in liters) or as a percentage of an unspecified maximum capacity. Combining such measures in a convincing way seems impossible. Indeed, the distinction is increasingly being made between the systematic review, which collects the information, and the meta-analysis, which computes a quantitative summary. It is acknowledged that it may not always be possible or desirable to apply a meta-analysis to a given systematic review.

## Exercises

1. Compute the fixed and random effects and their confidence intervals for the data in Table 12.1.

2. Show that $E(\hat{\sigma}^2) = \sigma^2$ in Equation 12.1. It may be useful to split the calculation into two. First, compute the expected value of $Q$, given the random effects $\{\theta_i\}$ and then take the expectation over the distribution of the random effects.

3. Explain, mathematically and intuitively, why the case $\sigma^2 = \infty$ corresponds to a summary that gives equal weight to all the trials.

4. Show that the fixed-effects estimate $\hat{\theta}_F$ is the slope of the regression through the origin for the Galbraith plot.

# *Further Reading*

This book has attempted to provide a broad view of the statistical issues underlying RCTs. However, it should by now be clear that running any sizable RCT is a major undertaking requiring close collaboration between workers from many disciplines. All investigators will need some knowledge of the medical, administrative, ethical, and statistical issues that underpin the trial, as well as a deeper knowledge of their own speciality. This book has not attempted to cover many of these facets, and those wishing to be more closely involved with actual trials will need to take their study further.

Fortunately, there are many excellent books that will cater for the needs of those wishing to extend their knowledge, and some of these are mentioned in the following text. This is, however, a highly selected and personal view of an extensive literature.

## Books on Clinical Trials in General

One of the most valuable books in this field is still

Pocock, S.J., *Clinical Trials: A Practical Approach*, Wiley, Chichester, 1983.

A comprehensive and more recent reference is

Piantadosi, S., *Clinical Trials: A Methodologic Perspective,* 2nd ed., Wiley, Chichester, 2005.

The following book is more idiosyncratic than either of the preceding books, but it is important for the view it propounds on the explanatory and pragmatic aspects of clinical trials.

Schwartz, D., Flamant, R., and Lellouch, J., *Clinical Trials* (translated by Healy, M.J.R.), Academic Press, London, 1980.

Many of the terms that are encountered in this field can be found as entries in the excellent book:

Armitage, P. and Colton, T. (Eds.), *Encyclopedia of Biostatistics*, 2nd ed., Wiley, Chichester, 2005.

## Books on More Specialized Topics

The main reference on sequential trials is

Armitage, P., *Sequential Medical Trials*, 2nd ed., Blackwell, Oxford, 1975.

A much more recent publication is

Whitehead, J., *The Design and Analysis of Sequential Clinical Trials*, 2nd ed., Ellis Horwood, Chichester, 1992.

A very comprehensive reference for crossover trials is

Jones, B. and Kenward, M.G., *Design and Analysis of Cross-Over Trials*, 2nd ed., Chapman & Hall/CRC Press, Boca Raton, FL, 2003.

A more personal view can be found in:

Senn, S.J., *Cross-Over Trials in Clinical Research*, 2nd ed., Wiley, Chichester, 2002.

A substantial reference for cluster-randomized trials is

Murray, D.M., *Design and Analysis of Group-Randomized Trials*, Oxford University Press, Oxford, 1998.

Many of the issues that attend meta-analyses are covered in a collection of articles that are published in:

Egger, M., Smith, G.D., and Altman, D.G., *Systematic Reviews in Health Care: Meta-Analysis in Contest*, BMJ Publishing, London, 2001.

A comprehensive treatise is

Whitehead, A., *Meta-Analysis of Controlled Clinical Trials*, Wiley, Chichester, 2002.

Interesting discussions of many of the ethical issues involved in RCTs can be found in:

Silverman, W.A., *Human Experimentation: A Guided Step into the Unknown*, Oxford University Press, Oxford, 1985.

Many groups of investigators use RCTs and most of the books cited do not assume the point of view of any particular group. However, the pharmaceutical industry is a large and important user of RCTs, and a book which largely takes this perspective is

Senn, S., *Statistical Issues in Drug Development*, Wiley, Chichester, 1997.

# Solutions to Exercises

## Chapter 1

1.
   a. The data are set in column C1 and are drawn from a single population. Labels for two treatments are given in column C2 in systematic order. The first part of the macro generates 100 random numbers in a third column and then sorts this in ascending order. The permutation required to do this is a random permutation and is applied to column C2, placing the resulting set of treatment labels in column C4. This set of treatment labels is an allocation of the outcomes that would have occurred from randomizing the 100 patients into two groups.

   b. The macro computes a signed $t$-statistic in k4 and assigns it to the next available row of column C5. In this way, the result of performing repeated randomizations and forming the $t$-statistic can be investigated. Although the data do not have a normal distribution, they have been divided into two groups at random and the $t$-statistics should still follow the $t$-distribution on 98 degrees of freedom.

   c. The data in column 1 are a sample from the distribution of exp(Z), where Z is a standard normal variable, having sample mean 1.85 and standard deviation 2.11. Running the macro in the question, evaluating the cumulative distribution function of the $t$-distribution on 98 degrees of freedom at C5, and plotting the result as suggested in the question gives the following graph. The null distribution of the $t$-statistic is the $t$-distribution (despite the marked nonnormality of the data) as the straight line in the graph on the following page demonstrates.

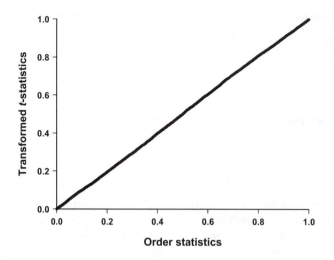

## Chapter 2

1. The comparison is biased because we are not comparing groups
   formed by randomization. The groups to receive antibiotics or *T*
   were comparable when randomized, but patients in the antibiotic
   group who did not test positive for *H. pylori* were excluded. It is at
   least plausible that these individuals may be less seriously diseased,
   so we are leaving a group of such patients in the *T* group but
   excluding them from the antibiotic group, thereby biasing the comparison (plausibly in favor of *T*).

Four possible alternatives are as follows:

- Perform the breath test before randomization and only randomize
  those with a positive breath test. All patients receiving antibiotics
  are compared with all patients receiving *T* and the comparison is
  unbiased. This is probably the best option but has the disadvantage
  that entry to the trial depends on the results of a test that is not 100%
  accurate; some patients with *H. pylori* will test negative and not be
  offered a treatment that would help.

- Randomize patients before the breath test and give antibiotics to all
  randomized to that group, regardless of the outcome of the breath
  test. Again, comparison of the groups receiving antibiotics and *T*
  would be as formed by randomization and therefore comparable.
  The disadvantage is that antibiotics would be given to patients in
  whom there is no infection; antibiotic treatment can lead to problems

and the doctor may feel he needs some evidence of infection before exposing a patient to such a risk, however small.

- Perform the test as described in the question, but compare all those randomized to antibiotics with all those randomized to $T$, regardless of whether or not they actually received antibiotics. Again, this would be unbiased because we are comparing groups as formed by randomization. However, the trial would need to decide what treatment should be offered to those randomized to antibiotics who had negative breath tests. If they were given $T$, then the trial would be less powerful than it might have been because of the presence of a proportion of identically treated patients in both groups.

- Perform the trial as in the question but perform the breath test in the $T$ group too, and then compare only those with positive breath tests. Although this is probably far better than the suggestion in the question, the groups being compared (allocated to antibiotics and then found to have positive breath test vs. allocated to $T$ and then found to have positive breath test) have not been formed solely by randomization, so this comparison cannot be claimed to be unbiased.

---

## Chapter 3

1.

    a. Here, $\sigma = 2.3$ mm, $\tau_M = 0.5$ mm and, if each group contains $n$ patients, $\lambda = \sqrt{2/n}$. To find the size of each group in a trial with power $1 - \beta$ at the two-sided $100\alpha\%$ level, we need to solve:

$$\frac{\tau_M}{\sigma\lambda} = \frac{0.5}{2.3}\sqrt{\tfrac{1}{2}n} = 1.96 + z_\beta$$

    which gives:

$$2n = \left\{4 \times 2.3 \times (1.96 + z_\beta)\right\}^2$$

    For $1 - \beta = 0.9, 0.8$, we obtain $z_{0.1}, z_{0.2} = 1.28, 0.84$ and substituting in the preceding equation gives the total number of patients as 889 (90%) or 664 (80%).

    b. The smallest difference detectable with 80% power from 300 patients occurs when both groups contain 150 patients. Hence $\lambda^{-1} = \sqrt{75} = 5\sqrt{3}$ and

$$\frac{\tau_M}{\sigma\lambda} = \tau_M \frac{5\sqrt{3}}{2.3} = 1.96 + z_{0.2} = 1.96 + 0.84$$

giving $\tau_M \approx 0.744$ mm

c. Here, we simply repeat the calculation for 80% power in question 1 (a) with $\tau_M = 1$, i.e., we find $n$ satisfying:

$$\frac{1}{2.3}\sqrt{\tfrac{1}{2}n} = 1.96 + 0.84$$

giving $2n = \left\{2 \times 2.3 \times (1.96 + 0.84)\right\}^2 = 166$

d. If using 2.3 mm underestimates $\sigma$ by 20% then we replace 2.3 in the preceding equation by $2.3 \div 0.8$, or if using 2.3 mm overestimates $\sigma$ by 20% then 2.3 goes to $2.3 \div 1.2$, so the preceding sample size estimate changes by a factor of $0.8^{-2}$ or $1.2^{-2}$, i.e., 166 changes to 260 or 116. This illustrates how sensitive sample size calculations are to apparently slight changes in the values used for the parameters in the formulae.

e. Assume the smaller group contains $n$ patients and the larger, $2n$, and so $\lambda^{-1} = \sqrt{(2n)/3}$. For 80% power to detect a 1-mm difference at the 5% level we need:

$$\frac{\sqrt{2n}}{2.3\sqrt{3}} = 1.96 + 0.84 \quad \Rightarrow \quad n = \tfrac{3}{2}\left[2.3 \times (1.96 + 0.84)\right]^2$$

giving groups of 62 and 124.

2. Write $\pi_T, \pi_P$ for the proportions believed to respond favorably on, respectively, the new treatment and placebo. We are looking for sample sizes that give 80% power to detect a change $\pi_T - \pi_P = 0.1$ at the 5% level when $\pi_P = 0.3$ or 0.2 or 0.6. Thus, we need to solve the following equation for $n$:

$$\frac{2\left(\arcsin(\sqrt{0.1 + \pi_P}) - \arcsin(\sqrt{\pi_P})\right)}{\sqrt{2/n}} = z_{0.2} + 1.96 = 0.84 + 1.96 = 2.8$$

Hence $n = 2.8^2 / [2(\arcsin(\sqrt{0.1 + \pi_P}) - \arcsin(\sqrt{\pi_P}))^2] = 355$ or 195 when $\pi_P = 0.3$ or 0.1. When $\pi_P = 0.6$ we obtain $n = 355$, so the number required to detect a difference of 0.3 to 0.4 is the same as for 0.6 to 0.7. We are looking to detect a change in the proportion of successes, but the definition of success in terms of the binary variable is essentially arbitrary, so if we had decided to determine the size of the trial based on reducing the proportion with unfavorable outcomes by 0.1, from 0.7 to 0.6, we would have been determining the sample size for the same trial. So a change from 0.7 to 0.6 must give the same sample size as a change from 0.3 to 0.4.

3. Let $\theta = \arcsin(\sqrt{x})$, $0 \le \theta \le \frac{1}{2}\pi$, so $x = \sin^2\theta$ and hence $1 - x = \cos^2\theta = \sin^2(\frac{1}{2}\pi - \theta)$; thus $\arcsin(\sqrt{1-x}) = \frac{1}{2}\pi - \arcsin(\sqrt{x})$. Applying this formula to the two terms in $f(1-y, 1-x)$ gives the required result.

   An alternative way of saying that you want to determine the sample size needed to detect a change in the proportion of successes from $\pi_A$ to $\pi_B$ is to say you want to determine the sample size needed to detect a change in the proportion of failures from $1 - \pi_A$ to $1 - \pi_B$. As what is labeled success and failure is arbitrary from a mathematical point of view, the sample size obtained starting from $\pi_A$ and $\pi_B$ in the usual formula must coincide with that obtained starting from $1 - \pi_A$ and $1 - \pi_B$. This is guaranteed by the identity proved in this question.

4. The RCT was planned to have power 90% at the 5% significance level, so we know $\tau_M/(\sigma\lambda) = z_{1\alpha} + z_\beta = 1.96 + 1.28 = 3.24$. When the data are collected, we calculate the $t$-statistic, $(\bar{x}_1 - \bar{x}_2)/(s\lambda)$, and we are told that the numerator is numerically equal to $\tau_M$ and that $s \approx \sigma$, thus the $t$-statistic is approximately $\tau_M/(\sigma\lambda) = 3.24$. Consequently, the two-sided $P$-value is

$$P = \Phi(-3.24) + 1 - \Phi(3.24) = 0.0012$$

   If $\bar{x}_1 - \bar{x}_2 = \frac{1}{2}\tau_M$ then $P = \Phi(-3.24/2) + 1 - \Phi(3.24/2) = 0.105$.

5. No. The trial may have been designed to provide a high probability of giving a significant result if the true difference between treatments was $\tau_M$, but if the true difference is less than this, there may still be a substantial chance of having a significant result. A more precise analysis is possible. Suppose the trial is designed to have power $1 - \beta$ to detect a difference of $\tau_M$ at the 5% level but the actual difference is $\zeta\tau_M$, a difference less than the minimal clinically important but nonzero difference corresponds to $0 < \zeta < 1$. The probability of a significant difference at the 5% level is then

$$\Pr(\tilde{Z} > z_{\frac{1}{2}\alpha}) + \Pr(\tilde{Z} < -z_{\frac{1}{2}\alpha}) = 1 - \Phi\left(z_{\frac{1}{2}\alpha} - \frac{\zeta\tau_M}{\lambda\sigma}\right) + \Phi\left(-z_{\frac{1}{2}\alpha} - \frac{\zeta\tau_M}{\lambda\sigma}\right)$$

where $\tilde{Z}$ is a normal random variable with mean $(\zeta\tau_M)/(\lambda\sigma)$ and variance 1. By the planning of the trial, we know that $(\zeta\tau_M)/(\lambda\sigma) = \zeta(1.96 + z_\beta)$, so the preceding probability is

$$1 - \Phi(-\zeta z_\beta + 1.96(1-\zeta)) + \Phi(-1.96(1+\zeta) - \zeta z_\beta)$$

For 90% power, i.e., $z_\beta = 1.28$, this can be plotted as a function of $\zeta$.

The graph below shows, for example, that even when the true effect is only 60% of that used in planning the trial, there is still about a 50% chance of obtaining a significant result.

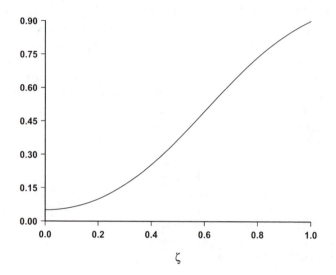

6. As $\bar{x}_1 - \bar{x}_2$ is independent of $s$, it follows that it is also independent of $1/s$, hence:

$$E(D) = \frac{E(\bar{x}_1 - \bar{x}_2)E(s^{-1})}{\lambda}$$

and if we approximate $E(s^{-1})$ by $\sigma^{-1}$ then we obtain $E(D) = \tau / \lambda\sigma$.

7. To obtain the exact expectation of $D$, we need to obtain an exact expression for $E(s^{-1})$ and use it to replace $\sigma^{-1}$ in the formula in question 6. Now, $(vs^2)/\sigma^2$ has a $\chi^2$ distribution with $v = m + n - 2$ degrees of freedom. Therefore, $E(\sigma / (s\sqrt{v})) = (\sigma/\sqrt{v})E(s^{-1}) = E(X^{-\frac{1}{2}})$ where $X$ has a $\chi^2$ distribution with $v$ degrees of freedom. This expectation can be evaluated as

$$K(v)^{-1} \int_0^\infty x^{-\frac{1}{2}} x^{\frac{1}{2}v-1} e^{-\frac{1}{2}x} dx = K(v)^{-1} \int_0^\infty x^{\frac{1}{2}(v-1)-1} e^{-\frac{1}{2}x} dx = \frac{K(v-1)}{K(v)}$$

and from the definition of $K$, we find that this is

$$\frac{2^{\frac{1}{2}(v-1)}}{2^{\frac{1}{2}v}} \frac{\Gamma(\frac{1}{2}(v-1))}{\Gamma(\frac{1}{2}v)} \approx \frac{1}{\sqrt{v-2}}$$

from which we obtain $E(s^{-1}) = \sigma^{-1}\sqrt{v}/(v-2)$. Thus the exact expectation of $D$ is $E(D) = (\tau/(\lambda\sigma))\sqrt{(v/(v-2))}$. Our approximation is thus a slight underestimate, by about 3.5% for two groups each of size 15 falling to 0.5% with two groups of 100. Note that use of the approximation will give sample sizes that are slightly too large, so the error is conservative (as well as very slight).

8. Write $f(u) = \arcsin(\sqrt{u})$. Then, applying a first-order Taylor expansion of $R/N$ about its mean, we obtain $E(f(R/N)) \approx f(\pi) + (\frac{R}{N} - \pi)f'(\pi)$. Hence, to first-order $E(f(R/N)) = f(\pi)$. However, we can go further by using a second-order Taylor expansion to obtain $E(f(R/N)) \approx f(\pi) + (\frac{R}{N} - \pi)f'(\pi) + \frac{1}{2}(\frac{R}{N} - \pi)^2 f''(\pi)$, and hence $E(f(R/N)) \approx f(\pi) + \frac{1}{2}\frac{\pi(1-\pi)}{N}f''(\pi)$.

    Evaluating the second derivative gives

$$E(\arcsin(\sqrt{R/N})) \approx \arcsin(\sqrt{\pi}) - \frac{1}{8}\frac{1-2\pi}{N\sqrt{\pi(1-\pi)}}$$

Note that the new correction vanishes when $\pi = \frac{1}{2}$, so the original formula is correct to second order in this case. Note also that the sign of correction changes as $\pi$ changes from below to above $\frac{1}{2}$ and that the magnitude of the correction increases as $\pi$ tends to its limit of 0 or 1.

9. The exercise is perhaps most efficiently performed by setting k99 = 0 and then executing the following macro 9 times:

```
let k99=k99+1
let k98=k99+3
let k10=pi(k99)
let k11=nn(k99)
base 401
random 10000 c3;
binomial k11 k10.
let c3=asin(sqrt(c3/k11))
let k1=mean(c3)
let k2=asin(sqrt(k10))
let k3=k2-(1-2*k10)/(8*k11*sqrt(k10*(1-k10)))
let k4=stdev(c3)
let k5=1/(2*sqrt(k11))
```

```
copy k1-k5 ck98
end
```

with column pi being 0.05 0.05 0.05 0.2 0.2 0.2 and 0.5 0.5 0.5 and nn containing 10 30 100 10 30 100 10 30 100. Note that the line `base 401` is not really necessary as it simply ensures that each run is based on the same underlying string of pseudorandom numbers. This essentially exists so that readers can reproduce the results in the following table exactly.

|            |   | $N = 10$ | $N = 30$ | $N = 100$ |
|------------|---|----------|----------|-----------|
|            | a | 0.142    | 0.194    | 0.220     |
| $\pi = 0.05$ | b | 0.226    | 0.226    | 0.226     |
|            | c | 0.174    | 0.208    | 0.220     |
|            | a | 0.428    | 0.456    | 0.462     |
| $\pi = 0.2$  | b | 0.464    | 0.464    | 0.464     |
|            | c | 0.445    | 0.457    | 0.462     |
|            | a | 0.786    | 0.786    | 0.786     |
| $\pi = 0.5$  | b | 0.785    | 0.785    | 0.785     |
|            | c | 0.785    | 0.785    | 0.785     |

Line a is the mean of the 10000 arcsin($\sqrt{R/N}$) values, b is arcsin($\sqrt{\pi}$), and c is the second-order correction from question 8. The approximations look very good for all $N$ when $\pi$ is 0.5 and also when it is 0.2 or 0.05 unless $N = 10$ when the approximation appears poorer.

|            |   | $N = 10$ | $N = 30$ | $N = 100$ |
|------------|---|----------|----------|-----------|
| $\pi = 0.05$ | a | 0.180    | 0.117    | 0.053     |
|            | b | 0.158    | 0.091    | 0.050     |
| $\pi = 0.2$  | a | 0.195    | 0.094    | 0.050     |
|            | b | 0.158    | 0.091    | 0.050     |
| $\pi = 0.5$  | a | 0.171    | 0.092    | 0.050     |
|            | b | 0.158    | 0.091    | 0.050     |

Here a is the standard deviation of the 10000 arcsin($\sqrt{R/N}$) values and b is the theoretical standard deviation, $1/(2\sqrt{N})$. The approximation is good for $N = 30$ and $N = 100$, provided $\pi > 0.05$. The approximation is less good for $N = 10$ and $\pi = 0.05$.

# Chapter 4

1. $N_1$ has a binomial distribution with parameters $N$ and $\frac{1}{2}$. From

$$\lambda(N_1, N_2) = \sqrt{\frac{1}{N_1} + \frac{1}{N_2}}$$

we see that $\lambda^{-2} = N_1 N_2 / N = (\frac{1}{2}N + X)(\frac{1}{2}N - X)/N = \frac{1}{4}N - \frac{X^2}{N}$.
The distribution of $N_1$ is well approximated by the normal distribution with mean $\frac{1}{2}N$ and variance $\frac{1}{4}N$, so $X$ has an approximate normal distribution with mean 0 and the same variance.
Hence $Z = 2X / \sqrt{N}$ has a standard normal distribution. $Z^2$ has a $\chi^2$ distribution with one degree of freedom and, as $\lambda^{-2} = \frac{1}{4}N - \frac{Z^2}{4}$, the result follows. Also, $\Pr(\lambda < L) = \Pr(\lambda^{-2} > L^{-2}) = \Pr(N - 4\lambda^{-2} < N - 4L^{-2}) = \Pr(\chi_1^2 < N - 4L^{-2})$. Setting this equal to 0.95 and noting that the 95% point of a $\chi^2$ distribution with one degree of freedom is 3.84, we find $L = 2 / \sqrt{N - 3.84}$. Thus, as the size of the trial increases, the value of $\lambda$ is 95% certain to be less than an amount that gets smaller, thereby increasing the power of the trial. Moreover, as the minimum value of $\lambda$ occurs when the groups have the same size, we know that $\lambda$ is 95% certain to be between $(2 / \sqrt{N}, 2 / \sqrt{N - 3.84})$, so the width of the range over which $\lambda$ is likely to vary decreases with $N$.

2. $\lambda(N_1, N_2) = \sqrt{N_1^{-1} + N_2^{-1}} = \sqrt{N / (N_1 N_2)}$. Writing $N_1 = \frac{1}{2}N - X$, $N_2 = \frac{1}{2}N + X$ this becomes $\lambda(N_1, N_2) = \sqrt{N / (\frac{1}{4}N^2 - X^2)}$, which is clearly minimized when $X = 0$ and $\lambda_{min} = 2 / \sqrt{N}$. If we approximate the distribution of the number of patients in group 1 by a normal distribution, we find we can approximate the distribution of $X$ by that of $\frac{1}{2}Z\sqrt{N}$, where $Z$ has a standard normal distribution. It follows that $\lambda^{-2} = \frac{1}{4}N - \frac{1}{4}Z^2$. Hence $(\lambda/\lambda_{min})^{-2} = 1 - Z^2/N$ and $\Pr(\lambda/\lambda_{min} > \xi) = \Pr([\lambda/\lambda_{min}]^{-2} < \xi^{-2}) \approx \Pr(Z^2/N > 1 - \xi^{-2})$.

Setting this equal to 0.05, we obtain $N(1 - \xi^{-2}) = 3.84$ because $\Pr(Z^2 > 3.84) = 0.05$.

Setting $\xi$ successively to 1.5 and 1.1 and solving gives $N = 6.9$ and 22.1, respectively.

3. Using RPBs with blocks of length six or less means that the numbers of patients allocated to the two treatments cannot differ by more than three, so the probability that the numbers differ by four is 0. The numbers on the two treatments can differ by more than two only if at least one of the blocks generated is either AAABBB or BBBAAA. Call these bad blocks. The probability that the ten blocks generated do not include a bad block is $(1 - p)^{10}$ where $p$ is the probability that a generated block is bad. Now $p = \Pr(\text{generate bad block})$

= Pr($AAABBB$ or $BBBAAA$ | choose block length 6)Pr(choose block length 6); Pr(choose block length 6) = 1/2, and first factor is 1/10 because there are 20 possible blocks, 2 of which are bad. Hence, required probability is $(1-\frac{1}{20})^{10}$ =0.599.

4. The allocation of the next two patients can be predicted when (1) the treatments already allocated are known (so trial cannot be double blind), (2) $4r+2$ patients have already been allocated, for some non-negative integer $r$, and (3) the last two patients received the same treatment. Assuming (1) is satisfied, then after recruiting $4r+2$ patients, two of the six possible blocks (AABB or BBAA) would allow prediction, so the probability of being able to predict the next two treatments is 1/3.

5. The first four cells of C4 contain random numbers uniformly distributed on (1,2), the second four are distributed on (2,3) and so on, with the last four uniformly distributed on $(N, N+1)$. Thus, the permutation that places the elements of C4 in ascending order must keep the first four rows in the first four rows, albeit possibly in a different order, the second group of four will similarly stay in the second group of four rows, etc. When this permutation is applied to C1, the two As and Bs in the first four rows will be permuted in a uniform random way (i.e., any of the 4! permutations is equally likely). Similarly, the two As and two Bs in rows 5 to 8 will be randomly permuted back into rows 5 to 8, and so on. C1 will contain As and Bs in random order, with rows $4r-3,\ldots,4r$ $(r > 0)$ containing two As and two Bs, i.e., it is an RPB allocation.

6. As $p > \frac{1}{2}$, $r > 1$, so each of the terms in the question is positive. It remains to show that the sum of the terms is one and this will be accomplished if we show

$$(r^2 - 1)\sum_{k=1}^{\infty} \frac{1}{r^{2k}} = 1$$

The summation is simply an infinite geometric progression with first term and common ratio both equal to $r^{-2}$, so the sum is $r^{-2}(1 - r^{-2})^{-1}$ = $(r^2 - 1)^{-1}$, as required. As $p$ tends to 1, $r$ increases without limit, so the distribution tends to that which places all its probability on the case of exact balance (as would be expected from the definition of a biased coin design with $p = 1$).

The mean is found by evaluating

$$2\frac{(r^2 - 1)}{r}\sum_{k=1}^{\infty} \frac{k}{r^{2k}}$$

and using the standard result (for $a < 1$) that

$$\sum_{i=1}^{\infty} ia^i = a(1-a)^{-2}$$

we see that the mean is $2r(r^2 - 1)^{-1} = 2p(1 - p)/(2p - 1)$. If $p = \frac{1}{2}$, the mean imbalance is $4/3$ but this value increases markedly as $p$ tends to $\frac{1}{2}$, as shown in the following figure.

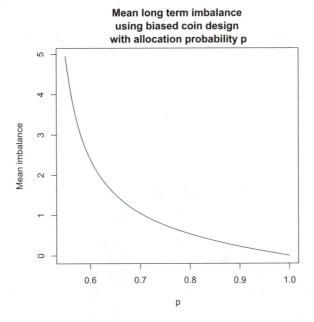

**Mean long term imbalance
using biased coin design
with allocation probability p**

7. Part of the problem here is to work out what is required. The whole point of the urn scheme is that during the trial some patients will be allocated to A with probability greater than $\frac{1}{2}$ and some with a lower probability. However, these are conditional probabilities, conditioned on the state of the trial just before a patient is allocated. The question asks for the probability of allocation to A of any future patient at the outset of the trial. This is interpreted to mean the *unconditional probability* of allocation of the $n$th patient (say) to A. Let $R(n)$ denote the allocation of the $n$th patient. The proof that $\Pr(R(n) = A) = \frac{1}{2}$ proceeds by induction on $n$. It is clear that $\Pr(R(1) = A) = \frac{1}{2}$ and we assume that $\Pr(R(m) = A) = \frac{1}{2}$ for all $m \le n$. If the number allocated to B among the first $n$ patients is $N_B(n)$ then

$$E(N_B(n)) = E \sum_{m=1}^{n} I(R(m) = B)$$

where $I(Q)$ is the indicator function for event $Q$ (i.e., it is 1 or 0 as $Q$ is true or false) and where the expectation is taken over all possible allocations $R(m)$, $m = 1, \ldots, n$. Under the assumption $\Pr(R(m) = A) = \frac{1}{2} = \Pr(R(m) = B)$, this sum is $\frac{1}{2}n$. Now from the definition of the UD($r,s$) scheme $\Pr(R(n+1) = A)$ can be found from

$$\Pr(R(n+1) = A \,|\, N_B(n)) = \frac{r + sN_B(n)}{2r + sn}$$

The expectation of this over all possible values of $N_B(n)$ is simply $\Pr(R(n+1) = A)$ because

$$\Pr(R(n+1) = A) = \sum_k \Pr(R(n+1) = A \,|\, N_B(n) = k)\Pr(N_B(n) = k)$$

$$= \sum_k \frac{r + sk}{2r + sn}\Pr(N_B(n) = k) = \frac{r + sE(N_B(n))}{2r + sn} = \frac{r + \frac{1}{2}sn}{2r + sn} = \frac{1}{2}$$

So, the inductive step has been proved, and the result that at the outset, each patient is equally likely to be allocated to A or B has been established.

8. Under simple randomization, the distribution of $D(n) = 2N_A(n)-n$ is approximately normal with mean 0 and variance $n$. Therefore, $|D(n)| > r$ corresponds to $|Z| = |D(n)|/\sqrt{n} > r/\sqrt{n}$ where $Z$ has a standard normal distribution so

$$\Pr(|Z| > r/\sqrt{n}) = 1 - \Phi\left(\frac{r}{\sqrt{n}}\right) + \Phi\left(-\frac{r}{\sqrt{n}}\right) = 2\left[1 - \Phi\left(\frac{r}{\sqrt{n}}\right)\right]$$

This is same expression as for the urn scheme but for the factor of $\sqrt{3}$ in the numerator. Consequently, the probability of a given imbalance is smaller for the urn scheme than for simple randomization because of this factor. Setting $r = n/10$, we compare $2(1 - \Phi(0.1\sqrt{n}))$ with $2(1 - \Phi(0.1\sqrt{3n}))$. The results are given in the following text. As seen in Chapter 3, the power is related to sample size through the quantity $\lambda$. For an imbalance of $r$ and total trial size $n$, we have

$$\lambda = \sqrt{\frac{1}{\frac{1}{2}(n-r)} + \frac{1}{\frac{1}{2}(n+r)}} = \sqrt{\frac{4n}{n^2 - r^2}} = 2\sqrt{\frac{1}{n(1 - 0.1^2)}} \cong \frac{2}{\sqrt{n}}(1 + 0.005)$$

when $r = n/10$.

The factor 1.005 becomes 1 when $r = 0$. So an imbalance of 10% will have a minimal effect on power. The following plot shows that even for trials as small as 50, there is only a very small chance of an imbalance this large if an urn scheme allocation is used. For simple randomization, even for trials as large as 100, there is still a probability of more than 0.3 of a larger imbalance and a good chance of an imbalance that will have a noticeable effect on power.

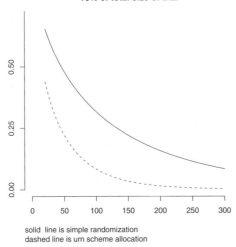

**Probability of an imbalance more than 10% of total size of trial**

solid line is simple randomization
dashed line is urn scheme allocation

9. If the minimum clinically important difference is a standard deviation, then $\tau_M/\sigma = 1$ and the equation for finding the sample size that has power of $1-\beta$ and two-sided significance level $\alpha$ is

$$\lambda^{-1} = z_\beta + z_{\frac{1}{2}\alpha} = \sqrt{nm/(m+n)}$$

where $m$ and $n$ are the sizes of the two groups. Setting $\alpha = 0.05$, $\beta = 0.1$ or 0.2 we obtain $\lambda^{-1} = 1.28 + 1.96$ (power = 0.9) or $\lambda^{-1} = 0.84 + 1.96$ (power = 0.8). Putting $m = n$ and solving we obtain a total sample size, $2n$, of 42 for a power of 0.9 and 31 (which we would round to 32 in practice) for a power of 0.8.

If now we decide that $m = \theta n$, so the (fixed) total number of patients is $N = n(1+\theta)$, then the power $1-\beta = \Phi(z_\beta)$ is now determined by

$$\lambda^{-1} = z_\beta + z_{\frac{1}{2}\alpha} = \sqrt{n\theta/(1+\theta)} = \sqrt{N\theta}/(1+\theta) \text{ or } 1-\beta = \Phi(-1.96 + \sqrt{N\theta}/(1+\theta))$$

This can be evaluated for $\theta = 1, 2, 3$ (1 is as a check on the powers we were supposed to achieve), to give the following powers

| Planned power for equal group sizes | Actual Powers | | |
|---|---|---|---|
| | $\theta = 1$ | $\theta = 2$ | $\theta = 3$ |
| 0.9 | 0.9 | 0.86 | 0.80 |
| 0.8 | 0.8 | 0.75 | 0.68 |
| 0.8 (if you rounded $N$ to 32) | 0.81 | 0.76 | 0.69 |

10. Write $n_A \left( = \sum_{i,j} n_{ijA} \right)$ for the number of patients allocated to treat-

ment A. The expectation of $n_A \bar{X}_A$ is $\sum_{i,j} n_{ijA}(\delta_i + \alpha_j + \tau_A)$ which can

be written as

$$\left( \sum_i n_{i+A}\delta_i \right) + \left( \sum_j n_{+jA}\alpha_j \right) + n_A\tau_A$$

with a similar expression for the expectation of $n_B \bar{X}_B$ and where a + sign in place of a subscript denotes summation over that subscript. The required expectation is, therefore:

$$\left( \sum_i \left[ \frac{n_{i+A}}{n_A} - \frac{n_{i+B}}{n_B} \right] \delta_i \right) + \left( \sum_j \left[ \frac{n_{+jA}}{n_A} - \frac{n_{+jB}}{n_B} \right] \alpha_j \right) + (\tau_A - \tau_B)$$

If condition * is satisfied then $n_A = n_B$ and so (*) ensures that the coefficients of the $\alpha$ and $\delta$ terms are all zero and the estimator is unbiased.

The condition * can be satisfied by the following arrangement in which $n_{ijA} \neq n_{ijB}$:

| | $i = 1$ | | $i = 2$ | | $n_{+jA}, n_{+jB}$ |
|---|---|---|---|---|---|
| $j=1$ | A:10 | B:5 | A:5 | B:10 | 15,15 |
| $j=2$ | A:5 | B:10 | A:10 | B:5 | 15,15 |
| $n_{i+A}, n_{i+B}$ | 15 | 15 | 15 | 15 | |

(There are many other possible configurations.)

Minimization attempts to achieve balance by trying to satisfy (*), whereas stratification looks to obtain balance by ensuring for each pair $(i, j)$ that $n_{ijA} = n_{ijB}$.

## Chapter 5

1. A single-blind trial is one in which the patient is unaware of the treatment they are receiving. In a double-blind trial, neither the patient nor the doctor* knows what treatment is being given. (It may be that the doctors involved in the clinical management of the patient know which treatment has been allocated and it is the doctor assessing the outcome who is unaware of treatment being administered.)

   It is important to take account of the element of subjectivity in the outcome measure before deciding on the necessity of making a trial double blind. If the outcome could clearly be subject to bias, such as a blood pressure measurement or a clinical assessment (for example, how much of the body is covered with plaques in psoriasis or size of a goiter), then it is important that, if at all possible, the trial be conducted double blind. However, if the outcome is, for example, a laboratory result such as serum sodium concentration, then blindness may be less important. However, other aspects may be important: in some diseases, the attitude of the doctor treating the patient may have an effect on the progress of the patient, so it may be inappropriate to describe the trial as double-blind if the doctor treating the patient knows what treatment they receive, even if the outcome is assessed by an independent doctor who is unaware of the allocated treatment.

2. Suppose the tablets to be given twice a day are green and those three times per day are red. It is supposed that each manufacturer will supply placebos that appear identical to the active red or green tablets. The trial can be made double blind by administering the following regimen.

| | Allocated Treatment | |
|---|---|---|
| | **Twice a Day** | **Three Times a Day** |
| Morning | Green active: Placebo red | Red active: Placebo green |
| Midday | Placebo red: *Placebo green** | Red active: *Placebo green** |
| Evening | Green active: Placebo red | Red active: Placebo green |

   *Note:* It is a matter of judgment whether you need to include green placebo tablets at midday; the trial would remain double-blind in their absence. It might help to maintain a blind. Suppose a patient feels dizzy half an hour after taking the tablets, then feeling dizzy half an hour after midday may lead them to infer that the red tablets were active. On the other hand, the administration of a scheme with a green placebo tablet at midday may be unworkable, as it would require patients in the twice-a-day group to have two sorts of green tablets.

## Chapter 6

1. For bivariate normal variables $Y$, $X$, we know $E(Y \mid X = x) = \mu_Y + \beta(x - \mu_X)$, where $\beta = \rho\sigma_Y / \sigma_X$. If, in the situation described in the question, the response on patient $i$ is $X_i$ and the observed baseline is $b_i$, then

$$E(X_i \mid b_i) = \mu + \beta(b_i - \mu_B) \qquad \text{Group C}$$

$$E(X_i \mid b_i) = \mu + \tau + \beta(b_i - \mu_B) \qquad \text{Group T}$$

with $\beta = \rho\sigma_X / \sigma_B$. We can take means of these expressions within each treatment group and obtain

$$E(\bar{X}_T - \bar{X}_C \mid \bar{b}_T, \bar{b}_C) = \tau + \rho\frac{\sigma_X}{\sigma_B}(\bar{b}_T - \bar{b}_C)$$

2.

a. The derivatives of the sum of squares are as follows:

$$\frac{\partial S}{\partial \mu} = -2\left\{ \sum_{i \text{ in } T}(x_i - \mu - \tau - \gamma b_i) + \sum_{i \text{ in } C}(x_i - \mu - \gamma b_i) \right\}$$

$$= -2\left\{ \sum(x_i - N\mu - N_T\tau - \gamma\sum b_i) \right\}$$

$$\frac{\partial S}{\partial \tau} = -\left\{ \sum_{i \text{ in } T}(x_i - \mu - \tau - \gamma b_i) \right\}$$

$$= -2\left\{ \sum_{i \text{ in } T}x_i - N_T\mu - N_T\tau - \gamma\sum_{i \text{ in } T}b_i \right\}$$

$$\frac{\partial S}{\partial \gamma} = -2\left\{ \sum_{i \text{ in } T}b_i(x_i - \mu - \tau - \gamma b_i) + \sum_{i \text{ in } C}b_i(x_i - \mu - \gamma b_i) \right\}$$

$$= -2\left\{ \sum x_i b_i - N\bar{b}\mu - N_T\bar{b}_T\tau - \gamma\sum b_i^2 \right\}$$

The estimators of the parameters are solution to the system of equations, which results when these quantities are set equal to zero, and it is this system that is shown in matrix notation in the question.

b. Substitute the given expressions for $\hat{\mu}, \hat{\tau}$ in the first two of these equations to see that they provide solutions for any $\hat{\gamma}$.

c. Substituting the given expressions for $\hat{\mu}, \hat{\tau}$ in the third of these equations and solving for $\hat{\gamma}$ gives the required solution. In order to obtain the exact form printed in the question, recall that for any bivariate sample of size $n$ $\Sigma(\xi_i - \bar{\xi})(\eta_i - \bar{\eta}) = \Sigma\xi_i\eta_i - n\bar{\xi}\bar{\eta}$.

d. The correction in population terms for baseline imbalance is to use

$$E(\bar{X}_T - \bar{X}_C \mid \bar{b}_T, \bar{b}_C) = \tau + \rho \frac{\sigma_X}{\sigma_B}(\bar{b}_T - \bar{b}_C),$$ so the corrected estimate of $\tau$

is $(\bar{X}_T - \bar{X}_C) - \rho \frac{\sigma_X}{\sigma_B}(\bar{b}_T - \bar{b}_C)$ and the coefficient of the baseline dif-

ference is $\text{cov}(X,B)/\text{var}(B)$, which is essentially the expression in (c), once we allow different means in the two treatment groups.

3.

a. $\text{cov}(\bar{x}, \sum \lambda_i x_i) = E(\sum \lambda_i \bar{x} x_i) - E(\bar{x})E(\sum \lambda_i x_i)$. Now the second

term vanishes because $E(\sum \lambda_i x_i) = \sum \lambda_i E(x_i) = \mu \sum \lambda_i = 0$. The

first term also vanishes because $E(\bar{x} x_i) = E(\bar{x} x_1)$, as all the $x$s have

the same distribution, hence $E(\sum \lambda_i \bar{x} x_i) = \sum \lambda_i E(\bar{x} x_i) =$

$\sum \lambda_i E(\bar{x} x_1) = 0$.

b. Start by noting that

$$\hat{\gamma} = \frac{\displaystyle\sum_{i \text{ in T}} x_i(b_i - \bar{b}_T) + \sum_{i \text{ in C}} x_i(b_i - \bar{b}_C)}{\displaystyle\sum_{i \text{ in T}}(b_i - \bar{b}_T)^2 + \sum_{i \text{ in C}}(b_i - \bar{b}_C)^2} = \hat{\gamma}_T + \hat{\gamma}_C$$

where $\hat{\gamma}_T$ depends only on the $x$s in group T and similarly for $\hat{\gamma}_C$. Then $\text{cov}(\bar{x}_T - \bar{x}_C, \hat{\gamma}) = \text{cov}(\bar{x}_T - \bar{x}_C, \hat{\gamma}_T + \hat{\gamma}_C) = \text{cov}(\bar{x}_T, \hat{\gamma}_T)$ $- \text{cov}(\bar{x}_C, \hat{\gamma}_C)$, as $\bar{x}_T$ is independent of $\hat{\gamma}_C$ as they depend on data from different groups (and similarly for $\bar{x}_C$ and $\hat{\gamma}_T$). Now, $\hat{\gamma}_T$ can be seen to be of the form $\Sigma \lambda_i x_i$ where $\Sigma \lambda_i = 0$, so the application of the result from (a) shows that the first term in

$\mathrm{cov}(\bar{x}_T, \hat{\gamma}_T) - \mathrm{cov}(\bar{x}_C, \hat{\gamma}_C)$ vanishes, and a similar observation for $\hat{\gamma}_C$ shows that the second term vanishes.

c.  From question 2 (b) $\hat{\tau} = (\bar{x}_T - \bar{x}_C) - \hat{\gamma}(\bar{b}_T - \bar{b}_C)$ and from part (b) of this question we obtain

$$\mathrm{var}(\hat{\tau}) = \mathrm{var}(\bar{x}_T - \bar{x}_C) + (\bar{b}_T - \bar{b}_C)^2 \, \mathrm{var}(\hat{\gamma}) = \sigma^2(N_T^{-1} + N_C^{-1}) + (\bar{b}_T - \bar{b}_C)^2 \, \mathrm{var}(\hat{\gamma})$$

$$\hat{\gamma} = \frac{\displaystyle\sum_{i \text{ in T}} x_i(b_i - \bar{b}_T) + \sum_{i \text{ in C}} x_i(b_i - \bar{b}_C)}{\displaystyle\sum_{i \text{ in T}} (b_i - \bar{b}_T)^2 + \sum_{i \text{ in C}} (b_i - \bar{b}_C)^2} =$$

$$\frac{\displaystyle\sum_{i \text{ in T}} (\mu + \tau + \gamma b_i + \varepsilon_i)(b_i - \bar{b}_T) + \sum_{i \text{ in C}} (\mu + \gamma b_i + \varepsilon_i)(b_i - \bar{b}_C)}{\displaystyle\sum_{i \text{ in T}} (b_i - \bar{b}_T)^2 + \sum_{i \text{ in C}} (b_i - \bar{b}_C)^2}$$

$$= \gamma + \frac{\displaystyle\sum_{i \text{ in T}} \varepsilon_i(b_i - \bar{b}_T) + \sum_{i \text{ in C}} \varepsilon_i(b_i - \bar{b}_C)}{\displaystyle\sum_{i \text{ in T}} (b_i - \bar{b}_T)^2 + \sum_{i \text{ in C}} (b_i - \bar{b}_C)^2}$$

Now the variance of left-hand side is the variance of the second term on the right, which is

$$\frac{\displaystyle\sum_{i \text{ in T}} \mathrm{var}(\varepsilon_i)(b_i - \bar{b}_T)^2 + \sum_{i \text{ in C}} \mathrm{var}(\varepsilon_i)(b_i - \bar{b}_C)^2}{\left(\displaystyle\sum_{i \text{ in T}} (b_i - \bar{b}_T)^2 + \sum_{i \text{ in C}} (b_i - \bar{b}_C)^2\right)^2}$$

using the independence of the residuals, and substituting var(E:) $= \sigma^2$ gives

$$\mathrm{var}(\hat{\gamma}) = \frac{\sigma^2}{\displaystyle\sum_{i \text{ in T}} (b_i - \bar{b}_T)^2 + \sum_{i \text{ in C}} (b_i - \bar{b}_C)^2}$$

4.  The means and SDs of the $\log_{10}$ of the numbers of polyps at 12 months in the two treatment groups are as follows:

| Treatment | $n$ | Mean | SD |
|---|---|---|---|
| Sulindac | 9 | 0.944 | 0.462 |
| Placebo | 10 | 1.630 | 0.434 |

A two-sample *t*-test gives $P = .004$ and the 95% confidence interval for the mean when treated with Sulindac — mean when given placebo is $(-1.12, -0.25)$. Thus there is good evidence of an effect of Sulindac. However, the data are compatible with a true mean effect $\tau$ anywhere between $-1.12$ and $-0.25$.

Although the logarithm of the number of polyps is a more suitable quantity for analysis, the actual number of polyps is a more familiar and interpretable quantity for the clinician. It is therefore helpful to recast the preceding analysis in terms of numbers of polyps. To do this, note that the arithmetic mean of the logarithms of the number of polyps is the logarithm of the geometric mean of the number of polyps. Therefore, if the true geometric means of the number of polyps on Sulindac and placebo are, respectively, $\mu_S^G, \mu_P^G$, then the preceding difference in arithmetic means, $0.944 - 1.630 = -0.686$, is an estimate of $\log(\mu_S^G / \mu_P^G)$, and the interval is a 95% confidence interval for $\log(\mu_S^G / \mu_P^G)$. Consequently, the estimate of $\mu_S^G / \mu_P^G$ is $10^{-0.686} = 0.21$ and the 95% confidence interval is $(10^{-1.12}, 10^{-0.25}) = (0.076, 0.56)$. Thus, we estimate that the number of polyps when treated with Sulindac is 21% of the number when given placebo, but this factor could be between 8% and 56%.

5. The outcome from using analysis of covariance with the log(number of polyps) at 12 months as the response and the log(number of polyps) at baseline as the covariate with treatment as the "model," is

**General Linear Model: log1012 months versus Rxn**

```
Factor Type Levels Values
Rxn Fixed 2 Placebo, Sulindac
```

Analysis of Variance for log1012months, using Adjusted SS for Tests

| Source | DF | Seq SS | Adj SS | Adj MS | F | P |
|---|---|---|---|---|---|---|
| log10baseline | 1 | 2.1212 | 1.6552 | 1.6552 | 15.15 | 0.001 |
| Rxn | 1 | 1.7641 | 1.7641 | 1.7641 | 16.14 | 0.001 |
| Error | 16 | 1.7485 | 1.7485 | 0.1093 | | |
| Total | 18 | 5.6339 | | | | |

$S = 0.330578$  R-Sq $= 68.96\%$  R-Sq(adj) $= 65.08\%$

| Term | Coef | SE Coef | T | P |
|---|---|---|---|---|
| Constant | 0.4249 | 0.2341 | 1.82 | 0.088 |
| log10baselin | 0.6598 | 0.1695 | 3.89 | 0.001 |

```
Least Squares Means for log1012months

Rxn            Mean    SE Mean
Placebo       1.5959    0.1049
Sulindac      0.9812    0.1106
```

The $P$-value for the difference between treatments is now 0.001, whereas before the baseline differences were taken into account, it was $P = 0.004$. Although in practical terms the change in the $P$-value is unimportant, it is instructive to consider the baseline means, which are 1.25 (Sulindac) and 1.36 (placebo). The difference in means if the baseline is ignored is $0.944 - 1.630 = -0.686$, whereas the difference in the adjusted means is $0.981 - 1.596 = -0.615$, so when the initial imbalance is taken into account, i.e., that the placebo group had a slightly higher mean log(number of polyps), the treatment effect is reduced slightly. It might be thought that this would increase the $P$-value, but the analysis of covariance estimates $\sigma$ as $\sqrt{0.1093} = 0.331$, whereas the $t$-test used a pooled SD of 0.447. It is this increase in precision that is responsible for the reduction in the $P$-value. Once the variability in the baseline is taken into account, the residual variability in the outcome is also reduced.

If the change from baseline is computed in the column "change" and the analysis of covariance performed on this variable as the response but other features of the analysis unchanged, then an edited version of the output from Minitab is as follows:

**General Linear Model: Change versus Rxn**

```
Factor Type Levels Values
Rxn Fixed 2 Placebo, Sulindac

Analysis of Variance for change, using Adjusted SS for
Tests
```

| Source | DF | Seq SS | Adj SS | Adj MS | F | P |
|---|---|---|---|---|---|---|
| log10baseline | 1 | 0.2576 | 0.4400 | 0.4400 | 4.03 | 0.062 |
| Rxn | 1 | 1.7641 | 1.7641 | 1.7641 | 16.14 | 0.001 |
| Error | 16 | 1.7485 | 1.7485 | 0.1093 | | |
| Total | 18 | 3.7702 | | | | |

```
S = 0.330578 R-Sq = 53.62% R-Sq(adj) = 47.83%
```

| Term | Coef | SE Coef | T | P |
|------|------|---------|---|---|
| Constant | 0.4249 | 0.2341 | 1.82 | 0.088 |
| log10baselin | -0.3402 | 0.1695 | -2.01 | 0.062 |

Least Squares Means for change

| Rxn | Mean | SE Mean |
|-----|------|---------|
| Placebo | 0.2870 | 0.1049 |
| Sulindac | -0.3277 | 0.1106 |

The *P*-value for the treatment effect is unchanged, the coefficient for the baseline has been reduced by 1. The difference between the adjusted means is unchanged, although the individual means have reduced by 1.309, which is the mean of all the baseline values in the analysis. These changes could be predicted because if the outcome at 12 months obeys the model $x_i = \mu + \tau + \gamma b_i + \varepsilon_i$ (in the treated group, $\tau$ omitted in placebo group), then the change, $d_i = x_i - b_i$, obeys $d_i = \mu + \tau + (\gamma - 1)b_i + \varepsilon_i$, etc. The *P*-value for the coefficient $\gamma$ changes because the estimate is closer to 0 after subtracting 1 but its standard error remains unchanged.

# Chapter 7

1. Starting with

$$G^2 = 2\sum_{i=1}^{4} o_i \log\left(\frac{o_i}{e_i}\right)$$

we want to get to an expression that does not involve logs and does use squared terms. This suggests that an expansion might be useful. We know $\log(1+x) \approx x - \frac{1}{2}x^2$ for small $x$ but the expression for $G^2$ is not obviously in the required form. However, under the null hypothesis, $o/e$ will not, at least for larger samples, deviate too far from one. It might be thought that writing $o/e = 1+(d/e)$ where $d = o - e$ and applying the expansion would be the way forward. It should also be noted that the method of construction for $d$ means that $\Sigma d = 0$. In fact this direct approach does not work (do you see why not?) and it is necessary to follow the hint in the question and apply this approach to alternative expression for $G^2$:

$$2\sum e\log(\tfrac{o}{e})+2\sum(o-e)\log(\tfrac{o}{e})=2\sum e\log(1+d/e)+2\sum d\log(1+d/e)$$

$$\approx 2\sum-\tfrac{1}{2}\frac{d^2}{e}+2\sum\left(\frac{d^2}{e}-\tfrac{1}{2}\frac{d^3}{e}\right)=\sum\frac{d^2}{e}=X^2$$

where terms in $d^3$ have been neglected.

2. First of all, note that $\sqrt{a^2+b^2}\leq|a|+|b|$. The upper limit for the interval for the difference in proportions by Newcombe's method is $p_P-p_T+\sqrt{[(p_T-l_T)^2+(u_P-p_P)^2]}$ and by the result just noted this must be less than or equal to $p_P-p_T+(p_T-l_T)+(u_P-p_P)=u_P-l_T$. This difference must lie in $[-1,1]$ because by the method of their construction both $u_P$ and $l_T$ lie in $[0,1]$. A similar argument shows that the lower limit is also in $[-1,1]$.

3. The recalculated table is

Point and Interval Estimates for the Different Measures of Discrepancy for Real and Reduced PUVA vs. TL-01 Trial: Reversing Direction of Comparison from Table 7.4

| Measure of Discrepancy | Full Trial (*P* = 0.018) | | Reduced Trial (*P* = 0.208) | |
| | Point Estimate | 95% Confidence Interval | Point Estimate | 95% Confidence Interval |
| --- | --- | --- | --- | --- |
| ARD (Equation 7.6) | −0.209 | −0.378, −0.041 | −0.160 | −0.405, 0.085 |
| ARD (Newcombe) | −0.209 | −0.367, −0.035 | −0.160 | −0.384, 0.088 |
| NNT* | 4.78 | 2.65, 24.39 | 6.25 | $(2.47,\infty)\cup(-\infty,-11.78)$ |
| RR | 0.438 | 0.212, 0.907 | 0.556 | 0.217, 1.425 |
| OR | 0.329 | 0.128, 0.847 | 0.444 | 0.124, 1.592 |

*Note:* Formally the signs here would reverse but it is not sensible to talk in terms of a negative NNT, and the way to express the change is that the NNTB on one treatment would change to an NNTH on the other treatment.

Essentially this table is unchanged from Table 7.4. The *P*-values are unchanged and the point and interval estimates for ARD change sign — this is sensible if one treatment clears a larger proportion than the other (a positive ARD) then it will fail to clear a smaller proportion than the poorer treatment. The NNT is also essentially unchanged. The OR in the above table (and the corresponding confidence intervals) can be obtained from the corresponding quantities in Table 7.4 by taking reciprocals. This is a consequence of using the odds, rather than the probability, to measure risk. The relabeling essentially maps $\pi\to 1-\pi$ and, under this transformation, OR $\to 1/$OR.

The only difference is that the RR under one labeling is not simply related to the RR for the other labeling. Using simpler figures, if the probability of cure on treatment A is 0.2 and on treatment B is 0.1, then the RR of cure on A relative to B is 2. However, the RR of failure to cure on A relative to B is $0.8/0.9 = 0.89$. Indeed, if the RR of cure were still 2 but arising from individual cure probabilities of 0.4 and 0.2, then the RR of failure to cure would not be 0.89 but $0.6/0.8 = 0.75$.

As the labeling is mathematically arbitrary, some statisticians have argued that this dependence of the RR on an arbitrary feature of the problem limits the usefulness of the RR. Although the RR should not be used without realizing this property, it must be conceded that the symmetry between cured and not cured, survived and died, is not all that apparent, and the labeling chosen may well reflect the clinical nature of the problem under study and not simply a mathematical formalism.

4. The unadjusted log OR and its confidence interval can be found by using the logistic regression with a general mean $x_{i0} = 1$ and $x_{i1} = 1$ if treatment P is given and $x_{i1} = 0$ if treatment T is given. No adjusting variables $x_{is}$ ($s > 1$) are used. The estimate of $\beta_1$ is the estimate of the log OR we require. The normal equations are

$$\sum_{i=1}^{n}(y_i - \pi_i)x_{ir} = 0, \quad r = 0,\ldots,q$$

In this model $\pi_i$ has just two possible values: $\pi_P = \exp(\beta_0+\beta_1)/[1+\exp(\beta_0+\beta_1)]$ if patient $i$ received P and $\pi_T = \exp(\beta_0)/[1+\exp(\beta_0)]$ if patient $i$ received T. The preceding equation for $r = 1$ gives

$$\sum_i(y_i - \pi_P) = 0 = r_P - n_P\pi_P$$

where the summation is over those patients receiving P. This gives the usual estimator for $\pi_P$. The equation for $r = 0$ gives

$$\sum_i(y_i - \pi_i) = 0 = r - n_P\pi_P - n_T\pi_T$$

where the summation is now over all patients. Combining this with the previous result shows that the usual estimator for $\pi_T$ is also obtained. Solving the equations relating the $\pi$ and $\beta$ parameters shows that the estimator of $\beta_1$ is $\log(\{r_P(n_T-r_T)\}/r_T(n_P-r_P)\})$.

The $(r, s)$ element of the information matrix of $\beta_0$ and $\beta_1$ is given by

$$\sum_{i=1}^{n} \hat{\pi}_i(1-\hat{\pi}_i)x_{ir}x_{is}, \quad r,s=0,\ldots,1$$

which is

$$\begin{pmatrix} n_p\hat{\pi}_p(1-\hat{\pi}_p)+n_T\hat{\pi}_T(1-\hat{\pi}_T) & n_p\hat{\pi}_p(1-\hat{\pi}_p) \\ n_p\hat{\pi}_p(1-\hat{\pi}_p) & n_p\hat{\pi}_p(1-\hat{\pi}_p) \end{pmatrix} =$$

$$\begin{pmatrix} \dfrac{r_p(n_p-r_p)}{n_p}+\dfrac{r_T(n_T-r_T)}{n_T} & \dfrac{r_p(n_p-r_p)}{n_p} \\ \dfrac{r_p(n_p-r_p)}{n_p} & \dfrac{r_p(n_p-r_p)}{n_p} \end{pmatrix}$$

The inverse of this is

$$\frac{n_p n_T}{r_p r_T(n_p-r_p)(n_T-r_T)}\begin{pmatrix} \dfrac{r_p(n_p-r_p)}{n_p} & -\dfrac{r_p(n_p-r_p)}{n_p} \\ -\dfrac{r_p(n_p-r_p)}{n_p} & \dfrac{r_p(n_p-r_p)}{n_p}+\dfrac{r_T(n_T-r_T)}{n_T} \end{pmatrix}$$

The variance of $\hat{\beta}_1$ is the bottom right element of this matrix, i.e.,

$$\frac{n_T r_p(n_p-r_p)+n_p r_T(n_T-r_T)}{r_p r_T(n_p-r_p)(n_T-r_T)} = \frac{n_T}{r_T(n_T-r_T)}+\frac{n_p}{r_p(n_p-r_p)}$$

$$= \frac{1}{r_T}+\frac{1}{(n_T-r_T)}+\frac{1}{r_p}+\frac{1}{(n_p-r_p)}$$

which agrees with the formula in Section 7.3.

5. The variance of the hypergeometric distribution is $V = E(R^2) - M^2$ where $R$ is a random variable with the hypergeometric distribution specified in Subsection 7.4.4 and $M$ is the mean of the distribution $= n_T r/n$. The smallest possible value of $R$ is $a_0 = \max\{0, r - n_p\}$ and the maximum value is $a_S = \min\{r, n_T\}$: define $a_2 = \max\{a_0, 2\}$.

Rather than evaluate $V$ directly from the previous expression, it is easier to note that the variance can be expressed as $V = E(R(R - 1)) + M - M^2$. The expectation on the right-hand side of this expression is

$$\sum_{a=a_0}^{a_S} a(a-1) \frac{\dbinom{n_T}{a}\dbinom{n_P}{r-a}}{\dbinom{n}{r}} = \sum_{a=a_2}^{a_S} a(a-1) \frac{\dbinom{n_T}{a}\dbinom{n_P}{r-a}}{\dbinom{n}{r}}$$

$$= \sum_{a=a_2}^{a_S} n_T(n_T-1) \frac{\dbinom{n_T-2}{a-2}\dbinom{n_P}{r-a}}{\dbinom{n}{r}}$$

$$= n_T(n_T-1) \frac{\dbinom{n-2}{r-2}}{\dbinom{n}{r}} = n_T(n_T-1) \frac{r(r-1)}{n(n-1)}$$

Adding $M - M^2$ to the preceding equation and simplifying gives the result $V = [n_T n_P r(n-r)]/[n^2(n-1)]$.

6. The density of an exponential survival time is $\lambda e^{-\lambda t}$ and the survival function is $-e^{-\lambda t}$, so the hazard function, which is the ratio $f(t)/S(t)$ is $\lambda$.

Writing $\lambda_T = \psi\lambda_P$, the log likelihood becomes

$$\ell(\lambda_P, \psi) = m_P \log \lambda_P - \lambda_P t_{+P} + m_T \log(\psi\lambda_P) - \lambda_P \psi t_{+T}$$

so the score function is

$$\frac{\partial \ell}{\partial \lambda_P} = \frac{m_P}{\lambda_P} - t_{+P} + \frac{m_T}{\lambda_P} - \psi t_{+T} = \frac{m}{\lambda_P} - t_{+P} - \psi t_{+T}$$

$$\frac{\partial \ell}{\partial \psi} = \frac{m_T}{\psi} - \lambda_P t_{+T}$$

Setting these equal to zero and solving, you obtain $\hat{\psi} = (m_T t_{+P})/(m_P t_{+T})$, which is the ratio of the estimates of the $\lambda$ parameters found in the text. The numerical value is 0.510. This is the hazard ratio of clearance on TL-01 relative to PUVA, i.e., the comparison is the opposite way round to that in the test. The comparison in this direction can be recovered by taking the reciprocal of this, which is 1.96, which is slightly closer to 1 than the value found from the nonparametric analysis.

The information matrix is

$$
\begin{pmatrix}
-\dfrac{\partial^2 \ell}{\partial \lambda_P^2} & -\dfrac{\partial^2 \ell}{\partial \lambda_P \partial \psi} \\[3mm]
-\dfrac{\partial^2 \ell}{\partial \lambda_P \partial \psi} & -\dfrac{\partial^2 \ell}{\partial \psi^2}
\end{pmatrix}
=
\begin{pmatrix}
\dfrac{m}{\lambda_P^2} & t_{+T} \\[3mm]
t_{+T} & \dfrac{m_T}{\psi^2}
\end{pmatrix}
$$

and the bottom right-hand element of its inverse is $(m\psi^2)/(m_T m_P)$ at the maximum likelihood estimator. Therefore, a standard 95% confidence interval is found as $\hat{\psi}[1 \pm 1.96\sqrt{m / (m_T m_P)}]$. This interval is (0.28, 0.75).

An alternative is to use profile likelihood methods. This considers the function $p(\psi) = \ell(\hat{\lambda}_{P\psi}, \psi)$ where $\hat{\lambda}_{P\psi}$ is the value of $\lambda_P$ that maximizes the log likelihood when the hazard ratio has the value $\psi$. Fixing the hazard ratio at $\psi$ and differentiating the log likelihood with respect to $\lambda_P$, we get

$$
\frac{\partial \ell}{\partial \lambda_P} = \frac{m}{\lambda_P} - t_{+P} - \psi t_{+T} = 0 \Rightarrow \hat{\lambda}_{P\psi} = \frac{m}{t_{+P} + \psi t_{+T}}
$$

(noting that the second derivative is negative, so this turning point is a maximum) and hence

$$
p(\psi) = m \log \hat{\lambda}_{P\psi} + m_T \log \psi - \hat{\lambda}_{P\psi}(\psi t_{+T} + t_{+P})
$$

$$
= m_T \log \psi - m \log(\psi t_{+T} + t_{+P}) - m + m \log m
$$

General likelihood theory indicates that a 95% confidence interval for $\psi$ is $\{\psi \mid p(\hat{\psi}) - p(\psi) \le 1.92\}$ where 1.92 features because it is half of 3.84, which is the 95% point of a $\chi^2$ distribution on one degree of freedom. The profile log likelihood for $\psi$, which is the name for $p(\psi)$, in this example is, therefore, $p(\psi) = 32 \log \psi - 73 \log(1154\psi + 754)$ (the terms not involving the argument can be omitted). This is plotted in the following figure. The maximum occurs at 0.510, and from the plot the 95% profile likelihood interval is (0.32, 0.81), which is similar to the interval obtained from the ordinary likelihood. The confidence interval for the comparison in the opposite direction is simply the reciprocal interval, namely (1.23, 3.13).

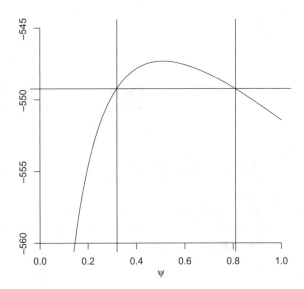

7. Note that because $E_1 + E_2 = O_1 + O_2$, we have $(O_1 - E_1)^2 = (O_2 - E_2)^2$ and, therefore, the simplified version of the log-rank statistic can be written as $(O_1 - E_1)^2(E_1^{-1} + E_2^{-1}) = (O_1 - E_1)^2(E_1 + E_2)/(E_1 E_2) = L_S$, say. We seek to show that $L_S \leq U^2 / V$, but the hint in the question shows that $U^2 / V' \leq U^2 / V$ where $V' = \Sigma v'_j$, so if we show that $L_S \leq U^2 / V'$ the desired result follows. On noting that $L_S = U^2(E_1 + E_2)/(E_1 E_2)$, this latter inequality amounts to $V'(E_1 + E_2) \leq E_1 E_2$. Is this true?

Note that $E_1 + E_2 = \Sigma d_j$ and $V' = \Sigma d_j x_j (1 - x_j)$ where $x_j = n_{1j}/n_j$. Therefore, the inequality holds if and only if

$$\sum w_j x_j (1 - x_j) \leq \sum w_j x_j \sum w_j (1 - x_j)$$

where $w_j = d_j / \Sigma d_i$ are positive numbers that sum to one. The right-hand side of the above inequality is $\Sigma w_j x_j - (\Sigma w_j x_j)^2$, and so the inequality holds if and only if

$$\left(\sum w_j x_j\right)^2 \leq \sum w_j x_j^2 = \left(\sum w_j x_j^2\right) \sum w_j$$

This does hold because it follows from the Cauchy-Schwartz inequality.

8. Stirling's approximation states that for large $n$, $n! \cong \sqrt{2\pi n}\, n^n e^{-n}$. The size of the first set is

$$\binom{4n}{2n}$$

and of the second is $6^n$, because there are 6 blocks of length 4 comprising 2 of each treatment. Applying Stirling's approximation gives

$$\binom{4n}{2n} = \frac{(4n)!}{((2n)!)^2} \approx \frac{\sqrt{8\pi n}\,4^{4n}n^{4n}e^{-4n}}{(4\pi n)2^{4n}n^{4n}e^{-4n}} = \frac{4^{4n}}{\sqrt{2\pi n}\,2^{4n}} = \frac{16^n}{\sqrt{2\pi n}}$$

and dividing this by $6^n$ gives the required ratio as $(8/3)^n / \sqrt{2\pi n}$. This increases without limit as $n$ increases. For a trial with 400 patients, $n = 100$, this ratio is approximately $1.6 \times 10^{41}$.

---

## Chapter 8

1. From Table 8.2 a group sequential trial with $N = 5$, $\alpha = 0.05$, and $1 - \beta = 0.9$ has $\mu = (\tau\sqrt{n})/(\sigma\sqrt{2}) = 1.592$. If $n = 20$ then $\tau/\sigma = 0.503$, that is, a difference of about $\frac{1}{2}$ a standard deviation can be detected. If a trial with $N = 10$ is used then $\mu = (\tau\sqrt{n})/(\sigma\sqrt{2}) = 1.156$ and using $\tau/\sigma = 0.503$ we obtain $n = 10.56$; so we would need to recruit 11 patients to each arm of each group in the new trial. The total number of patients that might be needed, $2nN$, is 200 for $N = 5$ and 220 for $N = 10$, although the rounding of $n$ in the latter means that the power is now likely to be slightly more than 90%.

2. In the development of the theory of group sequential trials, it is important that

$$S_M = \sum_{j=1}^{M} \bar{\delta}_j$$

comprises independent increments with mean $\mu$ and unit variance. If the definition

$$S_M = \sum_{j=1}^{M} \frac{\bar{d}_j}{\sqrt{2\sigma^2/n}} = \sum_{j=1}^{M} \bar{\delta}_j$$

is used when the groups have sizes $n$ and $2n$, then the $\bar{\delta}_j$ will not have unit variance, so a scale factor must be introduced. If each $\bar{\delta}_j$ is multiplied by $2/\sqrt{3}$ then the scaled $\bar{\delta}_j$ will have unit variance and the previous theory will apply, although in power calculations you now use $\mu = [\tau \sqrt{(2n)}]/[\sigma \sqrt{(3)}]$. The test can be based on the $S_M$ for trials with equal group size (with $n$ now interpreted as the size of the smaller group), provided the continuation region is $|S_M| \le b_M$, where $b_M = a_M \sqrt{(3)}/2$.

3. The case $N = 2$ involves the equation

$$f_2(s) = \int_{-a_1}^{a_1} f_1(u)\phi(s - u)du$$

and on the right-hand side $f_1(u)\phi(s - u)du$ is, ignoring infinitesimals, $\Pr(S_1 = u,$ and $\bar{\delta}_2 = s - u)$. This is summed not over all possible $u$ but over those with modulus less than $a_1$. The summation, therefore, yields $\Pr(S_2 = s,$ and $|S_1| \le a_1)$ or, slightly more precisely,

$$f_2(s)ds = \Pr(S_2 \in (s, s + ds), \text{ and } |S_1| \le a_1)$$

In general $f_M(s)ds = \Pr(S_M \in (s, s + ds),$ and $|S_j| \le a_j, j = 1, ..., M - 1)$. It follows, for example, that

$$\int_{-\infty}^{\infty} f_N(u)du = \Pr(|S_M| \le a_M, M = 1, ..., N - 1)$$

which explains the inequality in the question and why the $f$s are not densities.

4. From the answer to question 3, it is clear that

$$\int_{-\infty}^{-a_N} f_N(u)du + \int_{a_N}^{\infty} f_N(u) = \Pr(|S_N| > a_N \text{ and } |S_M| \le a_M, M = 1, ..., N - 1)$$

i.e., the probability that a significant result was found at the final analysis.

5. If $M$ is the random variable that records the number of groups recruited by termination, then the expected number of patients is $2nE(M)$, so an expression for $E(M)$ will suffice. This is plainly

$$\sum_{m=1}^{N-1} m \Pr(|S_m| > a_m; |S_k| \le a_k) + N \Pr(|S_m| \le a_m, m = 1, ..., N - 1)$$

where the final term arises because N groups are recruited if the trial has not terminated by the (N −1)th group, regardless of the result at the final analysis. This can be written as

$$\sum_{m=1}^{N-1} m \int_{R(m)} f_m(u;\mu)du + N \int_{-\infty}^{\infty} f_N(u;\mu)du$$

where $R(m) = [-\infty, -a_m] \cup [a_m, \infty]$.

6. The trial recruits either $4n$ patients or $2n$ patients, the latter only if the trial terminates at the first interim analysis, which it does with probability $p$. The expected number of patients is therefore $2n(2(1 - p) + p) = 4n - 2np$. It only remains to evaluate $p$. This is

$$\int_{-\infty}^{-a_1} \phi(u - \mu)du + \int_{a_1}^{\infty} \phi(u - \mu)du$$

$$= \Phi(-a_1 - \mu) + 1 - \Phi(a_1 - \mu) = \Phi(-z_{\frac{1}{2}\alpha'} - \mu) + 1 - \Phi(z_{\frac{1}{2}\alpha'} - \mu)$$

This is $\alpha'$ if $\mu = 0$ and increases if $\mu$ is nonzero. The plot against $\mu$ is shown in the following figure.

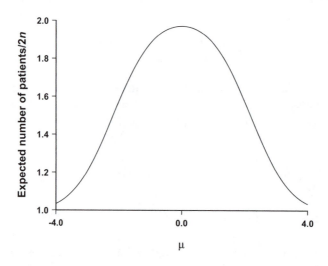

7. In the case $N = 2$, we have

$$f_2(s) = \int_{-a}^{a} \phi(u)\phi(s - u)du$$

where $a$ has been used for $a_1$ to save writing. Now rearrangement of the integrand gives this as

$$\frac{1}{2\pi} e^{-\frac{1}{4}s^2} \int_{-a}^{a} e^{-(u-\frac{1}{2}s)^2} du$$

In order to answer the question, we need to show that the integral of this over the whole real line is $\Pr(|S_1| \leq a)$. The expression is the product of the density of a normal random variable, $s$, with mean zero and variance 2 with the probability that a normal random variable with variance $\frac{1}{2}$ and mean $\frac{1}{2}s$ lies between $\pm a$, where $s$ is the first random variable. Thus, the integral required is the expectation of $\Phi((a - \frac{1}{2}S)\sqrt{2}) - \Phi((-a - \frac{1}{2}S)\sqrt{2})$ over the distribution of $S$. However, $\Phi((a - \frac{1}{2}S)\sqrt{2})$ is the probability that a standard normal variable $Z$, independent of $S$, is less than $(a - \frac{1}{2}S)\sqrt{2}$, so the required expression can be written as

$$E_S E_{Z|S}(I(Z < (a - \tfrac{1}{2}S)\sqrt{2})) - E_S E_{Z|S}(I(Z < (-a - \tfrac{1}{2}S)\sqrt{2}))$$

where $I(E)$ is the indicator function of event $E$. Now the repeated expectation is just the expectation over the joint distribution of $S$ and $Z$. The first indicator function is just $I(\frac{1}{\sqrt{2}}Z + \frac{1}{2}S < a)$ and the random variable $\frac{1}{\sqrt{2}}Z + \frac{1}{2}S$ is normal with mean 0 and variance $\frac{1}{2} + \frac{1}{2} \times 2 = 1$, so the repeated expectation is simply the probability $\Phi(a)$, and a similar calculation obtains for the term with $-a$ and so the required result is obtained.

## Chapter 9

1. No. Although the $P$-value of 0.03 provides evidence of an effect of treatment among males, the value of 0.4 does not demonstrate that there is no effect on females. The value of 0.4 means that the data from the females are compatible with a range of treatment differences, which will include a difference of zero. However, depending on the precision of the estimate for females, the range could be wide and encompass values that are compatible differences for the data from males.

2.

   a. The first step in this analysis is to compute the proportion of patients who clear in the trial in the four groups. These are shown in the following table:

| | Fair Skin | | Dark Skin | |
|---|---|---|---|---|
| | Treatment A | Treatment B | Treatment A | Treatment B |
| Proportion clearing | 0.35 | 0.19 | 0.40 | 0.13 |

There are at least two approaches to testing the null hypothesis of no treatment effect in the two subgroups. The first is to perform a $\chi^2$ test for the $2 \times 2$ table given in the question under each skin type. For patients with fair skin, we obtain $\chi^2 = 1.56$, $P = 0.21$, and for patients with dark skin $\chi^2 = 4.41$, $P = 0.04$.

An alternative approach is to compute $(p_A - p_B)/s.e.(p_A - p_B)$- and refer this to a standard normal distribution. The denominator is evaluated as the square root of $p_A(1-p_A)/n_A + p_B(1-p_B)/n_B$, where $p_A, n_A$ are, respectively, the proportion of patients clearing and the number of patients allocated to A, with similar definitions for treatment B.

For patients with fair skin, we obtain $p_A = 0.35$, $p_B = 0.19$, and $p_A(1-p_A)/n_A + p_B(1-p_B)/n_B = 0.121^2$; so $(p_A - p_B)/s.e.(p_A - p_B) = 1.32$, from which we obtain $P = \Phi(-1.32) + \{1 - \Phi(1.32)\} = 0.19$. (The result is similar to the $\chi^2$ test but not identical — if we had used a pooled proportion to calculate the preceding denominator then the results would have been exactly the same — see Section 7.2.)

For patients with dark skin, we obtain $p_A = 0.40$, $p_B = 0.13$ and $p_A(1-p_A)/n_A + p_B(1-p_B)/n_B = 0.120^2$, so $(p_A - p_B)/s.e.(p_A - p_B) = 2.25$, from which we obtain $P = \Phi(-2.25) + \{1 - \Phi(2.25)\} = 0.024$.

A naïve interpretation of these results is that there is an effect of treatment on patients with dark skin, but not on those with fair skin, hence the treatment affects the two types of patients differently. However, this is false. Although there is evidence that treatment A clears a higher proportion of patients with dark skin than does treatment B, there is no evidence that this is not the case in patients with fair skin. The $P$-value of 0.21 (or 0.19) for patients with fair skin means that there is no evidence against the null hypothesis, not that the null hypothesis is true — we may simply not have gathered sufficient data in this group to provide evidence against the null hypothesis.

b.  The appropriate way to test the null hypothesis that the treatment effect is the same for patients with fair and dark skin is first to compute the difference in the treatment effects, that is $\{p_A^{Dark} - p_B^{Dark}\} - \{p_A^{Fair} - p_B^{Fair}\} = \{0.40 - 0.13\} - \{0.35 - 0.19\} = 0.11$ and then to divide this by an estimate of its standard error, namely, $p_A^{Dark}(1-p_A^{Dark})/n_A^{Dark} + p_B^{Dark}(1-p_B^{Dark})/n_B^{Dark} + p_A^{Fair}(1-p_A^{Fair})/n_A^{Fair} +$

$p_B^{Fair}(1-p_B^{Fair})/n_B^{Fair} = 0.120^2 + 0.121^2 = 0.1704^2$. The test statistic is therefore $0.11 / 0.1704 = 0.65$, and the $P$-value is $P = \Phi(-0.65) + \{1 - \Phi(0.65)\} = 0.52$. There is, therefore, no evidence against the null hypothesis that the treatment effect is the same for patients with dark and fair skins. The difference in these treatment effects is 0.11 and the 95% confidence interval for this difference is $0.11 \pm 1.96 \times 0.1704 = (-0.22, 0.44)$. Thus, although there is no evidence that the treatment has different effects on the two groups of patients, the data are also compatible with there being quite a wide range of possible differences in the treatment effects.

# Chapter 10

1. Comparing those allocated to C with only those who did not withdraw from treatment with I is a comparison of groups not formed by randomization, hence the comparison cannot be claimed to be unbiased. You might wish to perform various analyses of these data, but one analysis that must be performed is the analysis that compares the groups as formed at randomization, with as complete follow-up as possible of those who had to stop taking indomethacin. Despite its obvious limitations, this analysis attempts to compare like with like. Indeed, the estimate obtained from this approach is an unbiased estimate of the overall effect of a policy of offering C or I. In practice, it may have been necessary to have an alternative to I available to offer to those unable to persist with taking this drug. This is the analysis by the dictum of intention to treat.

# Chapter 11

1. The first step in the analysis is to form the differences between the responses from a patient in the two periods. It is not important whether you take the differences (period 1 – period 2) or (period 2 – period 1) but you obviously need to make sure that the sign of your estimator accords with the direction you ascribe to the treatment difference you present. This solution follows the approach in Subsection 9.3.1, namely period 1 – period 2. This difference is calculated and stored in a column named difference.

The model used for the PEFRs is that given in Subsection 11.3.1, namely,

Sequence F then S

$$x_{i1} = \mu + \pi_1 + \tau_F + \xi_i + \varepsilon_{i1} \text{ (period 1) and } x_{i2} = \mu + \pi_2 + \tau_S + \xi_i + \varepsilon_{i2} \text{ (period 2)}$$

Sequence S then F

$$x_{i1} = \mu + \pi_1 + \tau_S + \xi_i + \varepsilon_{i1} \text{ (period 1) and } x_{i2} = \mu + \pi_2 + \tau_F + \xi_i + \varepsilon_{i2} \text{ (period 2)}$$

with *x*s denoting the appropriate PEFR. The treatment effect (formoterol – salbutamol) is defined as $\tau_F - \tau_S$ and the model for the within-patient differences implied by the preceding model is

$$d_i = x_{i1} - x_{i2} = \pi + \tau + \eta_i \quad \tau = \tau_F - \tau_S; \pi = \pi_1 - \pi_2 \text{ (sequence F then S)}$$

with $d_i = x_{i1} - x_{i2} = \pi - \tau + \eta_i$ in the other sequence.

So the difference in the means of the two groups is $2\tau$. A *t*-test comparing the sequences with respect to these differences tests the null hypothesis that $2\tau = 0$, which is obviously the same as a test of the hypothesis of no treatment effect, i.e., $\tau = 0$. The difference in means between the sequence groups and the associated confidence interval need to be divided by 2 to provide point and interval estimates of $\tau$. The result of applying a two-sample *t*-test (with variances assumed equal) to the column "difference" is

**Two-Sample T for Difference**

```
FS/SF   N     Mean    StDev   SE Mean
FS      7     30.7    33.0       12
SF      6    -62.5    44.7       18

95% CI for mu (FS)  -  mu (SF):  (46,  141)
T-Test mu (FS) = mu (SF) (vs not =):  T = 4.32 P = 0.0012
DF = 11
Both use Pooled StDev = 38.7
```

The *P*-value of 0.0012 indicates that there is clear evidence of a difference between the treatments. The difference in the means is 30.7 + 62.5 = 93.2 1/min, with 95% interval estimate (i.e., confidence interval) of (46, 141) 1/min. Dividing these by 2 gives the following point and interval estimates for $\tau$ of 46.7 1/min and (23.0 70.5) 1/min, respectively.

The data from the first period form a parallel group trial with the mean in the "F then S" group being $\mu + \pi_1 + \tau_F$ and that in the "S then F" group being $\mu + \pi_1 + \tau_S$. From this, it follows that the difference in the means of the two groups, using period 1 data only, is $\tau = \tau_F - \tau_S$, so a *t*-test on these two groups gives a *P*-value that tests the same null hypothesis as above and directly provides point and interval estimates for $\tau$.

**Two-Sample T for Period 1**

| FS/SF | N | Mean | StDev | SE Mean |
|-------|---|------|-------|---------|
| FS | 7 | 337.1 | 53.8 | 20 |
| SF | 6 | 283 | 105 | 43 |

95% CI for mu (FS) - mu (SF): (-46, 153)

T-Test mu (FS) = mu (SF) (vs not =): T = 1.19 P =0.26
DF = 11

Both use Pooled StDev = 81.4

The point estimate for $\tau$ is 54.1 l/min with 95% confidence interval from -46 l/min to 153 l/min. The *P*-value is 0.26. This analysis provides an estimate of the treatment effect that, though admittedly not all that close, is similar to the 46.7 l/min found from the analysis using both periods. However, the null hypothesis of no treatment effect, which was decisively rejected in the previous analysis, cannot now be rejected, and the confidence interval is much wider than that obtained before. The reason for this is that the first approach using the data from both periods has eliminated between-patient variability from the analysis; the pooled standard deviation is 38.7 l/min. The second approach does not remove this source of variability from the data, which in this instance is substantial, as can be seen from the pooled standard deviation of 81.4 l/min in the second analysis.

2.

a. The required expectation is calculated as the expectation of:

$$s_i = x_{i1} + x_{i2} = \mu + \pi_1 + \tau_F + \xi_i + \varepsilon_{i1} + \mu + \pi_2 + \tau_S + \gamma_F + \xi_i + \varepsilon_{i2}$$

$$= 2\mu + \pi_1 + \pi_2 + \tau_F + \tau_S + \gamma_F + 2\xi_i + \varepsilon_{i1} + \varepsilon_{i2}$$

The terms in $\xi$ and $\varepsilon$ are random variables with zero mean, so the required expectation is $\tilde{\mu} + \gamma_F$, where $\tilde{\mu} = 2\mu + \pi_1 + \pi_2 + \tau_F + \tau_S$. The corresponding expectation in the S then F group is obtained by interchanging the subscripts *F* and *S* in the preceding equation. This leaves $\tilde{\mu}$ unchanged so the expectation of the $s_i$ in the S then F group is $\tilde{\mu} + \gamma_S$.

b. The null hypothesis tested by comparing the $s_i$ in the S then F with the $s_i$ in the F then S group is that the means in the two groups are the same, namely $\gamma_S = \gamma_F$; that is, the carryover of S into F is the same as the carryover of F into S.

The *t*-test comparing the two sets of sums can be performed in Minitab and the output is shown in the following table, in which the column "sum" is the result of adding "period 1" to "period 2."

**Two-Sample T for Sum**

| FS/SF | N | Mean | StDev | SE Mean |
|-------|---|------|-------|---------|
| FS | 7 | 644 | 114 | 43 |
| SF | 6 | 629 | 174 | 71 |

95% CI for mu (FS) - mu (SF): (-163, 191)

T-Test mu (FS) = mu (SF) (vs not =): T = 0.18 P =0.86
DF = 11

Both use Pooled StDev = 145

The *P*-value is 0.86, implying that we cannot reject the null hypothesis that the carryover is the same for S and F. The estimate of $\gamma_F - \gamma_S$ is the difference in the means which is $644 - 629 = 15$ l/min, with 95% confidence interval $(-163, 191)$ l/min.

c. The estimator of the treatment effect using the data from periods 1 and 2 is $\frac{1}{2}(\bar{d}_{F\,then\,S} - \bar{d}_{S\,then\,F})$, and if the model with carryover is the true model, then $E[\frac{1}{2}(\bar{d}_{F\,then\,S} - \bar{d}_{S\,then\,F})] = (\tau_F - \tau_S) - \frac{1}{2}(\gamma_F - \gamma_S)$ (cf. Section 11.4). So if the analysis in question 1 is used, the bias is $-\frac{1}{2}(\gamma_F - \gamma_S)$. From the preceding entity we see that a 95% confidence interval for the bias term is $-\frac{1}{2} \times (-163, 191) = (-95.5, 81.5)$ l/min. Thus, the bias in our estimate of the treatment effect (46.7 l/min) could be very substantial. Testing for a carryover effect and, if the hypothesis of equal carryover effect cannot be rejected, proceeding as if it were genuinely absent is a procedure that can lead to very misleading results. Unless carryover can be excluded on nonstatistical grounds, then the AB/BA design is probably not to be recommended.

3.

a. The expectation of $\frac{1}{2}(\bar{d}_{AB} - \bar{d}_{BA})$ is equal to that of $\frac{1}{2}(d_1 - d_{2n})$ (or any two ds one from each sequence). Now $E[\frac{1}{2}d_1] = \frac{1}{2}(\mu + \pi_1 + \tau_A - \mu - \pi_2 - \tau_B) = \frac{1}{2}(\pi_1 - \pi_2 + \tau)$ and $E[\frac{1}{2}d_{2n}]$

$\frac{1}{2}(\pi_1 - \pi_2 - \tau)$; so required expectation is $\tau$. Also, $E[\bar{x}_{1AB} - \bar{x}_{1BA}] = (\mu + \pi_1 + \tau_A - \mu - \pi_1 - \tau_B) = \tau$, as required.

b. As the differences in the two sequences are independent,

$$\text{var}[\tfrac{1}{2}(\bar{d}_{AB} - \bar{d}_{BA})] = \tfrac{1}{4}\{\text{var}(\bar{d}_{AB}) + \text{var}(\bar{d}_{BA})\}$$

and

$$\text{var}(\bar{d}_{AB}) = \text{var}(d_1)/n = 2\sigma^2/n \text{ , } \text{var}(\bar{d}_{BA}) = \text{var}(d_{2n})/n = 2\sigma^2/n$$

so

$$\text{var}[\tfrac{1}{2}(\bar{d}_{AB} - \bar{d}_{BA})] = \tfrac{1}{4}\{\frac{2\sigma^2}{n} + \frac{2\sigma^2}{n}\} = \frac{\sigma^2}{n}$$

Again, $\bar{x}_{1AB}, \bar{x}_{1BA}$ are independent, so $\text{var}[\bar{x}_{1AB} - \bar{x}_{1BA}] = \text{var}[\bar{x}_{1AB}] + \text{var}[\bar{x}_{1BA}]$ and this is equal to

$$\text{var}[x_1]/n + \text{var}[x_{2n}]/n = (\sigma_B^2 + \sigma^2)/n + (\sigma_B^2 + \sigma^2)/n = 2(\sigma_B^2 + \sigma^2)/n$$

Hence $R = 2\{1 + (\sigma_B^2/\sigma^2)\}$.

c. If $\sigma_B^2 = 6\sigma^2$ then R = 14. Thus, if we chose to perform a parallel group trial (essentially use period 1 data only), then the standard error of the estimator of the effect of treatment would be $\sqrt{14} = 3.74$ times greater than that you would obtain using a crossover design if the between-patient variance was six times the within-patient variance. Thus, if there is the opportunity to run a crossover trial and there is substantially greater variation between patients than within, then a crossover trial can pay very worthwhile dividends.

4. Write $\xi(\tau) = \Phi\left(\dfrac{\delta - \tau}{\lambda\sigma} - z_{\frac{1}{2}\alpha}\right) - \Phi\left(\dfrac{-\delta - \tau}{\lambda\sigma} + z_{\frac{1}{2}\alpha}\right)$ and note (remembering

that $\Phi(-z) = 1 - \Phi(z)$) that

$$\xi(-\tau) = \Phi\left(\frac{\delta + \tau}{\lambda\sigma} - z_{\frac{1}{2}\alpha}\right) - \Phi\left(\frac{-\delta + \tau}{\lambda\sigma} + z_{\frac{1}{2}\alpha}\right)$$

$$= \left\{1 - \Phi\left(\frac{-\delta - \tau}{\lambda\sigma} + z_{\frac{1}{2}\alpha}\right)\right\} - \left\{1 - \Phi\left(\frac{\delta - \tau}{\lambda\sigma} - z_{\frac{1}{2}\alpha}\right)\right\}$$

$$= \xi(\tau)$$

Also note that

$$\xi(\tau) = \Phi\left(A - \frac{\tau}{\lambda\sigma}\right) - \Phi\left(-A - \frac{\tau}{\lambda\sigma}\right)$$

where

$$A = \frac{\delta}{\lambda\sigma} - z_{1\frac{1}{2}\alpha}$$

and so

$$\xi'(\tau) = \frac{1}{\lambda\sigma}\left\{\phi\left(-A - \frac{\tau}{\lambda\sigma}\right) - \phi\left(A - \frac{\tau}{\lambda\sigma}\right)\right\}$$

where $\phi$ is the standard normal density. Assuming that equivalence is possible, $A > 0$. As $\phi$ is symmetric about 0, with a maximum at 0 and decreases as its argument increases in magnitude, it can be seen that $\xi'(\tau) < 0$ for $\tau > 0$ and $\xi'(\tau) > 0$ for $\tau < 0$. Hence, $\xi(\tau)$ reaches a maximum over the region $\tau < -\delta$ at $\tau = -\delta$ and over the region $\tau > \delta$ at $\tau = \delta$. The result $\xi(-\tau) = \xi(\tau)$ shows that these maxima are equal, hence the required result.

5. The number of patients required on each treatment as found from Equation 11.8 is

$$N = \frac{2\sigma^2(1 + \rho(n_a - 1))(z_\beta + z_{1\frac{1}{2}\alpha})^2}{\tau_M^2}$$

If the cluster mean approach is taken, then the number of clusters on each treatment is estimated by Equation 11.9 to be

$$N_{Clusters} = \frac{2(\sigma_G^2 + \sigma_W^2 / n_a)(z_\beta + z_{1\frac{1}{2}\alpha})^2}{\tau_M^2}$$

so, given the average cluster size, $n_a$, the two estimates will be consistent if

$$n_a(\sigma_G^2 + \sigma_W^2 / n_a) = \sigma^2(1 + \rho(n_a - 1))$$

As the outcome follows Equation 11.7, $\rho = \sigma_G^2 / \sigma^2$ and $\sigma^2 = \sigma_G^2 + \sigma_W^2$. Hence, $n_a(\sigma_G^2 + \sigma_W^2 / n_a) = n_a \rho \sigma^2 + \sigma^2(1 - \rho) = \sigma^2(1 + \rho(n_a - 1))$ as required.

6. The variance of $\sum w_i \hat{\theta}_i$ is $\sum w_i^2 v_i$ and minimizing this subject to $\sum w_i = 1$ requires the unconstrained minimization of

$$\sum w_i^2 v_i - \lambda(\sum w_i - 1)$$

where $\lambda$ is a Lagrange multiplier. Differentiating with respect to the weights and setting to zero gives $w_i = \frac{1}{2}\lambda v_i^{-1}$, that is the weights for the minimum variance estimator are proportional to the reciprocal of the corresponding variance. The variance of $\left(\sum v_i^{-1}\right)^{-1} \left(\sum v_i^{-1} \hat{\theta}_i\right)$ can also be found as $\left(\sum v_i^{-1}\right)^{-1}$.

7. The estimator of the treatment effect is $\bar{X}_A^W - \bar{X}_B^W$, where each term is the weighted mean of the cluster means that receive, respectively, treatment A or B. The variance of this estimator is $V_A + V_B$ where $V_T = \mathrm{var}(\bar{X}_T^W)$ for $T = A$ or $B$. The minimum variance estimator of the treatment effect is, from question 6, when the weight applied to the $i$th cluster mean is proportional to $(\sigma_G^2 + \sigma_W^2 / n_i)^{-1}$. Also,

$$V_T = \left(\sum (\sigma_G^2 + \sigma_W^2 / n_i)^{-1}\right)^{-1}$$

where the sum is over clusters receiving treatment $T$. A test of the null hypothesis of no treatment effect can be made by referring $\left(\bar{X}_A^W - \bar{X}_B^W\right)/\sqrt{V_A + V_B}$ to a standard normal distribution.

These results are exact provided that the weights are known, which entails knowledge of $\sigma_G^2, \sigma_W^2$. Estimates will be available from standard techniques for variance components, but the properties of weighted analyses, which may be optimal when weights are known, can be much poorer when the weights themselves are estimated from the data.

## Chapter 12

1. The procedure is an application of the formulae in Subsection 12.2.2 and Subsection 12.2.3. As a check, some of the intermediate steps are shown here.

| Trial | Log Odds Ratio | $\sqrt{v_i}$ | $w_i$ | $w_i\hat{\theta}_i$ | $\tilde{w}_i$ | $\tilde{w}_i\hat{\theta}_i$ |
|-------|------|---------|---------|----------|----------|----------|
| 1 | −0.54226 | 0.21916 | 20.8203 | −11.290 | 9.20088 | −4.98925 |
| 2 | −1.49188 | 0.93850 | 1.1354 | −1.6938 | 1.06221 | −1.58468 |
| 3 | −1.55255 | 0.63520 | 2.4784 | −3.8479 | 2.15455 | −3.34504 |
| 4 | −0.08507 | 0.59167 | 2.8565 | −0.2430 | 2.43470 | −0.20712 |
| 5 | −1.83116 | 0.72561 | 1.8993 | −3.4779 | 1.70310 | −3.11865 |
| 6 | 0.09885 | 2.01234 | 0.2469 | 0.0244 | 0.24330 | 0.02405 |
| 7 | −0.34628 | 0.36711 | 7.4202 | −2.5694 | 5.11712 | −1.77194 |
| 8 | −0.02703 | 0.24500 | 16.6597 | −0.4503 | 8.28635 | −0.22397 |
| 9 | −0.61434 | 0.47446 | 4.4423 | −2.7291 | 3.49938 | −2.14980 |
| 10 | −1.29928 | 0.93640 | 1.1404 | −1.4818 | 1.06666 | −1.38589 |
| 11 | −1.31985 | 0.75342 | 1.7617 | −2.3251 | 1.59159 | −2.10066 |
| 12 | −0.10725 | 0.65975 | 2.2974 | −0.2464 | 2.01643 | −0.21625 |
| Total | | | 63.159 | −30.330 | 38.376 | −21.069 |

Consequently, $\hat{\theta}_F = -30.330 / 63.159 = -0.4802$ and $\hat{\theta}_R = -21.069/38.376 = -0.5490$, with standard errors of $1/\sqrt{63.159} = 0.1258$ and $1/\sqrt{38.376} = 0.1614$, respectively.

2. Note that

$$Q = \sum w_i(\hat{\theta}_i - \hat{\theta}_F)^2 = \sum w_i\hat{\theta}_i^2 - \left(\sum w_i\right)\hat{\theta}_F^2$$

Given the $\{\theta_i\}$, $E(\hat{\theta}_i^2 \mid \{\theta_i\}) = \theta_i^2 + w_i^{-1}$. Also,

$$E(\hat{\theta}_F^2 \mid \{\theta_i\}) = \left(\sum w_i\right)^{-2} E\left[\left(\sum w_i\hat{\theta}_i\right)^2\right]$$

Now, this can be written as

$$E(\hat{\theta}_F^2 \mid \{\theta_i\}) = \left(\sum w_i\right)^{-2} E\left[\sum_i w_i^2\hat{\theta}_i^2 + \sum_{i \neq j} w_i w_j\hat{\theta}_i\hat{\theta}_j\right]$$

and as the sampling errors on the different trials are independent this is

$$\left(\sum w_i\right)^{-2} E\left[\sum_i w_i^2(\theta_i^2 + w_i^{-1}) + \sum_{i \neq j} w_i w_j \hat{\theta}_i \hat{\theta}_j\right] =$$

$$\left(\sum w_i\right)^{-1} + \left(\sum w_i\right)^{-2}\left(\sum w_i \theta_i\right)^2$$

Therefore,

$$E(Q|\{\theta_i\}) = k - 1 + \sum w_i \theta_i^2 - \left(\sum w_i\right)^{-1}\left(\sum w_i \theta_i\right)^2$$

Now, $E(Q) = E(E(Q|\{\theta_i\}))$, where the outer expectation is taken over the distribution of the $\{\theta_i\}$. Using

$$E\left(\sum w_i \theta_i\right)^2 = \text{var}(\sum w_i \theta_i) + \theta^2\left(\sum w_i\right)^2 = (\sum w_i^2)\sigma^2 + \theta^2\left(\sum w_i\right)^2$$

and $E(\theta_i^2) = \sigma^2 + \theta^2$, we find

$$E(Q) = k - 1 + \theta^2(\sum w_i) + \sigma^2(\sum w_i) - \left(\sum w_i\right)^{-1}\left[\sigma^2\sum w_i^2 + \theta^2\left(\sum w_i\right)^2\right]$$

The terms in $\theta^2$ cancel and the expectation of

$$\frac{Q - (k-1)}{\sum w_i - (\sum w_i^2)/\sum w_i}$$

is seen to be $\sigma^2$. It can occur that $Q < k - 1$, in which case the estimate would be negative, which would not be sensible and this explains why the maximum is included in Equation 12.1.

3. Intuitively, if the between-trial variation is very large compared with any of the sampling variation, then the sampling variation is unimportant, and as each trial is affected equally by the between-trial variation, equal weighting of the trials is appropriate. Mathematically, it is noted that the overall estimate is

$$\frac{\sum \hat{\theta}_i(\sigma^2 + v_i)^{-1}}{\sum (\sigma^2 + v_i)^{-1}} = \frac{\sum \hat{\theta}_i(1 + \sigma^{-2}v_i)^{-1}}{\sum (1 + \sigma^{-2}v_i)^{-1}}$$

and as $\sigma^2 \to \infty$, each of the weights tends to one.

4. If the model $y = \beta x + e$ is fitted, then the estimate of $\beta$ is

$$\left(\sum y_i x_i\right) \big/ \left(\sum x_i^2\right)$$

Applying this to a Galbraith plot, $y_i = \hat{\theta}_i / se(\hat{\theta}_i) = \hat{\theta}_i / \sqrt{v_i}$ and $x_i = 1 / \sqrt{v_i}$. Substituting in the preceding equation gives the estimate of slope as

$$\left(\sum \hat{\theta}_i v_i^{-1}\right) \big/ \left(\sum v_i^{-1}\right) = \hat{\theta}_F$$

as required.

# References

Altman, D.G. (1991), *Practical Statistics for Medical Research*, Chapman & Hall/CRC, London.

Altman, D.G. (1998), Confidence intervals for the number needed to treat, *British Medical Journal*, 317, 1309–1312.

Appelman, Y.E.A., Piek, J.J., Strikwerda, S., Tijssen, J.G.P., de Feyter, P.J., David, G.K., Serruys, P.W., Margolis, J.R., Loelemay, M.J., Montauban van Swijndregt, E.W.J., Koolen, J.J. (1996), Randomised trial of excimer laser angioplasty versus balloon angioplasty for treatment of obstructive coronary artery disease, *Lancet*, 347, 79–84.

Armitage, P. (1975), *Sequential Medical Trials*, 2nd ed., Blackwell, Oxford.

Armitage, P., Berry, G., Matthews, J.N.S. (2002), *Statistical Methods in Medical Research*, 4th ed., Blackwell, Oxford.

Armitage, P., Hills, M. (1982), The two-period crossover trial, *The Statistician*, 31, 119–131.

Armitage, P., McPherson, C.K., Rowe, B.C. (1969), Repeated significance tests on accumulating data, *Journal of the Royal Statistical Society: Series A*, 132, 235–244.

Begg, C.B. (1990), On inferences from Wei's biased coin design for clinical trials, *Biometrika*, 77, 467–484.

Brandjes, D.P.M., Buller, H.R., Heijboer, H., Huisman, M.V., de Rijk, M., Jagt, H., ten Cate, J.W. (1997), Randomised trial of effect of compression stockings in patients with symptomatic proximal-vein thrombosis, *Lancet*, 349, 759–762.

Chase, P.J. (1970), Combinations of $M$ out of $N$ objects, *Communications of the Association for Computing Machinery*, 13, 368.

Cockburn, F., Belton, N.R., Purvis, R.J., Giles, M.M., Brown, J.K., Turner, T.L., Wilkinson, E.M., Forfar, J.O., Barrie, W.J.M., McKay, G.S., Pocock, S.J. (1980), Maternal vitamin D intake and mineral metabolism in mothers and their newborn infants. *British Medical Journal*, 281, 11–14.

Collaborative Group on Antenatal Steroid Therapy (1981), Effect of antenatal dexamethasone therapy on prevention of respiratory distress syndrome, *American Journal of Obstetrics and Gynecology*, 141, 276–287.

Collett, D. (2002), *Modelling Binary Data*, 2nd ed., Chapman & Hall/CRC Press, Boca Raton, FL.

Collett, D. (2003), *Modelling Survival Data in Medical Research*, 2nd ed., Chapman & Hall/CRC Press, Boca Raton, FL.

Cox, D.R. (1972), Regression models and life-tables (with discussion), *Journal of the Royal Statistical Society: Series B*, 34, 187–220.

Crowley, P., Chalmers, I., Keirse, M.J.N.C. (1990), The effects of corticosteroid administration before preterm delivery: an overview of the evidence from controlled trials, *British Journal of Obstetrics and Gynaecology*, 97, 11–25.

Efron, B. (1971), Forcing a sequential experiment to be balanced, *Biometrika*, 58, 403–417.

Ellenberg, S.S., Fleming, T.R., DeMets, D.L. (2002), *Data Monitoring Committees in Clinical Trials: A Practical Perspective*, Wiley, Chichester.

European Coronary Surgery Study Group (1979), Coronary-artery bypass surgery in stable angina pectoris: survival at two years, *Lancet*, i, 889–893.

Eysenck, H.J. (1995), Problems with meta-analysis, in *Systematic Reviews*, Eds., Chalmers, I. and Altman, D.G., BMJ Publishing, London, pp. 64–74.

Fentiman, I.S., Rubens, R.D., Hayward, J.L. (1983), Control of pleural effusions in patients with breast-cancer — a randomized trial, *Cancer*, 52, 737–739.

Fisher, B., Redmond, C., Brown, A., Wickerham, D.L., Wolmark, N., Allegra, J., Escher, G., Lippman, M., Savlov, E., Wittliff, J., Fisher, E.R., Plotkin, D., Bowman, D., Wolter, J., Bornstein, R., Desser, R., Frelick, R. (1983), Influence of tumor estrogen and progesterone receptor levels on the response to tamoxifen and chemotherapy in primary breast cancer, *Journal of Clinical Oncology*, 1, 227–241.

Fleming, T.R., Harrington, D.P., O'Brien, P.C. (1984), Designs for group sequential tests, *Controlled Clinical Trials*, 5, 348–361.

Gail, M., Simon, R. (1985), Testing for qualitative interactions between treatment effects and patient subsets, *Biometrics*, 41, 361–372.

Giardiello, F.M., Hamilton, S.R., Krush, A.J., Piantadosi, S., Hylind, L.M., Celano, P., Booker, S.V., Robinson, C.R., Offerhaus, G.J. (1993), Treatment of colonic and rectal adenomas with Sulindac in familial adenomatous polyposis, *New England Journal of Medicine*, 328, 1313–1316.

Gordon, P.M., Diffey, B.L., Matthews, J.N.S., Farr, P.M. (1999), A randomized comparison of narrow-band TL-01 phototherapy and PUVA photochemotherapy for psoriasis, *Journal of the American Academy of Dermatology*, 41, 728–732.

Grosskurth, H., Mosha, F., Todd, J., Mwijarubi, E., Klokke, A., Senkoro, K., Mayaud, P., Changalucha, J., Nicoll, A., ka-Gina, G., Newell, J., Mugeye, K., Mabey, D., Hayes, R. (1995), Impact of improved treatment of sexually transmitted diseases on HIV infection in rural Tanzania: randomized controlled trial, *Lancet*, 346, 530–536.

Hacke, W., Kaste, M., Fieschi, C., von Kummer, R., Davalos, A., Meier, D., Larrue, V., Bluhmki, E., Davis, S., Donnan, G., Schneider, D., Diez-Tejedor, E., Trouillas, P. for the Second European-Australasian Acute Stroke Study Investigators (1998), Randomised double-blind placebo-controlled trial of thrombolytic therapy with intravenous alteplase in acute ischaemic stroke (ECASS II), *Lancet*, 352, 1245–1251.

Hackett, A.F., Court, S., Matthews, J.N.S., McCowen, C., Parkin, J.M. (1989), Do education groups help diabetics and their parents? *Archives of Disease in Childhood*, 64, 997–1003.

Haybittle, J.L. (1971), Repeated assessment of results in clinical trials of cancer treatment, *British Journal of Radiology*, 44, 793–797.

Hill, A.B. (1962), *Statistical Methods in Clinical and Preventive Medicine*, Livingstone, Edinburgh.

Hommel, E., Parving, H.H., Mathiesen, E., Edsberg, B., Damkjaer Nielsen, M., Giese, J. (1986), Effect of Captopril on kidney function in insulin-dependent diabetic patients with nephropathy, *British Medical Journal*, 293, 467–470.

Kinmonth, A.L., Woodcock, A., Griffin, S., Spiegal, N., Campbell, M.J. (1998), Randomised controlled trial of patient centred care of diabetes in general practice: impact on current well being and future disease, *British Medical Journal*, 317, 1202–1208.

Lan, K.K.G., DeMets, D.L. (1983), Discrete sequential boundaries for clinical trials, *Biometrika*, 70, 659–663.

Machin, D., Campbell, M.J., Fayers, P.M., Pinol, A.P.Y. (1997), *Sample Size Tables for Clinical Studies*, 2nd ed., Blackwell, Oxford.

Mantel, N., Haenszel, W. (1959), Statistical aspects of the analysis of data from retrospective studies of disease, *Journal of the National Institute of Cancer*, 22, 719–748.

McCullagh, P., Nelder, J.A. (1989), *Generalized Linear Models*, 2nd ed., Chapman & Hall/CRC Press, Boca Raton, FL.

McPherson, C.K., Armitage, P. (1971), Repeated significance tests on accumulating data when the null hypothesis is not true, *Journal of the Royal Statistical Society: Series A*, 134, 15–25.

MIST Study Group (1998), Randomised trial of efficacy and safety of inhaled zanamivir in treatment of influenza A and B virus infections, *Lancet*, 352, 1877–1881 (Erratum vol. 353, 504).

Newcombe, R.G. (1998), Interval estimation for the difference between independent proportions: comparison of eleven methods, *Statistics in Medicine*, 17, 873–890.

O'Brien, P.C. (1984), Procedures for comparing samples with multiple endpoints, *Biometrics*, 40, 1079–1087.

O'Brien, P.C., Fleming, T.R. (1979), A multiple testing procedure for clinical trials, *Biometrics*, 35, 549–556.

Peto, R., Pike, M.C., Armitage, P., Breslow, N.E., Cox, D.R., Howard, S.V., Mantel, N., McPherson, K., Peto, J., Smith, P.G. (1976), Design and analysis of randomized clinical trials requiring prolonged observation of each patient: I, Introduction and design, *British Journal of Cancer*, 34, 585–612.

Piantadosi, S. (2005), *Clinical Trials: A Methodologic Perspective*, 2nd ed., Wiley, Chichester.

Pocock, S.J. (1977), Group sequential methods in the design and analysis of clinical trials, *Biometrika*, 64, 191–199.

Pocock, S.J. (1993), Statistical and ethical issues in monitoring clinical trials, *Statistics in Medicine*, 12, 1459–1469.

Richards, S.H., Coast, J., Gunnell, D.J., Peters, T.J., Pounsford, J., Darlow, M.-A. (1998), Randomised controlled trial comparing effectiveness and acceptability of an early discharge, hospital at home scheme with acute hospital care, *British Medical Journal*, 316, 1796–1801 (Erratum vol. 317, 786).

Robins, J.M., Breslow, N., Greenland, S. (1986), Estimators of the Mantel-Haenszel variance consistent in both sparse and large-strata limiting models, *Biometrics*, 42, 311–323.

Robinson, L.D., Jewell, N.P. (1991), Some surprising results about covariate adjustment in logistic regression models, *International Statistical Review*, 58, 227–240.

Rosenberger, W.F., Lachin, J.M. (2002), *Randomization in Clinical Trials: Theory and Practice*, Wiley, Chichester.

Scandinavian Simvastatin Survival Study Group (1994), Randomised trial of cholesterol lowering in 4444 patients with coronary heart disease: the Scandinavian Simvastatin Survival Study *Lancet*, 344, 1383–1389.

Senn, S.J., Auclair, P. (1990), The graphical representation of clinical trials with particular reference to measurements over time, *Statistics in Medicine*, 9, 1287–1302 (Erratum: *Statistics in Medicine*, 10, 487).

Simes, R.J. (1986), An improved Bonferroni procedure for multiple tests of significance, *Biometrika*, 73, 751–754.

Smith, A.C., Dowsett, J.F., Russell, R.C.G., Hatfield, A.R.W., Cotton, P.B. (1994), Randomised trial of endoscopic stenting versus surgical bypass in malignant low bileduct obstruction, *Lancet*, 344, 1655–1660.

Spiegelhalter, D.J., Abrams, K.R., Myles, J.P. (2003), *Bayesian Approaches to Clinical Trials and Health-Care Evaluation*, Wiley, Chichester.

Tate, J.J.T., Dawson, J.W., Chung, S.C.S., Lau, W.Y., Li, A.K.C. (1993), Laparoscopic versus open appendectomy — prospective randomized trial, *Lancet*, 342, 633–637.

Thompson, S.G. (1993), Controversies in meta-analysis: the case of the trials of serum cholesterol reduction, *Statistical Methods in Medical Research*, 2, 173–192.

Ware, J.H. (1989), Investigating therapies of potentially great benefit: ECMO, *Statistical Science*, 4, 298–340.

Wei, L.J. (1977), A class of designs for sequential clinical trials, *Journal of the American Statistical Association*, 72, 382–386.

Wei, L.J. (1978), An application of an urn model to the design of sequential controlled clinical trials, *Journal of the American Statistical Association*, 73, 559–563.

Whitehead, J. (1992), *The Design and Analysis of Sequential Clinical Trials*, 2nd ed., Ellis Horwood, Chichester.

Winston, D.J., Wirin, D., Shaked, A., Busuttil, R.W. (1995), Randomised comparison of ganciclovir and high-dose acyclovir for long-term cytomegalovirus prophylaxis in liver-transplant recipients, *Lancet*, 346, 69–74.

# Index